Genital Skin Disorders

Diagnosis and Treatment

Genital
Skin Disorders

Diagnosis and Treatment

BENJAMIN K. FISHER, MD, FRCP(C)

Chief, Division of Dermatology
The Wellesley Hospital
Toronto, Ontario
Professor Emeritus of Dermatology
University of Toronto Medical School
Toronto, Ontario, Canada

LYNETTE J. MARGESSON, MD, FRCPC

Assistant Professor
Division of Dermatology
Queens University
Kingston, Ontario, Canada

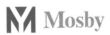 Mosby

St. Louis Baltimore Boston Carlsbad
Chicago Minneapolis New York Philadelphia Portland
London Milan Sydney Tokyo Toronto

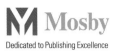

Mosby
Dedicated to Publishing Excellence

A Times Mirror
Company

Editor: Susie Baxter
Developmental Editor: Ellen Baker Geisel
Project Manager: Patricia Tannian
Senior Production Editor: Melissa Mraz Lastarria
Senior Composition Specialist: Chris Robinson
Book Design Manager: Gail Morey Hudson
Manufacturing Supervisor: Dave Graybill
Cover Design: Teresa Breckwoldt
Cover Image: Egyptian National Museum, Cairo Egypt/ET Archive,
            London/SuperStock

Printed in the United States of America
Composition by Mosby Electronic Publishing
Printing/binding by Walsworth Publishing Co.

Mosby, Inc.
11830 Westline Industrial Drive
St. Louis, Missouri 64146

Library of Congress Cataloging in Publication Data

Fisher, Benjamin K.
    Genital skin disorders : diagnosis and treatment/Benjamin K.
Fisher, Lynette J. Margesson.
        P.   Cm.
    Includes bibliographical references and index.
    ISBN 0-8151-2886-X
    1. Generative organs—Diseases. 2. Skin—Diseases. 3. Generative
organs—Diseases—Atlases. 4. Skin—Diseases—Atlases.
I. Margesson, Lynette J. II. Title.
    [DNLM: 1. Skin Diseases—atlases. 2. Genital Diseases, Female—
atlases. 3. Genital Diseases, Male—atlases. WR 17 F5332g 1998
RC877.F57 1998
616.6æ5—dc21
DNLM/DLC
for Library of Congress   97-35557
                                                            CIP

98 99 00 01 02 / 9 8 7 6 5 4 3 2 1

This book is dedicated to my patients
who allowed me to photograph their intimate body regions
so that we physicians could learn and in turn help.
BKF

This book is dedicated to my many steadfast vulvar patients,
who have taught me so much so that I can help others;
and to my enthusiastic mentors in vulvar disease
Drs. Marilynne McKay, Stephanie Pinkus, Maria Turner, and Libby Edwards.
LJM

Introduction

Three questions should be answered when confronted with a lesion in the genital area:

1. Is this lesion caused by sexually transmitted disease?
2. Is this lesion specific to the genitals?
3. Is this lesion a manifestation of a more generalized nature?

Genital lesions can be divided into those that are seen on the genitals and nowhere else, those that involve the genitals as part of a generalized skin or systemic disease or those that may appear anywhere on the skin, but happen to be localized to the genitals or the vulva alone.

For example, phimosis or pearly penile papules are conditions limited to the penis. Labial adhesions and vulvar vestibulitis are conditions limited to the vulva. Psoriasis or scabies frequently involves the penis or the vulva as part of a generalized eruption. Herpes simplex or fixed drug eruption may be seen anywhere on the skin but may be limited to the genitals alone.

A good history is extremely important at arriving at a proper diagnosis of any genital lesion. Questions relating to general health, sexual life style, regular habits, drug history, chronicle of traveling outside the country, and local application of medication or cosmetics, may all contain important clues for a correct diagnosis.

Patients with lesions in an intimate area are understandably quite anxious. They may be worried that the lesion may be transmitted to their sexual partners or that it may be a cancer. It is essential that a nonjudgmental, sympathetic attitude be conveyed to the patient, allowing him or her to relax and respond to your questions. If necessary, repeat your questions in different words to help jog the patient's memory. A little extra time spent on obtaining a good history may be crucial in arriving at the correct diagnosis and will save the patient unnecessary extra medical visits and needless expenses for ineffective medications.

Preface

This is not an in-depth text on genital diseases. It is intended to be an easily accessible text/atlas to acquaint readers with the morphologic presentation of diseases or disorders that afflict the genitals, to help readers arrive at an early diagnosis, and to help them select appropriate therapeutic modalities for their patients.

We present in these pages some 184 diseases and disorders seen by family practitioners, dermatologists, gynecologists, urologists, and sexually transmitted disease specialists. Along with clinical photographs, we have tried to combine a complete but concise written description of the conditions with the specific details to facilitate an accurate diagnosis. Recommended common therapeutic modalities are provided for each condition. Medications are referred to by their generic names. Exact details of the use of more esoteric medications is beyond the scope of this text/atlas, but we have included numerous references to help direct readers to additional information.

The clinical photographs have been chosen to best exemplify each condition to aid readers in making a visual comparison to recognize the disease. Where we deemed necessary, we have added useful information on histologic findings and therapeutic points. At the end of the text are appendices that provide further help in making the diagnosis and treating the various types of conditions such as ulcers and erosions.

We hope readers who seek to identify a specific lesion will find in this text/atlas a similar photograph or description that will help them to arrive at an accurate diagnosis and management of their patients.

ACKNOWLEDGMENTS

This book would not have been possible without the teaching of Dr. Ricky Schachter, the enthusiasm and support of my dear friend Dr. Ben Fisher, and the excellent and time-consuming editing of my husband, Dr. Bill Danby. I also wish to acknowledge the help of my partner in our Regional Vulvar Clinic, Dr. Peter Bryson.

Lynette J. Margesson, M.D.

I would like to thank here all those patients who willingly or almost willingly agreed to expose themselves to my camera. Special thanks are owed to many of my colleagues who referred cases to me for diagnosis or just for my interest. Thanks to those true friends who sent me interesting and unusual slides to help complete my collection. Special thanks to Mrs. Susie Baxter, Senior Editor at Mosby, for her helpful suggestions and wise advice. Without their support this book could have never been written.

Benjamin K. Fisher, M.D.

Contents

Detailed Contents

Genital Skin Disorders

Diagnosis and Treatment

PART I

THE PENIS

BENJAMIN K. FISHER

INTRODUCTION

This section is based on my 35-year experience in the dermatologic manifestations of penile lesions and their photographic recording. It started in 1962 as an assignment to photograph interesting skin lesions for the Dermatology Department of the Boston City Hospital where I was Chief-Resident. A few typical slides of penile lesions served as the basis for a growing collection that has been used over the years in various lectures for students and physicians. The reputation that I was an expert on penile lesions developed, which prompted many of my colleagues to refer patients with both common and unusual penile problems to me.

The penis is prone to trauma; infections caused by viral, bacterial, and yeast organisms; infestations; various inflammatory and vesicular conditions; degenerative and pigmentary changes; congenital abnormalities; benign and malignant tumors; and self-induced lesions. The following chapters deal with these and other conditions.

A cardinal principle that should always be kept in mind is that any lesion on the penis has to be suspected of being a result of a sexually transmitted disease (STD), especially if it is an ulcer or an erosion. It should be considered as an STD unless proven otherwise, either by a satisfactory, careful clinical history, the appropriate laboratory tests or a biopsy, or preferably a combination of these. ▲

CHAPTER 1

Normal Anatomy of the Penis

The penis is composed of three erectile longitudinal structures, the two corpora cavernosa situated laterally on the dorsum, and one corpus spongiosum situated ventrally, below and between the corpora cavernosa. The erectile tissue forming these structures is made up of numerous endothelially lined sinuses. The corpus spongiosum surrounds the urethra and expands at its distal end to form the rounded glans penis, having in its center the vertical urethral opening (meatus). The corpora cavernosa are surrounded and separated by a dense connective tissue layer known as the tunica albuginea or Buck's fascia. A similar but thinner layer surrounds the corpus spongiosum.

The base of the conical glans penis, also commonly referred to as "glans," is a ringlike, even structure, called the corona glandis, but commonly referred to as the "corona." On its ventral surface it curves anteriorly to form an inverted V-shaped angle pointing centrally toward the meatal opening. The corona is slightly more red-violaceous than the color of the glans penis and measures about 5 mm in width in the adult.

The base of the corona, at its junction with the distal part of the shaft of the penis, forms a shallow groove, referred to as the "neck" of the penis or the coronal sulcus. The skin of the penis becomes infolded distally to form the foreskin (prepuce), which covers the glans. The potential space between the glans penis and the foreskin is called the preputial sac. *Circumcision* is the term used for excision of the foreskin.

The ventral part of the penile shaft shows in its center a thin, vertical, barely raised line or fold, that stretches from the urethral opening through the penis, scrotum, and perineum to the anal opening. This is the remnant of the normal embryonic fusion in these areas. It is termed the *raphe,* and its penile part is referred to as the median raphe of the penis. Penis width and thickness vary greatly from individual to individual. The *frenulum* is a thickened skin fold that attaches from the distal part of the median raphe of the penis to anywhere between the ventral tip of the corona to the urethral meatus. In some individuals the frenulum may be missing (Fig. 1-1).

ARTERIES, VEINS, AND NERVES OF THE PENIS

The penis is richly supplied with arterial blood from the pudendal artery that branches into the four following arteries: the dorsal artery of the penis, the deep cavernous artery, the bulbar artery, and the urethral artery. These arteries supply the erectile tissues with large amounts of blood. Venous return is through three major veins: the cavernous vein, the deep dorsal vein, and the superficial dorsal vein. Sensory innervation is through the dorsal nerve of the penis, a branch of the pudendal nerve.

PILOSEBACEOUS UNITS

A small number of sebaceous glands and pilosebaceous units occur normally on the entire length of

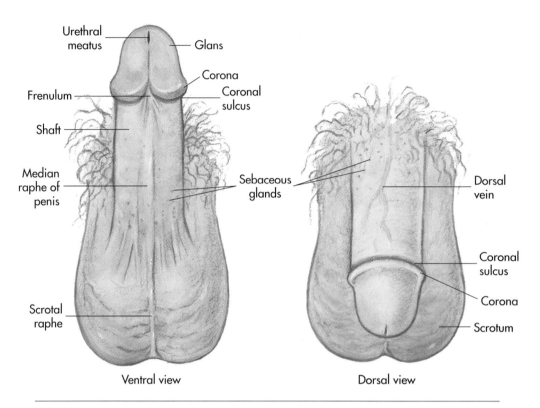

Ventral view

Dorsal view

FIG. 1-1
Normal Penis.

the shaft of the penis. They are small (1 to 2 mm), skin-colored, pink, or yellowish, barely raised papules that become more obvious when the surrounding skin is stretched. Their concentration is noticeably increased in the proximal quarter of the penile shaft. They are of no clinical significance, but in rare cases may cause anxiety to a patient who suddenly notices them and worries that these may be warts.

A few mature hairs may occasionally grow in the proximal third of the shaft of the penis. Tyson's glands are small preputial sebaceous glands that open directly into the preputial surface. Rarely these enlarge and may be mistaken for molluscum contagiosum lesions.[1]

REFERENCE

1. Piccinno R, Carrel CF, Menni S, Brancaleon W: Preputial ectopic glands mimicking molluscum contagiosum, *Acta Derm Venereol Suppl (Stockh)* 70:344-345, 1990.

CHAPTER 2

Congenital Malformations of the Penis

DOUBLE URETHRA

Double urethras are a fairly common condition (Fig. 2-1). Most of the time the patient is not even aware that he has a double urethra. It is usually an incidental finding during a routine examination. It has no pathologic significance and may be familial.

ACCRETION OF THE PENIS

The coronal sulcus is not complete, because of a congenital fusion of the glans to the distal part of the shaft of the penis. This fusion may be complete or partial (Fig. 2-2). The patient does not suffer from this condition, but it still may cause him some problems. For example, in a partial accretion there may be a persistent sinus that can harbor saprophytic spirochetes. On dark-field examination, these may be confused with *Treponema pallidium,* the causative organism of syphilis, and the patient may be treated for a disease that he does not have. These saprophytic spirochetes are similar to those that can be found in the normal mouth and are totally harmless.

Treatment consists of slitting the adhesion, actually a very simple procedure.

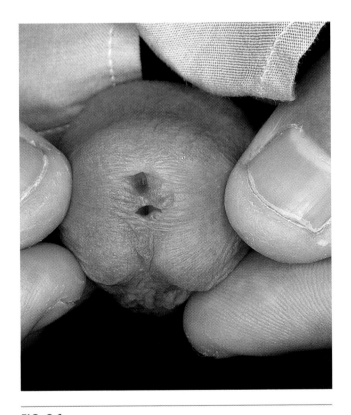

FIG. 2-1
Double Urethra. An incidental finding in a patient not aware of having this condition. His father had an identical finding.

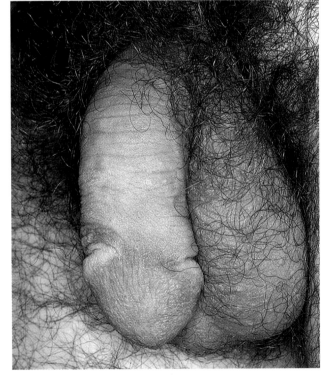

FIG. 2-2
Partial Accretion of the Penis. The corona is fused to the shaft in one small area on the dorsum of the penis.

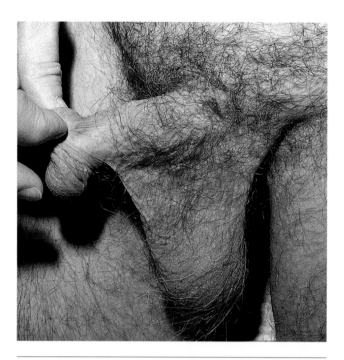

FIG. 2-3
Pterygium of the Scrotum to the Penis. The scrotal skin is fused to the proximal two thirds of the shaft. This is a benign anatomic aberration of no clinical significance.

PTERYGIUM OF THE PENIS

The scrotal skin adheres to the shaft of the penis (Fig. 2-3). It causes no problems and most frequently the patient is unaware that he has anything unusual. No treatment is necessary.

SCROTAL GLANS PENIS (GLANS PENIS PLICATUM)

This is a very rare condition manifested by thin, deep vertical furrows and tiny papillomas involving the entire glans penis. Separating the sides of the furrows by pulling the skin folds apart shows no cracks, bleeding, or any evidence of inflammation. The condition is very similar to the changes seen in scrotal tongue (lingua plicata), and in the one case that we have seen, both conditions were present in the same patient (Fig 2-4). The condition seems to be asymptomatic, although our patient complained of tenderness at the time of ejaculation. Whether this entity is related to the presence of scrotal tongue is impossible to say until more cases are recognized and reported.[1]

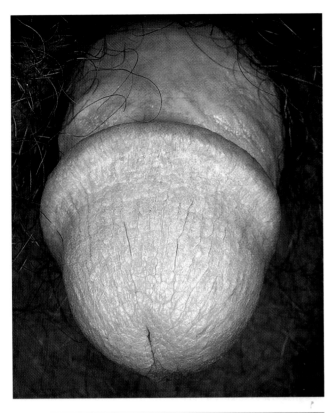

FIG. 2-4
Scrotal Glans Penis (glans penis plicatum). Multiple vertical, thin, deep furrows and tiny papillomas on glans penis. Changes very similar to those seen in scrotal tongue. The two conditions may coexist in the same patient.
(Courtesty Charlene D. Linzon, MD.)

REFERENCES
1. Fisher BK, Linzon CD: Scrotal glans penis (glans penis plicatum) associated with scrotal tongue (lingua plicata), *Int J Derm* 36:762-763, 1997.

CHAPTER 3

Traumatic Lesions of the Penis

Traumatic lesions are usually characterized by erosions or ulcers, frequently with linear or geometric borders (Fig. 3-1). Patients may be reluctant to give a good history of how these lesions occurred. The geometric or bizarre borders of the lesions are an important clue to the diagnosis.[1] Fig. 3-2 shows a traumatic ulcer in a drug addict who, having run out of veins, injected pentobarbital sodium (Nembutal) into the dorsal vein of the penis, causing a breakdown of the tissue. Borders of the ulcer are typically linear.

FRACTURE OF THE PENIS

A fracture is a frightening occurrence that happens when the erect penis sustains a severe blow, which is usually accidental, during intercourse. It can happen by "missing the target" or by falling against a hard object such as a bed's leg. A cracking noise may be audible, and the penis immediately loses its erection with the appearance of a hematoma, swelling, and pain (Fig. 3-3). This rare condition should be considered an emergency. The patient should be seen as soon as possible by a urologist, to decide whether surgery is necessary to evacuate the hematoma and to repair the torn tunica albuginea. Failure to do this may cause future scarring and deformity.[2,3]

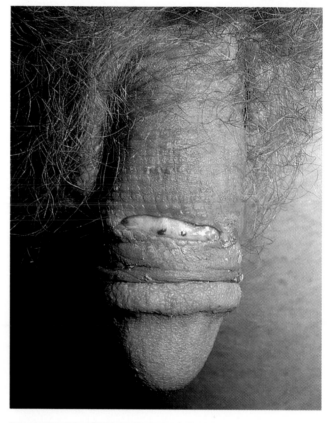

FIG. 3-2
Traumatic Ulcer in a Drug Addict. The borders of the ulcer are typically linear.

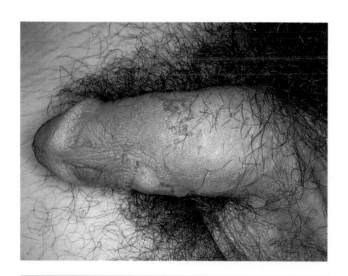

FIG. 3-1
Traumatic Erosions on the Shaft. One lesion shows linear borders; the other one has bizarre borders.

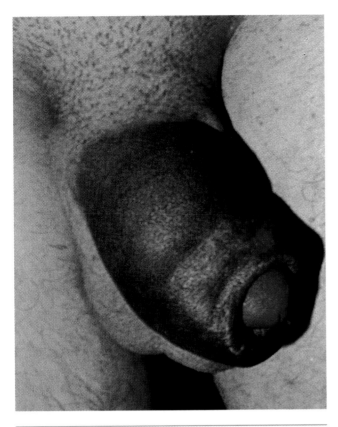

FIG. 3-3
Fracture of the Penis. A large hematoma and swelling involves most of the shaft. This condition requires emergency care.
(Courtesy Dr. Coleman Jacobson.)

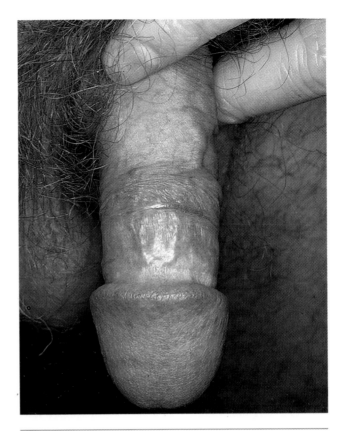

FIG. 3-4
Persistent Penile Painful Fissure. A horizontal crack with slight inflammation is located on the shaft of the penis. This condition may be seen in both circumcised and uncircumcised individuals.

PERSISTENT PAINFUL PENILE FISSURE

This is an exquisitely painful horizontal crack on the shaft of the penis that is aggravated by sexual intercourse. The area around the crack may at times show erythema secondary to inflammation (Fig. 3-4). The pain may be so severe, during and after intercourse, that the patient is reluctant to have normal sexual relations. It is usually seen in individuals between the ages of 30 and 50 years. The cause is unknown, but the friction of intercourse may split open a healed lesion. Biopsy shows a nonspecific inflammation.

Therapy with local steroid or antibiotic creams is not helpful. Occasionally Bowen's disease mimics this condition and can be cured by total excision (Fig. 3-5).

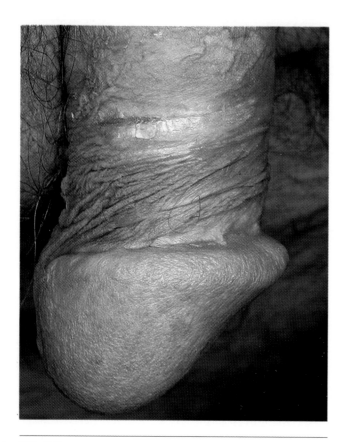

FIG. 3-5

Bowen's Disease (squamous cell carcinoma in situ). This condition presented as a pink, minimally infiltrated, horizontal, cracked plaque. The lesion was very tender and was misdiagnosed as persistent penile painful fissure. Excision of the lesion was curative.

REFERENCES

Traumatic Lesions of the Penis

1. Cass CA, Gleich P, Smith C: Male genital injuries from external trauma, *Br J Urol* 57:467-470, 1985.

Fracture of the Penis

2. Davies DM, Mitchell I: Fracture of the penis, *Br J Urol* 50:426, 1978.
3. Goh SH, Trapnell JE: Fracture of the penis, *Br J Surg* 67:680-681, 1980.

CHAPTER 4

Infectious Diseases of the Penis

VIRAL DISEASES

Warts

The synonyms for genital warts include venereal warts, condylomata acuminata, and human papillomavirus (HPV) infection. Its etiology involves HPV, a DNA papovavirus. Over 70 subtypes have been isolated; 90% of genital warts are caused by subtypes 6 and 11. Warts are mainly sexually transmitted. The age group most infected is young adults (16 to 30 years old), but all sexually active males are prone to infection. A patient's history involves exposure to a sexual partner with veneral warts, prior history of warts, or immunosuppression with an incubation period of weeks to months. The condition can be asymptomatic or occasionally mildly pruritic. Physical examination reveals papules and plaques, with a differential diagnosis of pearly penile papules, molluscum contagiosum, lichen planus, or lichen nitidus being made.

Diagnosis

Generally a diagnoses is easy clinically. A definite diagnosis can be made by biopsy.

Treatment

Often unsatisfactory, treatment is by local destructive measures. These include cryotherapy with liquid nitrogen, podophyllin resin, electrodesiccation, trichloracetic acid, and carbon dioxide laser.

Note: *Sexual partner should always be checked and treated if necessary.*

Etiologic Factors

Warts are caused by various types of HPV.[1,2] They are easy to diagnose but difficult to treat. The lesions may be small and skin-colored (Fig. 4-1, *A*) or raised and hyperpigmented (Fig. 4-1, *B*). They may also form plaques (Fig. 4-1, *C*) that mimic Bowen's disease. When in doubt, a biopsy of a small specimen confirms the proper diagnosis.

The moist variety of a penile wart is termed *condyloma acuminatum*. Lesions may be small or large, skin-colored or red, and may form cauliflower-like plaques (Fig. 4-2, *A* to *C*). They may also be intraurethral (Fig. 4-2, *D*).[3]

Of all anogenital warts, 5% to 10% are caused by HPV having an oncogenic potential (mainly subtypes 16 and 18; less commonly subtypes 31, 33, 35, 51 and 52). Hence the patient's sexual partner should be checked regularly for cervical carcinoma.[4]

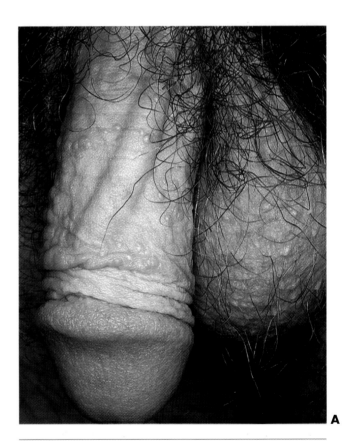

A

FIG. 4-1

Penile Warts. **A**, Multiple small, smooth, globular skin-colored, and pink papules on the shaft of the penis. Typical early lesions are shown.   *continued*

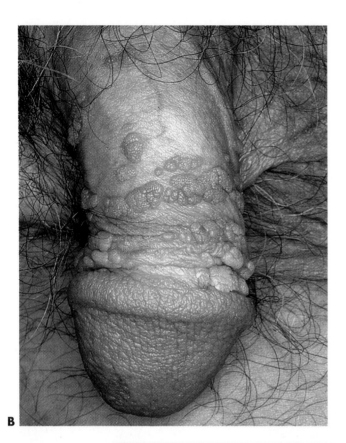

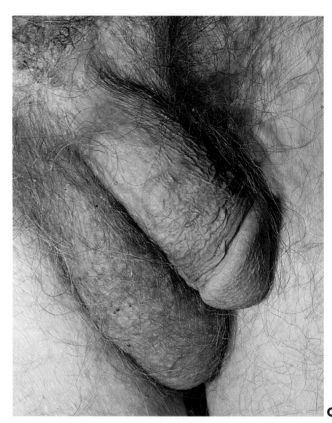

B

C

FIG. 4-1, cont'd
B, Numerous rough, raised, and hyperpigmented, small and large papules are located on the penile shaft. C, Pink, hyperkeratotic plaque located at the base of the penis. Clinically the plaque looked like Bowen's disease; histologically it was a typical wart.

Treatment may be difficult and prolonged. Many destructive measures have been tried to eradicate these lesions. None of the measures is ideal. The patient should be informed of the unpredictable course of the disease and the unpredictable duration of treatment. Cryotherapy with liquid nitrogen, podophyllin, and laser treatment are some of the most popular therapeutic modalities. ▼ **I prefer to start with cryotherapy. Using the spray gun, I freeze each wart 3 times, letting them thaw between each freezing. I repeat the treatment every 2 weeks.** ▲ Podophyllin 25%, in tincture of benzoin compound, works well for moist lesions. It is applied with a wooden applicator (the wooden side of a cotton-tip applicator will do) to the lesions, left to dry, and then washed off with soap and water after 3 to 4

hours. A 1% 5-fluorouracil solution seems to work well for intrameatal lesions. Resistant cases can be treated with gentle electrodesiccation or vaporization with the carbon dioxide laser using a low wattage. Any of the methods used may leave permanent hypopigmented flat scars. Foreskin involvement may be cured by circumcision. The patient's female sexual partner should always be checked by a gynecologist and treated if necessary.

Giant condyloma acuminatum of Buschke and Loewenstein clinically looks like a large aggregate of condylomata acuminata. It is most frequently located on the glans penis and on the foreskin of uncircumcised males. The term *giant condyloma* is a misnomer, because the condition is in reality a verrucous carcinoma that invades deeply into the

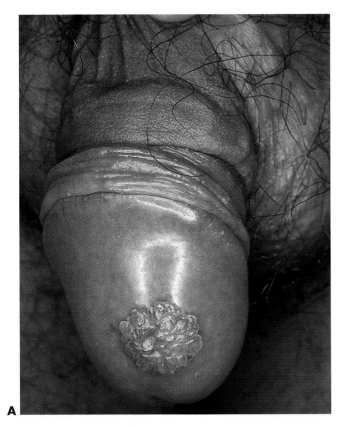

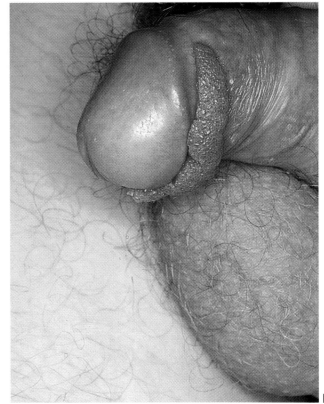

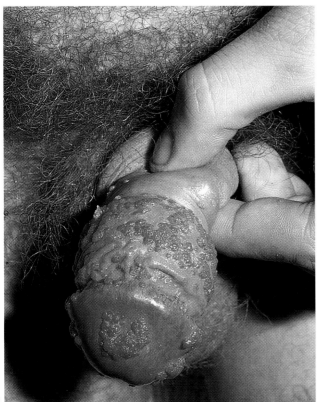

FIG. 4-2

A, Condyloma Acuminatum. Large, solitary, red, cauliflower-like papule located on glans penis. **B,** Condyloma Acuminatum. A large, red, "cock's comb"-like soft linear plaque located on distal shaft and corona. **C,** Condyloma Acuminata. Numerous red, moist papules and papular plaques located on glans penis and mucosal aspect of foreskin. Cases like the one shown here may respond dramatically to circumcision.

continued

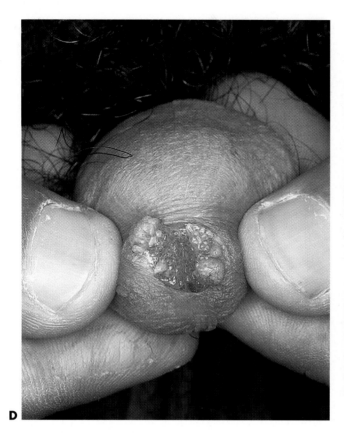

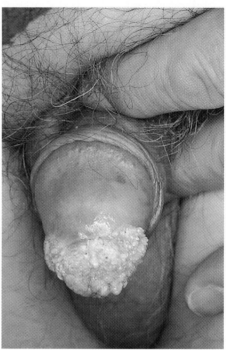

FIG. 4-2, cont'd
D, Intraurethral Condylomata Acuminata. Soft, whitish, moist papillomas are quite obvious when the sides of the meatal opening are pulled outward. **E**, Giant Condyloma Acuminatum of Buschke and Loewenstein. This is in reality a verrucous carcinoma. This asymptomatic, cauliflower-like, raised verrucous tumor on the glans penis has been growing slowly for 5 years. Three biopsies were done; two of which reported as "wart," and only one reported as verrucous carcinoma.
(**E**, Courtesy Dr. Charles Lynde.)

underlying tissues. Although it is a locally aggressive tumor, metastases to regional lymph nodes are a rare occurrence. Treatment is usually surgical.[5,6,7]

Bowenoid papulosis is another condition caused by several types of the human papillomavirus (usually subtypes 16, 18, 32, and 33). Clinically the lesions do not look like typical warts or condylomata. They may present as small papules that may be skin-colored, pink, or hyperpigmented and may involve the penis and the scrotum. They may be mistaken for flat warts, lichen planus, or psoriasis (Fig. 4-3). A biopsy confirms the accurate diagnosis.

The lesions may change with time. Their numbers may increase, decrease, or the lesions may disappear without treatment. They derive their name from the fact that, histologically, they are practically identical to Bowen's disease (intraepidermal squamous cell carcinoma). These lesions are considered precancerous and unless treated, may cause cervical carcinoma in the patient's female sexual partner.

Treatment of the lesions is with liquid nitrogen cryotherapy or with the carbon dioxide laser.[8]

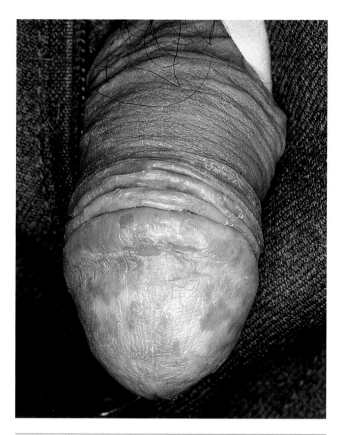

FIG. 4-3
Bowenoid Papulosis. Multiple pink flat papules of various sizes located on the glans penis. The papules are indistinguishable clinically from warts, psoriasis, or lichen planus. The histology of Bowenoid papulosis is identical to that of Bowen's disease.

Herpes Simplex

The synonyms for herpes simplex are herpes, genital herpes, herpes progenitalis, and cold sore. Age at occurrence is commonly among sexually active adults. Its etiology includes herpes simplex virus (HSV) type 2, less commonly type 1. The transmission is sexual with an incubation period of 2 to 20 days, with an average of 1 week. The history for herpes simplex involves recent sexual exposure. ▼ **Establish whether similar lesions have occurred in the past in the same area or neighboring sites. Also check if the patient's sexual partner has suffered from similar lesions. ▲**

Physical examination reveals grouped lesions (vesicles, pustules, scabs, erosions) with or without inflammation, anywhere on the penis or scrotum. Accompanying inguinal lymphadenopathy is a common finding. The differential diagnoses include syphilitic small chancres, traumatic erosions, gonococcal erosions, folliculitis, scabies, pemphigus, pemphigoid, fixed drug eruption, and foscarnet reaction.

Diagnosis

Painful recurrent lesions in same site, starting as small grouped vesicles, are clues used to reach a diagnosis. A definite diagnosis is determined from a Tzanck's smear (viral giant cells), a monoclonal antibody test, and/or a biopsy.

Treatment

Treatment includes the use of systemic antivirals: acyclovir, famciclovir, and valacyclovir.

Recurrent Genital Herpes

The vast majority of observed genital herpes (over 99.9%) is recurrent genital herpes. The eruption is preceded by a prodrome of an itching or burning sensation several hours to a day before a red patch, which soon develops clear grouped vesicles, appears. The amount of pain and discomfort varies from individual to individual.

Lesions of herpes simplex undergo an orderly evolution, provided they are not disturbed or traumatized. They start as a small group of clear vesicles (Fig. 4-4, *A*), which then become pustules (Fig. 4-4, *B*). When the pustules dry, scabs are formed. Older vesicles may show central necrosis or sagging, a very characteristic feature of viral vesicles (Fig. 4-4, *C*). The pustular phase does not signify a secondary bacterial infection; it is due to the normal appearance of neutrophils that invade the vesicle as a response to the viral infection. When the vesicles or the pustules, which are thinned-roofed, are torn by trauma or friction, moist small erosions or ulcers appear, which may be the presenting complaint to the physician (Fig. 4-5). The eruption heals within 1 to 2 weeks, at times leaving hypopigmented or hyperpigmented macules or superficial scars. Primary genital herpes denotes the first inoculation of the herpes virus into the affected

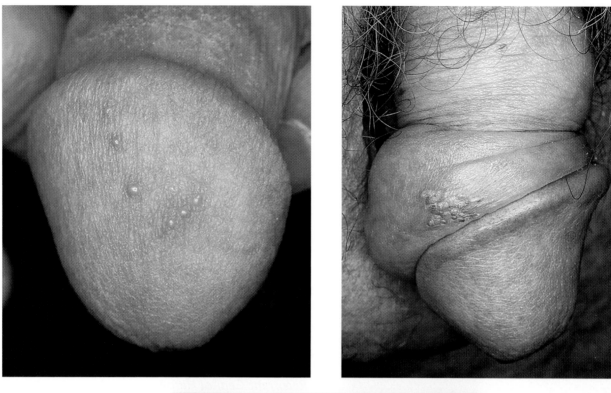

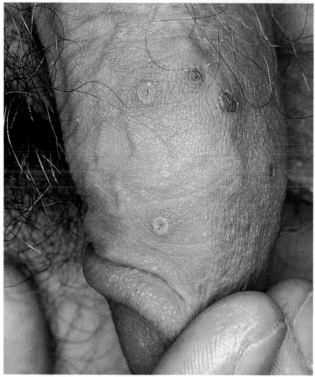

FIG. 4-4

A, Herpes Simplex. The earliest lesions show grouped clear vesicles. B, Grouped pustules. The concomitant inflammation has caused erythema and swelling. C, Two centrally depressed old pustules and three scabs are seen surrounded by erythema and slight swelling.

site. The skin lesions are similar to those seen in the recurrent type but are frequently larger in size and number. They are frequently accompanied by fever, headache, malaise, and myalgia that last 3 to 4 days. Tender inguinal lymphadenopathy, dysuria, and urethral discharge may be present. The eruption lasts 2 to 4 weeks. Future recurrent lesions usually appear at the same site or close to it.

The viral nature of the lesions can be confirmed by the finding of viral giant cells from scrapings of the bottom of the blisters stained with Wright's or Giemsa stain (Tzanck's smear). Testing these scrapings with monoclonal antibodies to the herpes simplex virus, if positive, confirms the presence of this virus. At present this is the most accurate test from which results can be obtained in less than 2 hours. Electron microscopy of blister fluid is another helpful method to identify the virus.

Grouped erosions or ulcers on the penis, such as those encountered in herpes, may also be a manifestation of multiple syphilitic chancres or may be a mixed infection of these two diseases. Hence a darkfield examination and serologic test for syphilis must be done in all cases of erosive or ulcerated lesions. The possibility of a concomitant HIV infection should be ruled out.

In immunosuppressed individuals the herpetic lesions may be quite altered and atypical. They may present as persistent papules (Fig. 4-6, *A*) or as chronic ulcers (Fig. 4-6, *B*).

Treatment of genital herpes simplex is with systemic antiviral agents such as acyclovir, famciclovir, and valacyclovir, all of which offer good control. Acyclovir (200 mg 5 times a day for 5 to 7 days) usually controls an acute attack. The dosage of famciclovir is 125 mg bid for 5 days, and for

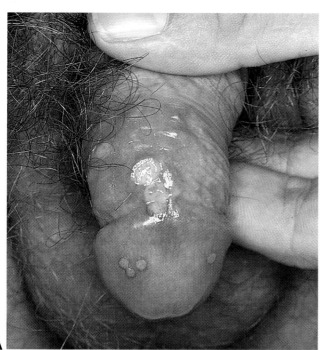

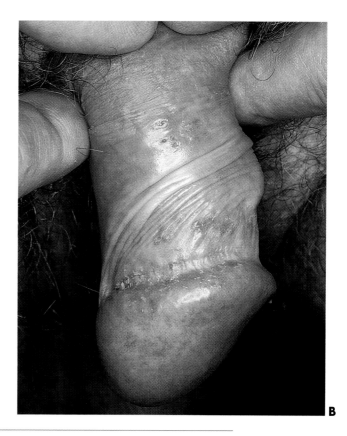

A

B

FIG. 4-5

A, Herpes Simplex. Grouped erosions are located on the glans, and larger ulcers are located on the shaft of penis. Multiple syphilitic chancres may look identical. **B,** Multiple tiny erosions and ulcers are shown on the mucosal aspect of foreskin.

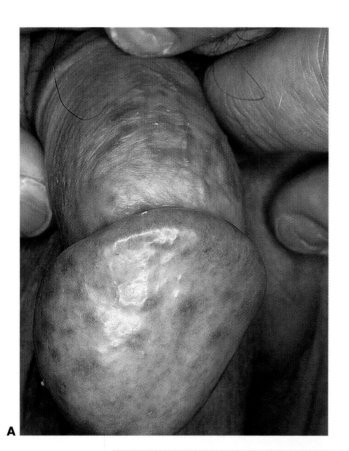
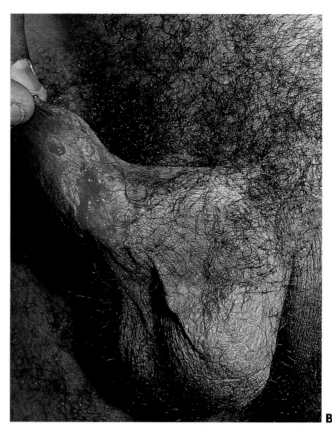

FIG. 4-6
A, Herpes simplex in the immunosuppressed patient. Multiple persistent papules are located on the glans penis in a patient undergoing chemotherapy for Hodgkin's disease. **B,** Nonhealing penile ulcers in a patient with AIDS.

valacyclovir the dosage is 500 mg bid for 5 days. Valacyclovir should not be used in immunosuppressed patients. The manufacturer's product monograph (GlaxoWellcome Inc., 1966) states that valacyclovir may cause thrombotic thrombocytopenic purpura/hemolytic uremic syndrome (TTP/HUS) in immunosuppressed patients, sometimes resulting in death.

Topical preparations are not useful in the treatment of genital herpes simplex.[9,10]

Herpes Zoster

Herpes Zoster is caused by the varicella zoster virus (VZV). There is a history of a sudden onset of unilateral, usually painful, vesicular eruptions. Onset usually occurs after the age of 60. The differential diagnoses include herpes simplex, cellulitis, contact dermatitis, and pemphigoid.

Diagnosis
Unilateral, grouped, dermatomal, vesicular, pustular, or scabby lesions are quite typical. A definite

diagnosis is made in finding monoclonal antibodies to herpes zoster in scrapings from the floor of the blister. Tzanck's smear, biopsy, and electron microscopy will not differentiate between herpes simplex and herpes zoster.

Treatment

In mild cases with few symptoms, patients should be treated symptomatically with saline compresses twice a day, followed by an antibacterial ointment application, such as Betadine ointment. In more severe cases or in immunosuppressed individuals early treatment with systemic antiviral agents (acyclovir, famciclovir, valacyclovir) is indicated. The dose for acyclovir is 800 mg 5 times a day for 7 to 10 days. Famciclovir is given 500 mg tid for 7 days, and valacyclovir is given 1000 mg bid for 7 days. Valacyclovir should not be used in immunosuppressed patients (see treatment for herpes simplex).

Areas of Involvement

Herpes zoster rarely involves the penis. It may be seen when dermatomes S1, S2, S3, and S4 are involved (Fig. 4-7).

The unilateral involvement of the penis and scrotum, the presence of lesions on the thigh and leg, and the presence of pain in these areas are all useful clues for diagnosis.

The individual skin lesions are identical to those seen in genital herpes simplex. The eruption lasts 3 to 4 weeks and may leave scars. In some individuals postherpetic neuralgia persists for an unpredictable time.

Molluscum Contagiousum

Molluscum contagiosum is caused by a DNA poxvirus. Lesions gradually appear over a few weeks. HIV infection is a risk factor. The lesions are usually asymptomatic or occasionally itchy, with onset usually occurring in young adults. Physical examination reveals umbilicated small round papules. The differential diagnoses include warts, sebaceous hyperplasia, and basal cell carcinoma, and, in the immunocompromised, lesions of *Cryptococcus neoformans* and *Histoplasma capsulatum*. A definite diagnosis can be made from a biopsy or from a Giemsa stain of expressed material from the lesion. Treatment options include cryotherapy with liquid nitrogen, electrodesiccation, and curettage.

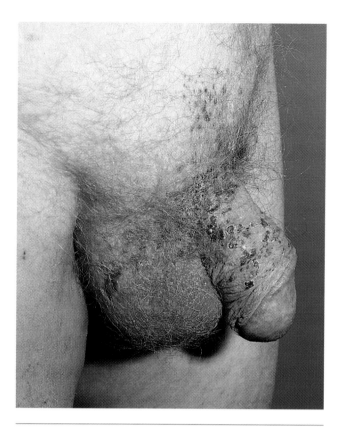

FIG. 4-7
Herpes Zoster. Healing grouped scabs located on the right side of the pubic area, scrotum, penis, and right thigh. Dermatomes involved were S1, S2, S3, and S4.

This poxvirus infection presents as small, skin-colored or pink, shiny, usually umbilicated, round papules that at times are flat-topped. They usually are easy to diagnose (Fig. 4-8, *A*), except when no umbilication is seen, at which time the lesions may be confused with genital warts. On rare occasions, these lesions will self-destroy, probably from an immunologic inflammatory reaction that causes erythema and scabbing (Fig. 4-8, *B*). This may cause difficulty in diagnosis, but careful examination of the area usually reveals a few intact typical umbilicated lesions.

The histologic picture of molluscum contagiosum is pathognomonic, demonstrating the typical inclusion bodies. If the content of a papule is squeezed out and smeared on a slide, a Giemsa stain will demonstrate the same inclusion bodies (molluscum bodies).

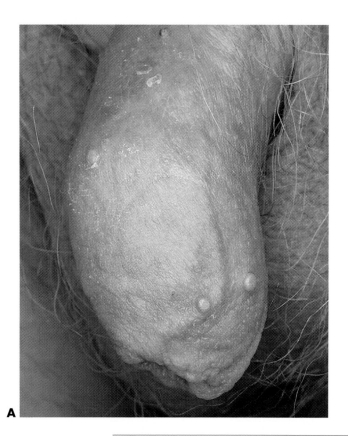
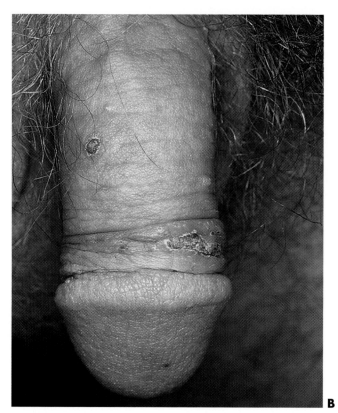

A

B

FIG. 4-8
Molluscum Contagiosum. **A**, Typical umbilicated skin-colored papules located on the foreskin. **B**, The lesions are self-destructing. Multiple scabs and rare small skin-colored papules are located on the shaft of the penis.

Treatment

Treatment options consist of freezing the lesions with liquid nitrogen, curetting them, or applying cantharidin to the lesions. The patient should be checked and treated every 2 to 3 weeks, because tiny lesions missed on previous visits will grow in the interim and will become obvious. The condition may be transmitted to sexual partners, and they should be examined and treated if necessary.[11,12]

BACTERIAL INFECTIONS
Acute Abscess

Penile abscess is a rare occurrence. When this happens, the involved area is red, hot, swollen, and tender like an abscess anywhere else (Fig. 4-9, *A*). In immunosuppressed individuals unusual bacteria may cause atypical abscesses that may be less inflammatory and less painful (Fig. 4-9, *B*).

Streptococcal Infections

Erysipelas or cellulitis is not uncommon and has to be treated aggressively and with a great deal of respect. Early lesions look like cellulitis elsewhere on the body. The involved area is swollen, red, hot, and painful. At times the portal of entry of the bacteria can be seen (Fig. 4-10, *A*). Edema and occasionally even a blister are present. Most of the time early systemic antibiotic treatment clears up the

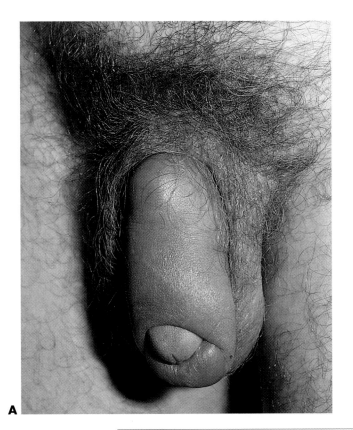
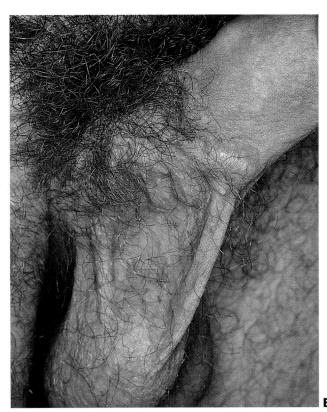

A

B

FIG. 4-9

A, Acute abscess caused by *E. coli*. A round mass located at the base of the penis is red and swollen with obvious edema of the foreskin. **B,** A bacterial abscess caused by *Staphylococcus lugdunensis* in a patient with AIDS. The lesion was a pink indolent nodule at the base of the penis of several months duration. Just under the nodule is a lesion of molluscum contagiosum.

infection, but in several instances, when the antibiotics are stopped, the cellulitis recurs. The cellulitis may extend from the penis to the scrotum and the pubic area.

Two major problems exist. First, this streptococcal infection may at times behave viciously and cause necrotic areas, which may advance rapidly and cause tissue destruction (Fig. 4-10, *B*). This calls for rapid therapeutic action with high doses of antibiotics. In my experience this may not always be enough. The addition of systemic steroids in addition to high doses of penicillin, such as penicillin V 300 mg 4 times a day for several weeks, seems to be necessary to rapidly reduce the edema and erythema. ▼ **I usually start my patients on 40 mg**

prednisone a day and taper this dosage gradually over several weeks. ▲

The second problem is, that like with cellulitis elsewhere, if it becomes recurrent, it may progress into chronic, irreversible lymphedema (Fig. 4-10, *C*). The severe cases may cause elephantiasis of the penis and of the scrotum with permanent deformity of the penis and loss of sexual function (Fig. 4-10, *D*). Usually very little can be done to help the long-standing cases of chronic lymphedema of the penis. For this reason early cases should be treated both with high doses of penicillin and with prednisone, which should be tapered off as the condition improves. If there is improvement with noticeable receding of the edema, corrective surgery may at times be helpful.

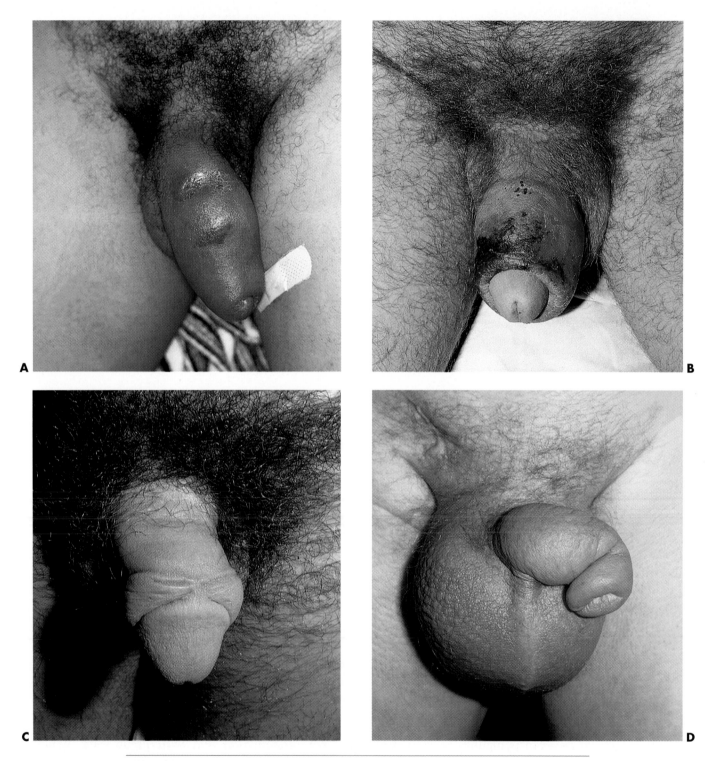

FIG. 4-10
For legend see opposite page.

Syphilis

Primary Syphilis (Chancre)

The chancre is the primary lesion of syphilis, caused by the spirochete *Treponema pallidum* at the point where the treponeme enters the body. The portal of entrance may be intact mucosa or abraded skin. The classic description of this lesion by John Hunter 300 years ago, the typical "Hunterian chancre," is the one best known to most physicians: presenting an indolent, punched out ulcer with a clean base and firm round borders (Fig. 4-11). This typical Hunterian chancre is still seen, but the more atypical forms are the ones more commonly encountered. These may be painful or superficial, and the base of the lesion may be dirty. Therefore any erosion or ulcer on the penis should be suspected of being syphilitic, unless proven to be caused by a different etiologic condition (Fig. 4-12). Such lesions should be tested by dark-field examination, biopsy, serology, or a combination of these. An early chancre may present as a papule, a healing chancre may show a scab, and at times the lesions may mimic a patch of dermatitis (Fig. 4-13, *A*).

The differential diagnoses are therefore vast and should include any condition causing an ulceration, such as trauma, genital herpes, lymphogranuloma venereum, granuloma inguinale, chancroid (mimics syphilitic chancre most closely), gonorrheal ulcer, fixed drug eruption, and aphthous ulcer. Remember two important points: (1) any of these lesions may coexist with syphilis thus being part of a mixed infection, and (2) do not be fooled by multiple lesions. Chancres may indeed be multiple (see Fig. 4-12, *A*, *C*, and *D*).

The chancre may be intraurethral, which may be missed on a cursory examination (Fig. 4-13, *B*).

FIG. 4-10

A, Erysipelas (cellulitis). The penis is red and swollen. The erosion on the proximal part of the shaft is probably the portal of entry of the bacteria. **B**, Necrotic lesions appeared on the penis a few days after the onset of infection. Two months of therapy with penicillin and prednisone were required to achieve a cure. The area has remained scarred. **C**, Early, irreversible lymphedema, caused by recurrent erysipelas, is shown. **D**, Elphantiasis of the penis and scrotum. Both areas are swollen and indurated. The penis is permanently distorted and has loss of sexual function. Aggressive therapy with penicillin and prednisone at the onset of the disease would have prevented this disastrous outcome.

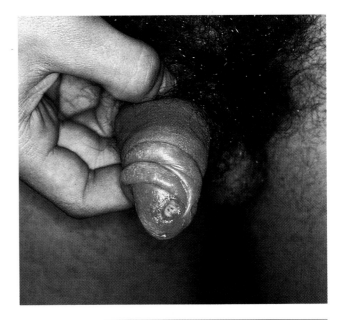

FIG. 4-11

Primary Syphilitic Chancre on Glans Penis. The lesion is a typical Hunterian chancre; showing a round, punched out ulcer with firm indurated borders.

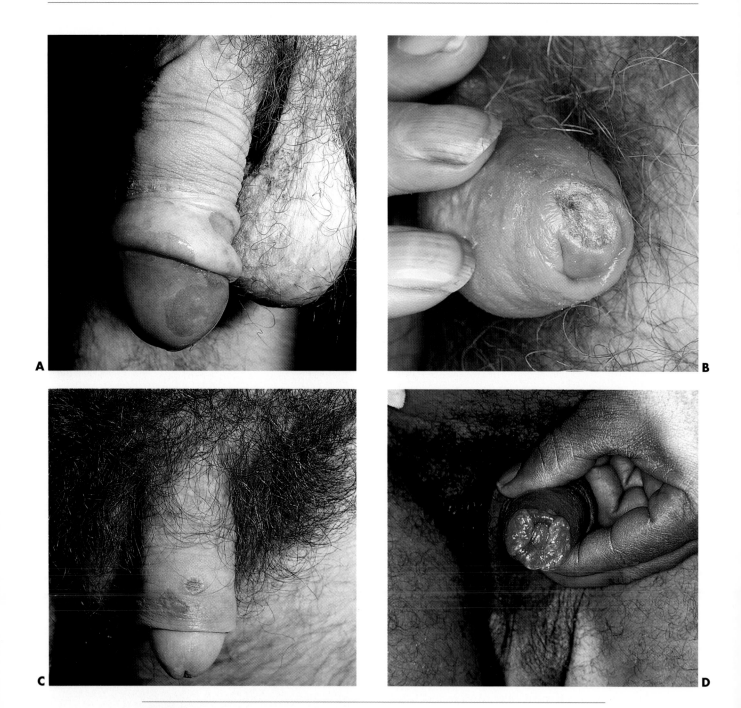

FIG. 4-12

A, Multiple syphilitic chancres. The lesions are superficial erosions, except for one superficial ulcer located on the left side of the foreskin. **B,** Primary syphilitic chancre. A superficial ulcer is shown on the tip of the penis. **C,** Two superficial ulcers of primary syphilitic chancre are located on the foreskin. One of the lesions has a raised shiny border mimicking herpes simplex vesicles. The two conditions may coexist. **D,** Two large ulcers of primary syphilitic chancre are located on the tip of the foreskin mimicking pyogenic granulomas.

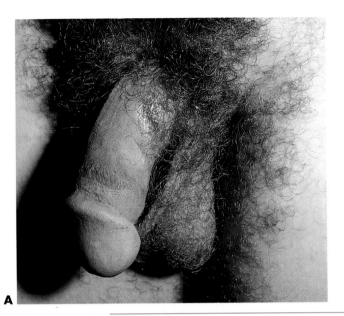
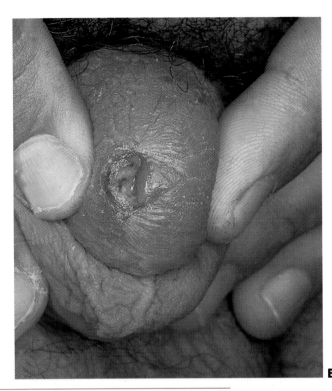

FIG. 4-13
A, Syphilitic chancre located at the base of the penis. The lesion is a moist eroded patch, mimicking an acute dermatitis. **B,** Intraurethatal syphilitic chancre. The ulcer is seen below the meatal opening on the right side.

A chancre heals with or without treatment and usually leaves a scar, which may remain obvious. While the chancre heals, secondary syphilitic lesions that frequently involve the penis may appear. These may be macules, papules, eroded papules or arciform, and annular lesions, the latter seen particularly in dark-skinned individuals (Fig. 4-14, *A* and *B*). The differential diagnoses of these secondary syphilitic lesions include a viral exanthema such as infectious mononucleosis or the exanthema seen in AIDS, papulosquamous conditions such as psoriasis, lichen planus, pityriasis rosea, and pityriasis lichenoides; drug eruption, tinea versicolor, condyloma acuminata and scabies. In patients with AIDS the lesions may be conspicuously numerous (Fig. 4-14, *C*).

Laboratory Aids in Syphilis

A positive dark-field examination result confirms the diagnosis of primary and secondary syphilis.

Biopsy
Biopsy is greatly helpful when it shows the two fundamental pathologic changes seen in syphilis: swelling and proliferation of endothelial cells, and a predominantly perivascular infiltration composed of lymphocytes and many plasma cells. It is the presence of these plasma cells that usually alerts the pathologist to the possibility of syphilis. Silver stain may demonstrate the presence of spirochetes.

Serologic Tests for Syphilis (STS)
The serologic tests for syphilis can be divided into two groups: nontreponemal or reagin tests and treponemal or specific tests.

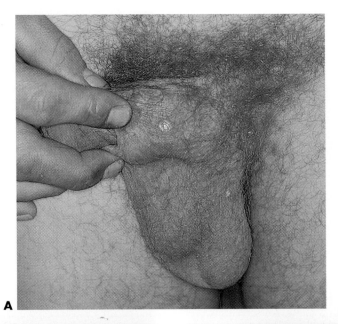

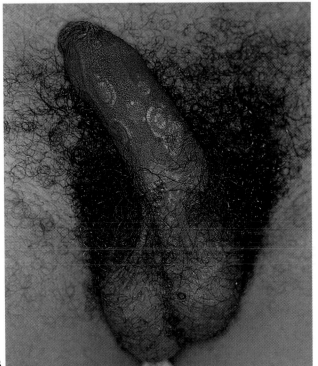

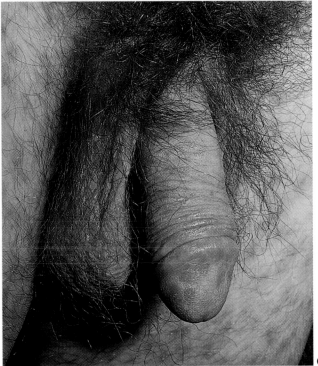

FIG. 4-14
Secondary syphilis. **A,** Papules, some of which are eroded, are seen on the penis, scrotum, and thighs. **B,** Several arciform and annular lesions are seen on the shaft of penis in a dark-skinned patient. The bleeding lesion is secondary to scraping by the physician for a dark-field examination. **C,** Secondary syphilis in a patient with AIDS. Several flat purplish-brown lesions are seen on the thighs.

The nontreponemal tests are screening tests that, if negative, will usually exclude the diagnosis of syphilis. The two most commonly used tests are the Venereal Disease Research Laboratory (VDRL) test and the Rapid Plasma Reagin (RPR) test. Both are flocculation tests. If these tests give a positive result, they must be confirmed by a positive treponemal test before a diagnosis of syphilis can be made.

The treponemal tests are confirming tests that are usually used when a nontreponemal screening test is reported as positive. The two most commonly used treponemal tests are the fluorescent treponemal antibody/absorption (FTA/ABS) test and the *treponema pallidum* hemagglutination (TPHA) test.

False-positive results may be caused by autoimmune or connective tissue disease, or by a concomitant viral infection.

Serology in Primary Syphilis

Approximately 25% of cases have a positive VDRL test result during the first week of the chancre appearance; 50% have a positive result during the second week of their chancre; 75% have a positive result during the third week; and 100% have a positive result when the chancre has been present for 4 weeks. In secondary syphilis virtually 100% of the cases are VDRL positive, except in those rare occasions when there is excessive production of antibody that interferes with normal flocculation or complement fixation process, causing a negative result (prozone phenomenon). When the prozone phenomenon is suspected, dilution of the serum will give a strong positive reaction.

Treatment

The generally accepted treatment of early syphilis (primary, secondary, and latent syphilis of not more than 2 years' duration) is penicillin G benzathine (Bicillin) 2.4 million units, given by intramuscular injection in a single session. This is usually given as 1.2 million units in each buttock to minimize pain. ▼ I personally prefer to follow the treatment recommendation suggested by Nicholas J. Fiumara, which repeats the same treatment after a 1 week interval. Thus the optimal tratment for early syphilis is a total dose of penicillin G benzathine 4.8 million units, given in two divided doses 1 week apart because the single dose of 2.4 million units has occasionally been proven insufficient.[13,14] ▲ Alternative treatment is aqueous penicillin G procaine, 600,000 units injected intramuscularly once daily for 10 consecutive days.

For those patients who are allergic to penicillin, use tetracycline by mouth 500 mg 4 times a day for 15 days.

Syphilis in AIDS patients has to be treated in an identical manner as treating an immunocompetent individual. There is no solid evidence to suggest that higher doses of antibiotics are required to treat AIDS patients infected with syphilis.

Sometimes secondary syphilitic lesions may be seen on the scrotum without any lesions on the penis. These may be papules and in dark-skinned individuals the lesions may be annular or circinate.[15]

Tertiary syphilis on the penis is extremely rare. Lesions are seen as gummas on the foreskin, glans, shaft, and scrotum.[16]

Gonorrhea

The most common manifestation of gonorrhea is gonococcal urethritis, but other lesions may be produced by the causative gram-negative diplococcus, *Neisseria gonorrhoeae*. The marked inflammation may cause paraphimosis (Fig. 4-15, *A*). Balanitis and erosive balanitis may be seen. The gonococcus may produce superficial pustules, as well as erosions and ulcers that may mimic syphilitic chancres (Fig. 4-15, *B*).[17,18] Syphilis and gonorrhea may coexist in the same patient (Fig. 4-15, *C*).

Diagnosis of gonorrhea can be confirmed by smears of the pus or secretion showing intracellular diplococci in neutrophils and by cultures of the gonococcus, which grows on specific culture media. Treatment of choice is one injection of ceftriaxone 250 mg given intramuscularly in a single dose or defixime 400 mg by mouth in a single dose. ▼ It is recommended that treatment for all sexually transmitted diseases be verified with the local health authorities for the current recommendations since resistant bacterial strains do develop and treatment recommendations change periodically. If there is any question or doubt as to the optimal treatment of any specific case, a telephone call to the local Health Officer is all that is needed. ▲

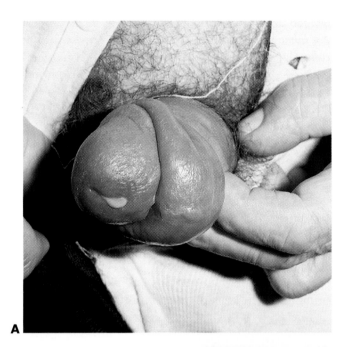

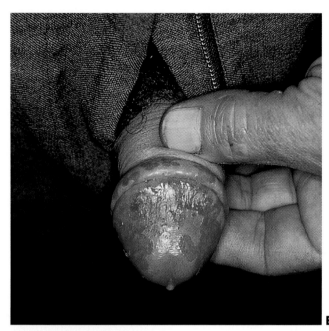

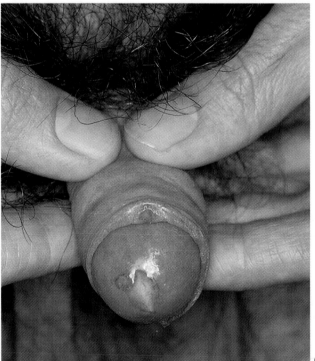

FIG. 4-15
A, Gonorrhea. Purulent urethritis and paraphimosis are shown. **B,** Erosive balanitis showing multiple erosions on the glans penis and corona. Purulent urethritis is present. **C,** Gonorrhea and syphilis coexisting in the same patient. Syphilitic chancres and gonorrheal urethritis are seen.

Chancroid

Also called "soft chancre," chancroid is caused by the gram-negative bacillus, *Haemophilus ducreyi*. It is characterized by one or more tender ulcers with a yellowish, dirty surface, frequently surrounded by erythema. A typical ulcer is associated with one or more, tender, regional inguinal lymph nodes ("buboes") (Fig. 4-16). By tradition a chancroid ulcer can be distinguished from a syphilitic ulcer, because the chancroid ulcer is soft and very tender, whereas the syphilitic chancre is firm and painless. In practice, however, these criteria are totally unreliable. Typical indolent syphilitic chancres are rarely seen, secondarily infected syphilitic chancres are frequently painful, and last but not least both syphilis and chancroid may coexist in the same ulcer as a mixed infection.

Differential diagnosis is the same as for syphilic chancre. The diagnosis is confirmed by demonstrating the typical "school-of-fish" gram-negative coccobacteria in smears or by positive cultures on specific culture media. This, however, is not always successful, because the organism is difficult to grow in culture. In these cases detection can be achieved by using the polymerase chain reaction.[19]

Treatment

Treatment is effective with azithromycin 1 gram orally in a single dose. Satisfactory alternate medications are ceftriaxone 250 mg intramuscularly in a single dose or erythromycin 500 mg orally 4 times a day for 10 days.[20]

Lymphogranuloma Venereum

The causative agent of lymphogranuloma venereum (LGV) is *Chlamydia trachomatis,* types L1, L2, and L3. The disease occurs most commonly in individuals between 20 and 50 years of age. The patient history includes sexual exposure to a possibly infectious partner, travel to an endemic area with sexual exposure, and the appearance of primary stage and secondary stage lesions. The incubation period for LGV is 3 to 20 days for the primary stage and 10 days to 6 months for the secondary stage.

Physical examination in the primary stage reveals a small papule, erosion, or ulcer that heals in a few days, sometimes leaving a small scale, which disap-

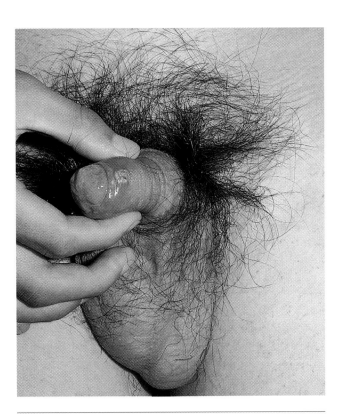

FIG. 4-16
Chancroid. A yellowish ulcer is seen on the foreskin. The inguinal lymph nodes are inflamed, red, and swollen (buboes).

pears rapidly, usually without leaving a scar. Patients in the secondary stage have systemic symptoms of fever and malaise associated with inguinal tender lymphadenopathy (bubo). Occasionally an association with erythema nodosum and erythema multiforme is discovered. Differential diagnoses for the primary stage include primary syphilis, chancroid, and genital herpes and for the secondary stage include genital herpes, syphilis, bacterial lymphadenitis, chancroid, Hodgkin's disease, bubonic plague, tuberculosis, tularemia, and incarcerated inguinal hernia.

Diagnosis

A complement-fixation test, if titer is greater than 1:64, confirms active LGV. The microimmunofluorescent test is proven to be a very sensitive and specific test.

Treatment

Doxycycline 100 mg bid for 21 days is the treatment of choice for LGV. An alternative treatment is erythromycin or tetracycline 500 mg qid for 21 days, or sulfisoxazole 500 mg qid for 21 days.

Etiologic Factors

Caused by chlamydia trachomatis, LGV is characterized by an early, transient primary lesion, usually a papule, followed by a tender unilateral inflamed inguinal lymph node (bubo), which may be associated with abdominal, rectal, and back pain. Bilateral lymph node involvement may be seen. The primary lesion may be seen as a small scale when the early papule has healed. A characteristic finding is the "groove sign of Greenblatt," caused by swollen lymph nodes just above and below Poupart's ligament in the groin (Fig. 4-17). The lymph nodes may rupture and form draining sinuses or produce fistulas into the penis and urethra, causing scars and irreversible deformities of

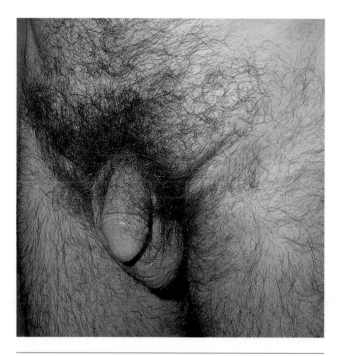

FIG. 4-17

Lymphogranuloma venereum: swollen left femoral and inguinal lymph nodes showing the "groove sign of Greenblatt" (separation of the femoral from the inguinal nodes by Poupart's ligament) are observed. A small healing primary lesion can be seen on the glans penis.

the penis. Elephantiasis of the penis and of the scrotum are rarely seen late complications.

Fluctuant buboes should be aspirated with a syringe and needle. They should not be incised and drained because of the risk of nonhealing fistulas. Early diagnosis and treatment are mandatory to prevent the multiple complications that LGV is known to cause.[21]

Granuloma Inguinale (Donovanosis)

Granuloma inguinale, caused by the gram-negative bacterium *Calymmatobacterium granulomatis*, is mainly seen in the tropics with small endemic foci in all continents except Europe. However, travelers or immigrants may harbor the disease, and therefore it may be seen anywhere.[22,23] The lesions are small ulcers that may coalesce and become larger lesions with fleshy surfaces. They heal in some areas, leaving scars, only to start again in adjacent sites (Fig. 4-18, *A*).

Diagnosis

The histiocytes in granuloma inguinale contain safety pin–like gram-negative bacteria, referred to as Donovan bodies, which may be seen easily in tissue smears stained with Giemsa, Wright's, or silver stains (Fig. 4-18, *B*). Another nice technique for demonstrating these bacteria is by doing an epon semi-thin section, as used for electron microscopy (Fig. 4-18, *C*). Both of these methods can be used to establish the diagnosis.

Treatment

The treatment of choice is tetracycline 500 mg 4 times a day for 21 days. If the lesions are not cured by that time, treatment should be continued until all lesions have completely healed. As with all sexually transmitted diseases, all sexual contacts must be traced, examined, and treated if needed. The possibility of concomitant HIV infection should always be considered and ruled out by doing an HIV-antibody test.

Tuberculous Lesions of the Penis

The tuberculous lesions may manifest themselves as painful ulcers or nontender nodules (Fig. 4-19).[24]

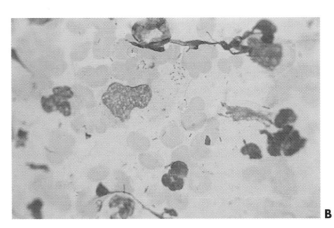

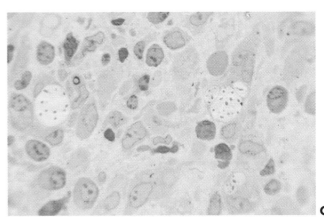

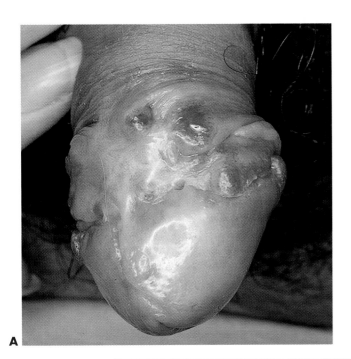

FIG. 4-18

A, Granuloma Inguinale. A plaque of active ulcers and scarring are located on the glans penis. **B,** Intracellular, "safety pin–like," bipolar-staining bacilli, also called Donovan bodies, are clustered within a histiocyte in a smear taken from a lesion of granuloma inguinale (upper center). Giemsa stain × 100. **C,** An epon-embedded, semithin section, demonstrating Donovan bodies in pale histiocytes.

(**C,** From Hacker P, Fisher BK, Dekoven J, et al: Int J Dermatol 31:696-699, 1992.)

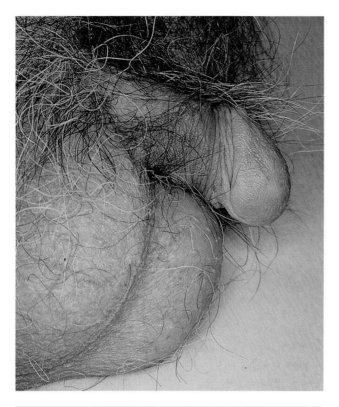

FIG. 4-19
Tuberculosis. Nontender, pink nodule located on the glans, adjacent to frenulum. The histology showed a typical tuberculous granuloma. The patient had a history of renal tuberculosis.
(Courtesy Dr. Robert N. Richards.)

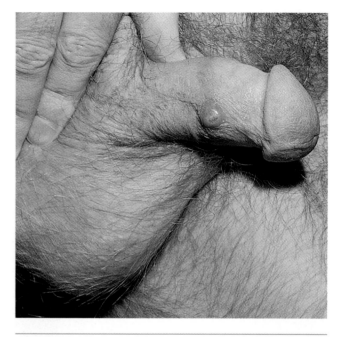

FIG. 4-20
Bacillary Angiomatosis in an AIDS Patient. A smooth, pink, slightly eroded papule is located on the shaft of the penis.

Papulonecrotic tuberculids may involve the penis in successive crops, causing scarring that may lead to a "worm-eaten" appearance.[25] Frequently the patient or a close family member has obvious tuberculosis in the lungs or in another organ. Typical tuberculous granulomas are seen histologically. Acid-fast bacteria may or may not be present in the histologic sections.

Treatment consists of triple therapy for tuberculosis and should be monitored by an expert familiar with the treatment of this disease.

Bacillary Angiomatosis

Although it may rarely affect immunocompetent patients, bacillary angiomatosis is mostly seen in immunosuppressed individuals. It is a systemic disease caused by the gram-negative, rickettsial-like bacilli, *Bartonella henselae* and *Bartonella quintana*. Usually in immunocompetent patients *Bartonella henselae* causes cat-scratch disease and *Bartonella quintana* causes Trench Fever. Bacillary angiomatosis can involve the skin, liver, spleen, bones, and lymph nodes. Skin lesions may be

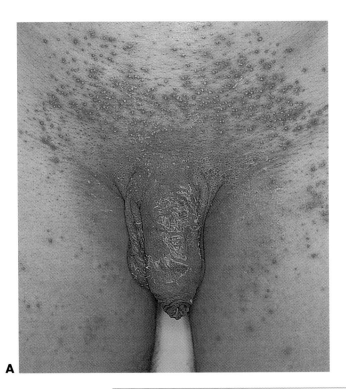

A

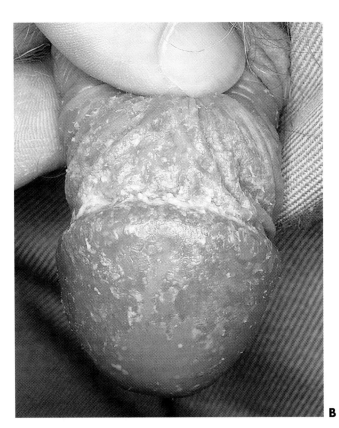

B

FIG. 4-21
A, Moniliasis. The penis is inflamed and scaly, with multiple papules and pustules located in the groin, pubic area, and base of the penis. Many typical satellite lesions can be seen. **B,** Erythema, whitish patches, and superficial erosions located on the glans penis and foreskin. The white patches represent monilial colonies.

solitary or multiple. They usually present as dark-red papules and nodules, which may look like hemangiomas, pyogenic granulomas, or lesions of Kaposi's sarcoma. They may be eroded with a yellowish surface mimicking a furuncle; or may present as pink, smooth papules (Fig. 4-20); or skin-colored subcutaneous nodules.

Several of these various skin lesions may coexist in the same patient. The histology is fairly typical, and the bacteria usually can be demonstrated with a silver stain such as the Whartin-Starry stain.

Occasionally this stain fails to show the organisms. In those cases, if bacillary angiomatosis is still suspected, electron-microscopy examination of the suspected tissue should be done. Bacilli, if present, will show up very clearly. It is important to diagnose the condition early, as failure to do so may lead to a fatal multisystem infection.

Treatment for the disease is with erythromycin 500 mg 4 times a day, for several weeks or several months. Alternative drugs are azithromycin and doxycycline. Relapses are known to occur.[26,27]

FUNGUS AND YEAST INFECTIONS
Candidiasis of the Penis

Candidiasis, a common condition, may be acquired from an infected sexual partner or may be precipitated by immunosuppression or diabetes. Clinical manifestations of the eruption consist of small papules and pustules with typical satellite lesions (Fig. 4-21, *A*) or a pattern of erythema with feathery whitish streaks, similar to the thrush lesions seen in the oral mucosa (Fig. 4-21, *B*). These white streaks are really colonies of candida that can rapidly be identified by taking a scraping and doing a KOH preparation for microscopic examination. At times erosions may be seen, sometimes with satellite lesions.

Treatment consists of identifying and treating the predisposing cause such as diabetes, and treating the skin eruption with an appropriate anticandidal topical medication, such as ketoconazole or nystatin. It is important to treat the sexual partner as well so that a "Ping-Pong" type reinfection does not occur. Effective local treatment can be carried out by using ketoconazole cream twice a day or 1% hydrocortisone in ketoconazole (Nizoral) cream twice a day. The addition of hydrocortisone to the antifungal preparation will reduce the existing inflammation and will promote healing.

In candidal septicemia, necrotic lesions with black eschars may rarely be seen on the penis.[28]

Tinea cruris

Superficial dermatophytes rarely affect the penis.[29] Occasionally, scaly patches may be seen on the base of the penis as part of a *Tinea cruris* infection, which so commonly involves the groin, pubic area, and buttocks. There is no adequate explanation as to why these fungal infections almost always spare the penis. They respond readily to treatment with ketoconazole or terbinafine (Lamisil) cream twice a day. For widespread infection, terbinafine by mouth is indicated (250 mg once a day for 6 to 12 consecutive weeks).

REFERENCES
Viral Diseases
1. Cobb MW: Human papilloma virus infection, *J Am Acad Dermatol* 22:547-567, 1990.
2. Seigel JF, Mellinger BC: Human papillomavirus in the male patient, *Urol Clin North Am* 19:83-91, 1992.
3. Oriel JD: Natural history of genital warts, *Br J Vener Dis* 47:1-13, 1971.
4. Quan MB, Moy RL: The role of human papilloma virus in carcinoma, *J Am Acad Dermatol* 25:698-705, 1991.
5. Eng AM, Morgan NE, Blekys I: Giant condyloma acuminatum, *Cutis* 24:203-206, 209, 1979.
6. Kanik AB, Lee J, Wax F, Bhawan J: Penile verrucous carcinoma in a 37-year-old circumcised man, *J Am Acad Dermatol* 37:329-331, 1997.
7. Ilkay AK, Chodak, GW, Voegelzang NJ, et al.: Buschke-Lowenstein tumor: therapeutic options including systemic chemotherapy, *Urology* 42:599-602, 1993.
8. Schwartz RA, Fanniger CK: Bowenoid papulosis, *J Am Acad Dermatol* 24:261-264, 1991.
9. Maccato ML, Kaufman RH: Herpes genitalis, *Dermatol Clin* 10:415-422, 1992.
10. Lavoie SR, Kaplowitz LG: Management of genital herpes infections, *Semin Dermatol* 13:248-255, 1994.
11. Brown ST, Nalley JF, Kraus SJ: Molluscum contagiosum, *Sex Trans Dis* 8:227-234, 1981.
12. Lewis EJ, Lam M, Crutchfield CE III: An update on molluscum contagiosum, *Cutis* 60:29-34, 1997.

Bacterial Infections
13. Fiumara NJ: The treatment of primary and secondary syphilis: the serologic response, *JAMA* 243:2500-2502, 1980.
14. Berger TG, Fiumara NJ, Whitfield M: Syphilis and the treponematoses. In Arndt KK, Leboit PE, Robinson JK, Wintraub BU, editors: *Cutaneous medicine and surgery*, vol 2, Philadelphia, 1996, Saunders, 949-963.
15. Chapel TA: Primary and secondary syphilis, *Cutis* 33:47-53, 1984.
16. Korting CW: *Practical dermatology of the genital region*, Philadelphia, 1981, Saunders, 174..
17. Landergren G: Gonorrheal ulcer of the penis: report of a case, *Acta Derm Venereol* 41:320-323, 1961.
18. Haim S, Merzbach D: Gonococcal penile ulcer, *Br J Venerol Dis* 46:336-337, 1970.

19. Webb RM, Hotchkiss R, Currier M, et al: Chancroid detected by polymerase chain reaction, *Arch Dermatol* 132:17-18, 1996.

20. Felman YM: Recent developments in sexually transmitted diseases: chancroid-epidemiology, diagnosis, and treatment, *Cutis* 44:113-114, 1989.

21. Hopsu-Havu VK, Sonck CE: Infiltrative, ulcerative and fistular lesions of the penis due to lymphogranuloma venereum, *Br J Vener Dis* 49:193-202, 1973.

22. Niemel PLA, Engelkens HJH, van der Meijden WI, Stolz E: Donovanosis (granuloma inguinale) still exists, *Int J Dermatol* 31: 244-246, 1992.

23. Hacker P, Fisher BK, Dekoven J, et al: Granuloma inguinale: three cases diagnosed in Toronto, Canada, *Int J Dermatol* 31:696-699, 1992.

24. Venkataramaiah NR, Dutta SN, van Raalte JA: Tuberculous ulcer of the penis, *Postgrad Med J* 58:59-60, 1982.

25. Jeyakumar W, Ganesh R, Mohanram F, et al.: Papulonecrotic tuberculids of the glans penis: case report, *Genitourin Med* 64:130-132, 1988.

26. Lipa J, Peters W, Fornasier V, Fisher B: Bacillary angiomatosis: a unique cutaneous complication of HIV infection, *Can J Plast Surg* 3(2):96-101, 1995.

27. Nosal JM: Bacillary angiomatosis, cat-scratch disease and bartonellosis: what's the connection? *Int J Dermatol* 36:405-411, 1997.

Fungus and Yeast Infections

28. Odds FC: Genital candidiasis, *Clin Exp Dermatol* 7:345-354, 1982.

29. Dekio S, Jidio J: Tinea of the glans penis, *Dermatologica* 178:112-114, 1989.

SCABIES

Scabies almost always involves the penis. The lesions are usually papules, vesicles, or scabs; less frequently small pustules, excoriations, and typical burrows (Fig. 5-1). Severe itch is usually present, but occasionally the patient may not be aware that he has lesions on his penis. Elsewhere on the skin the lesions may be few or multiple, but it is very rare not to have penile lesions in scabies. This is of great diagnostic importance in cases of itchy dermatoses of uncertain nature where scabies is also considered. If lesions are present on the penis, the diagnosis of scabies is virtually confirmed.

Scabietic lesions on the penis may at times be associated with lymphangitis or lymphadenitis caused by secondary bacterial infection, which requires systemic antibiotic treatment. This secondary infection is caused by bacteria that enter the skin through excoriations caused by the intense itch. Treatment with antibiotics such as penicillin or ciprofloxacin (Cipro) is indicated. Even when scabies has been adequately treated, residual "post-scabetic" lesions may persist for several months. These are usually manifested as raised papules, small purplish nodules, or hyperpigmented flat small plaques localized on the penis or scrotum (Fig. 5-2). With time these lesions disappear. A nonfluoridated steroid cream may help to hasten their evolution.

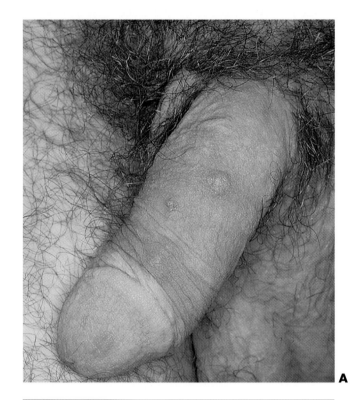

A

FIG. 5-1
Scabies. A, Papules of various sizes on the glans and shaft of the penis.

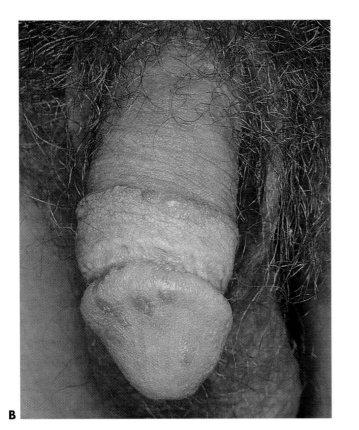

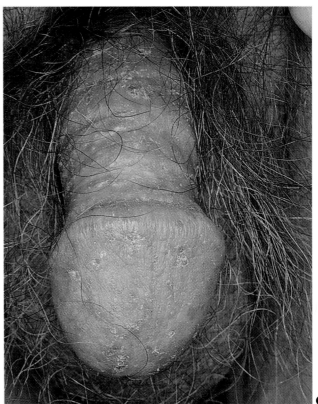

FIG. 5-1, cont'd
B, Numerous large papules mainly on the glans penis. **C,** Multiple typical scabetic burrows and small scaly lesions on the glans penis and shaft.

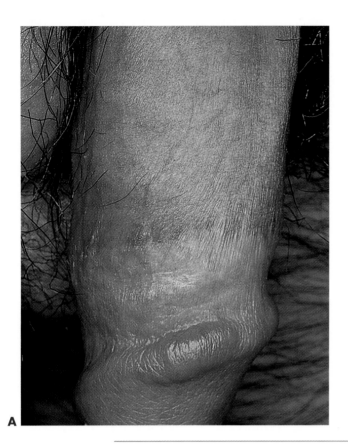 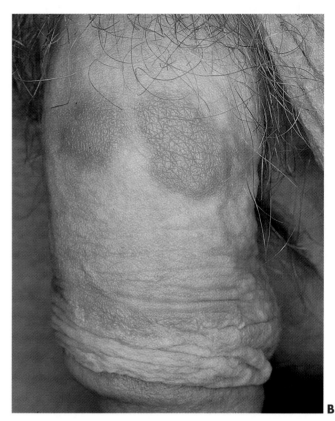

FIG. 5-2
A, A large post-scabetic nodule on the corona.   **B,** Two hyperpigmented, post-scabetic flat plaques on the shaft of the penis. These may be misdiagnosed as a fixed drug eruption.

A rare variety of scabies, Norwegian scabies, presents yellowish scaly patches that do not look like the typical scabetic lesions (Fig. 5-3). These lesions contain numerous scabies mites that are easily identified under the micropscope.

Treatment of scabies should be carried out by using topical 1% lindane (gamma-benzene hexachloride) or topical 5% permethrin (Nix). Because of the emergence of resistant strains of scabies mites to lindane, the use of permethrin in the treatment of scabies is increasing. In my opinion, the commonly practiced method of treating scabies with a one-time, 12-hour application of either lindane or permethrin is inadequate in many cases. ▼ **I instruct my patients to apply the cream (I never use a lotion or a shampoo) for 24 hours and then reapply it for another 24 hours, each time preceded by a 20-** **minute hot soapy bath. I often repeat the treatment once, after one week, especially if the patient has not responded to previous treatment(s). ▲** The cream should be applied to all skin areas below the neck. In infants and immunosuppressed individuals all of the skin surface should be treated, including the face and scalp. All household members of the scabetic patient, as well as any sexual partners, should be treated concomitantly.

Small children under 5 years of age should be treated with 10% precipitated sulfur in white petrolatum to avoid the rare occurrence of seizures. This ointment should be rubbed into all skin areas, face and scalp included, and left for 24 hours. The procedure should be repeated once or twice after 24 hours.[1,2,3]

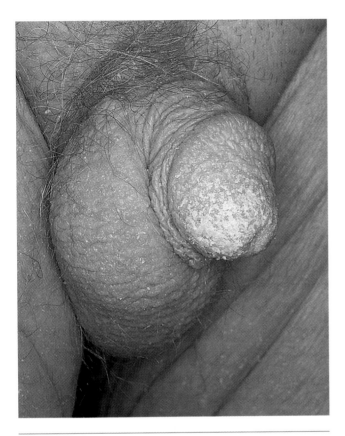

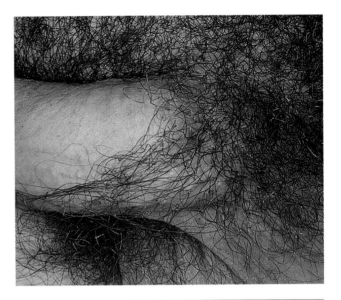

FIG. 5-3
Norwegian Scabies. Yellowish thick scales on the glans penis. The scales contain vast numbers of mites.

FIG. 5-4
In this case of pediculosis pubis, several crab-lice are seen on the base of the penis as specks of dark-brown dirt.

PEDICULOSIS PUBIS

The infestation of pediculosis pubis is caused by crab-lice, which attach themselves to the base of the hairs in the pubic area and in the groins. The lice look like small, dark-brown or black, specks of dirt. At times they are found on the base of the penis (Fig. 5-4). When these lice are pulled from their point of attachment with tweezers, their movement easily identifies their nature.

Treatment is with lindane or permethrin shampoo or lotion. These should be applied to the affected areas for 10 minutes and then washed off. Sexual partners should undergo the same treatment.[4]

REFERENCES

Scabies
1. Elgart M: Scabies, *Dermatol Clin* 8:253-263, 1990.
2. Orkin M, Maibach HI: Scabies therapy: 1993, *Semin Dermatol* 12:22-25, 1993.
3. Funkhouser ME, Omohundro C, Ross A, et al.: Management of scabies in patients with human immunodeficiency virus disease, *Arch Dermatol* 129:911-913, 1993.

Pediculosis Pubis
4. Elgart M: Pediculosis, *Dermatol Clin* 8:219-228, 1990.

CHAPTER 6

Inflammatory Lesions of the Penis

This chapter deals with a variety of lesions that are characterized by clinical and/or histologic inflammation. As can be expected in any inflammatory skin lesion, many of these lesions exhibit redness, at times oozing or scaling, and cause frequent itching or burning but rarely pain.

INFLAMMATORY LESIONS

Balanitis and Balanoposthitis

One of the most common inflammatory lesions of the penis is nonspecific balanitis or nonspecific balanoposthitis. Balanitis is defined as inflammation of the glans penis; posthitis is inflammation of the foreskin; and a combination of these is balanoposthitis (Fig. 6-1). Most of the time the cause for this inflammation is unknown.

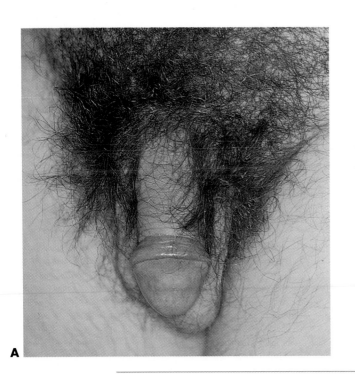
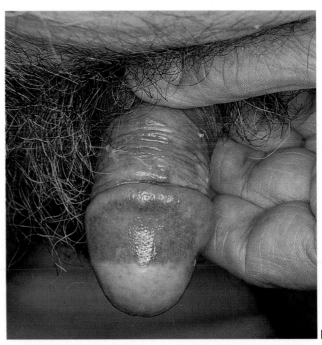

A

B

FIG. 6-1

Balanoposthitis. **A**, A few red patches on the glans penis. The mucosal aspect of the foreskin is inflamed and red. **B**, Erythema and oozing on the glans penis and on the mucosal aspect of the foreskin.

Diagnosis

Prevailing theories implicate seborrheic dermatitis, poor hygiene, a large amount of smegma, or a low-grade bacterial or yeast infection. At times balanitis may become erosive. This may be associated with diabetes or with chronic urinary incontinence. At times the lesion may suggest malignancy (Fig. 6-2).

Treatment

Temporary relief is usually achieved by topical steroid-antifungal mixture preparations. Circumcision will cure balanoposthitis. However, erosive balanitis may be seen without any obvious etiologic cause and responds frequently to symptomatic treatment with compresses and topical antibiotics. For compresses use a regular saline or vinegar solution (one-half teaspoon vinegar per glass of water) twice a day, followed by the application of an antibiotic ointment or cream such as fusidic acid (Fucidin) or 2% mupirocin ointment (Bactroban).

ACUTE CONTACT DERMATITIS OR CONTACT BALANITIS

Acute contact dermatitis is not an uncommon condition. Multiple allergens can cause it. Most of the time the allergen is transferred to the penis by the fingers while the patient is urinating.

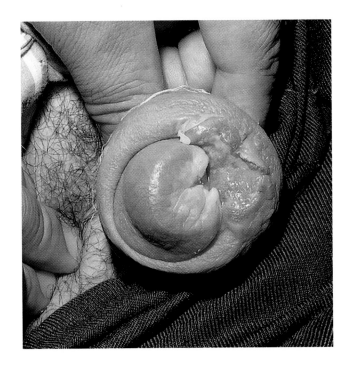

FIG. 6-2
Erosive balanoposthitis in a paraplegic with incontinence. The biopsy showed no malignant changes.

Diagnosis

Causative allergens may be poison ivy,[1] creams used to treat other body areas, antiseptics, and spermatocide creams (Fig. 6-3, *A*). Acute contact dermatitis may be associated with marked edema of the penis and foreskin (Fig. 6-3, *B*). If the dermatitis becomes chronic, the penis will show dry areas with scaly folded and wrinkled skin (Fig. 6-3, *C*). If the inflammation is severe enough, it can damage the melanocytes, which results in permanent loss of pigment in the area. For example, hypopigmentation is seen in patients who become allergic to rubber, secondary to the use of latex condoms. Patients who are employed in the rubber industry and who become allergic to rubber or one of its constituents (monobenzyl ether of hydroquinone) may also show hypopigmentation (Fig. 6-3, *D*). Severe irritating chemicals, such as nitrogen mustard used in chemical warfare, may cause severe inflammation and erosions of the penis and scrotum (Fig. 6-3, *E*).

Treatment

In severe cases of contact dermatitis, a short course of systemic steroids (prednisone 20 mg qam for 5 to 7 days, then tapered off gradually by 5 mg every 5 to 7 days) may have to be used in conjunction with soothing compresses with a saline or vinegar solution (one-half teaspoon regular vinegar per glass of lukewarm water).[2]

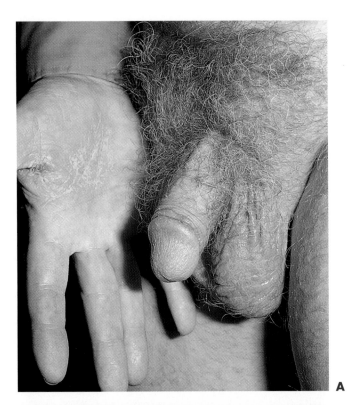

A

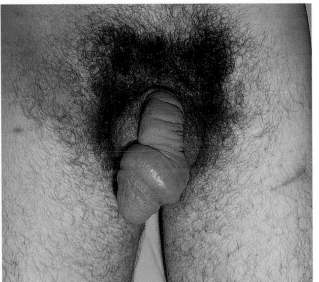

B

FIG. 6-3
A, Contact dermatitis of the penis and scrotum caused by a vitamin-A acid cream used to treat hyperkeratosis of the palms. Both the corona and scrotum are inflamed and red. **B,** Acute contact dermatitis of the thighs and penis, with marked redness and edema of the penis.

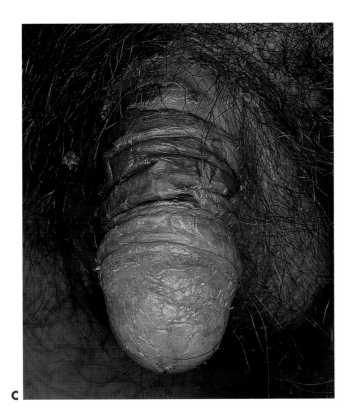

C

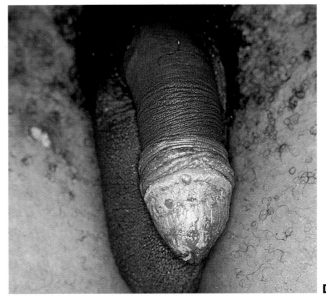

D

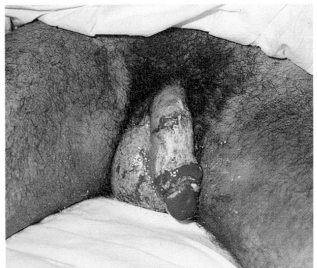

E

FIG. 6-3, cont'd

C, A patient with chronic contact dermatitis. The glans penis is red and scaly, and the shaft is dry with horizontal folds. **D,** Contact dermatitis of the penis with secondary hypopigmentation. **E,** Severe erosive contact dermatitis of the penis and scrotum caused by nitrogen mustard used in chemical warfare.

(**E,** Courtesy Dr. Yahya Dowlati.)

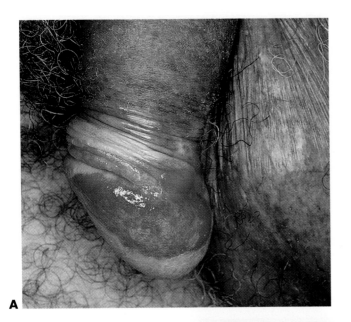

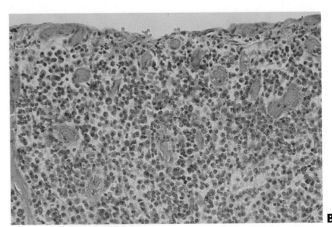

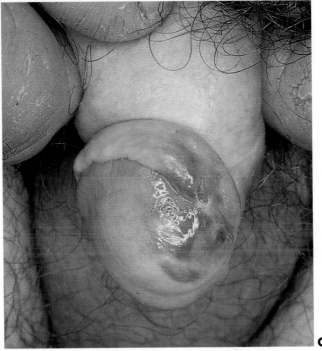

FIG. 6-4
A, A patient with plasma cell balanitis (balanitis circumscripta plasmacellularis). Red, shiny, well-circumscribed plaque is located on the glans penis and extends to the fore-skin. **B,** Histology of plasma cell balanitis. Numerous plasma cells and a few lympho-cytes are seen in the upper dermis. The epidermal cells have become eroded and have disappeared in this section. Several prominent blood vessels are present (H&E × 40). **C,** Reddish, glistening, well-circumscribed patch of plasma cell balanitis on the glans penis, extending to the corona. Several brown spots of various shades are present in the lesion suggestive of a melanocytic lesion, such as a melanoma. These brown spots are the manifestation of hemosiderin deposits. Biopsy is mandatory to rule out melanoma. (Courtesy Dr. Harvey G. Shapero.)

Balanitis Circumscripta Plasmacellularis (Zoon's Balanitis)

This plasma cell balanitis is characterized by a red, shiny, well-circumscribed patch or plaque that involves the glans penis, but may extend to the distal end of the shaft (Fig. 6-4, *A*). The etiology of this condition is unknown, and it frequently responds to the local application of antibiotics. The histopathology is characteristic, showing a thin or absent epidermis and a bandlike infiltrate composed of numerous plasma cells and dilated capillaries (Fig. 6-4, *B*). At times extravasation of red blood cells and deposition of hemosiderin may be seen.[3] When this occurrence is significant, the clinical lesion may show dark-brown pigmented spots that may cause a suspicion of a melanocytic lesion, such as a melanoma (Fig. 6-4, *C*). Clinically plasma cell balanitis should be differentiated from erythroplasia of Queyrat (squamous cell carcinoma in situ), and on those rare occasions when there is a heavy deposition of hemosiderin, from a melanocytic lesion such as melanoma.[4,5,6]

Juvenile Xanthogranuloma (Nevoxanthoendothelioma)

Juvenile xanthogranuloma is a rare benign lesion that presents as an asymptomatic pinkish-yellowish smooth nodule and may be mistaken for a neoplastic lesion. The histology is very typical, showing a dermal infiltrate composed of lymphocytes, eosinophils, histiocytes, foam cells, and Touton giant cells.

Sclerosing Lymphangitis of the Penis

The lesion is a cordlike, usually horizontal, subcutaneous linear nodule that corresponds to a thrombosed or sclerosed lymphatic vessel. It is usually seen in young adults who are overactive sexually. Honeymooners are good candidates for this condition, which is entirely benign and disappears on its own within a few weeks (Fig. 6-5). No treatment is necessary.[7]

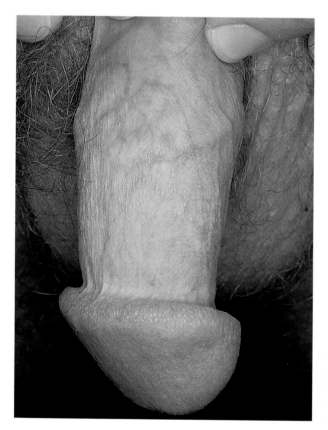

FIG. 6-5
Sclerosing Lymphangitis of the Penis. A horizontal, cordlike, skin-colored, asymptomatic nodule seen on the mid shaft of the penis.

GANGRENOUS LESIONS

Ordinary pyoderma gangrenosum is an uncommon, severe, progressive, ulcerative condition. It usually starts as a pustule that breaks down and becomes an enlarging ulcer, usually with a typical violaceous, frequently raised, undermined border. An associated systemic disease may be found in about 50% of cases. Penile pyoderma gangrenosum is extremely rare and only a handful of cases have been reported.[8] Biopsy is very helpful.

Treatment consists of moderate doses of systemic steroids (40 to 60 mg of prednisone daily), to be tapered off as the patient improves. In selected cases, where the lesions are relatively small, intralesional injections of triamcinolone acetonide, 10 mg/ml, may clear up the lesions.

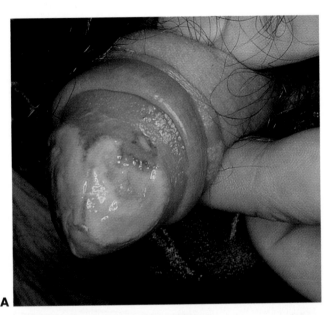

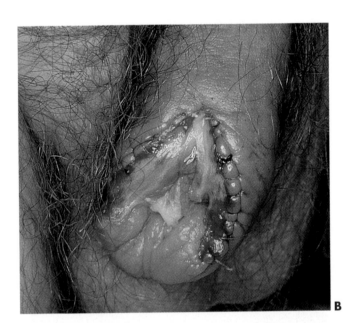

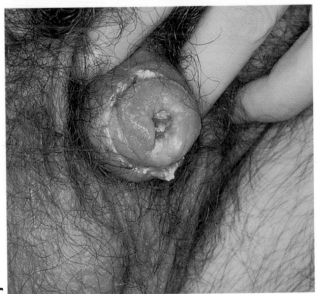

FIG. 6-6

Destructive Pyoderma Gangrenosum of the Penis. **A,** Necrotic, grayish-yellowish, moist patch on the glans penis. **B,** Forty-eight hours after surgical excision of the lesion. Gangrene in the center of the surgical site has reappeared as a dark gray patch. **C,** Three weeks following reexcision of the gangrenous site and institution of therapy with high-dose systemic steroids and azathioprine (Imuran). The condition has settled down, but the patient lost half of his penis.

(Courtesy Dr. Brock Kirkpatrick.)

Destructive Pyoderma Gangrenosum of the Penis

Destructive pyoderma gangrenosum is an extremely rare, rapidly destructive, necrotizing condition and does not look nor behave like the ordinary pyoderma gangrenosum. A black necrotic soft patch appears on the glans penis and progresses rapidly with severe tissue destruction. Surgical treatment is usually not helpful (Fig. 6-6). This grave condition should be treated aggressively with both systemic steroids (prednisone 60 to 80 mg a day) and immunosuppressive agents, such as azathioprine (Imuran) 100 mg a day. When improvement is evi-

dent these drugs can be tapered off very gradually; otherwise the entire penis will be destroyed (Fig. 6-7). The condition should be distinguished from dry necrosis of the glans penis seen in diabetic patients with end-stage renal disease, which carries a poor prognosis, with the patient usually dying within a few months. Cryoglobulinemia may cause a similar lesion with the same fatal outcome. Clinically a black eschar develops and persists on the glans penis for weeks without any change. It does not respond to symptomatic treatment (Fig. 6-8).[9]

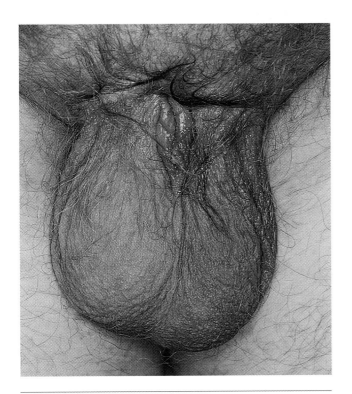

FIG. 6-7
Destructive Pyoderma Gangrenosum of the Penis. This patient's condition had been misdiagnosed, first as a bacterial infection, then as a deep fungal infection. Treatment with various antibiotics did not help. The patient lost his entire penis within several weeks.

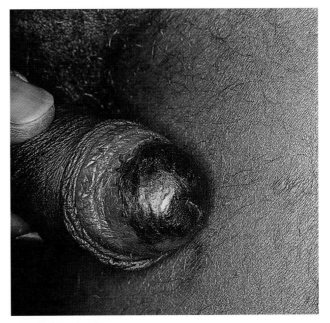

FIG. 6-8
Dry necrosis of the glans penis in a patient with diabetes diagnosed with end-stage renal disease. Persistent black eschar is observed on the glans penis. The patient died a few weeks after the appearance of the lesion.

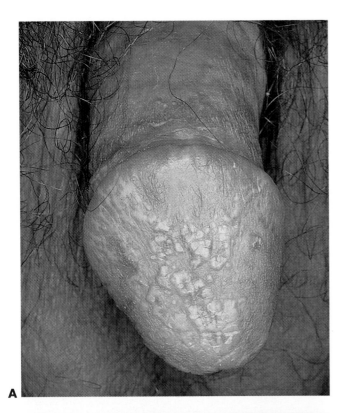

A

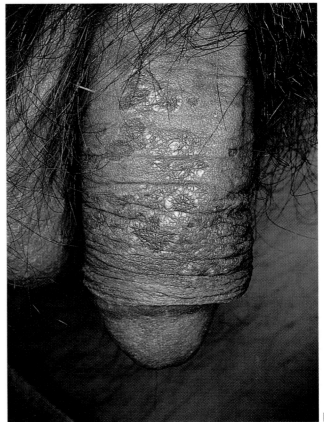

B

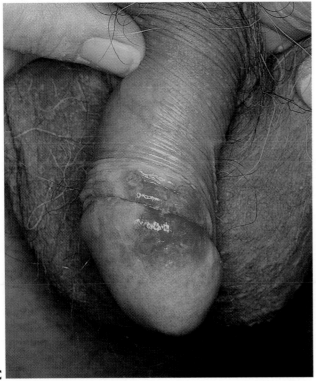

C

FIG. 6-9

Lichen Planus. **A,** Several violaceous polygonal, flat-topped, shiny papules, some with fine scales, are observed on the glans penis. **B,** Several annular, shiny, violaceous papules with hyperpigmented centers. Hyperpigmented lesions are common in dark-skinned individuals. **C,** Erosive lichen planus. Eroded patches on the glans and foreskin. The lesion looks very similar to plasma cell balanitis, fixed drug eruption, and erythroplasia of Queyrat. A biopsy will differentiate between these entities.

PAPULOSQUAMOUS CONDITIONS

The papulosquamous diseases commonly involve the penis. In this group of diseases, lichen planus and psoriasis are encountered most frequently. The lesions on the penis may be part of a generalized skin eruption, or the lesions may be confined to the penis alone.[10]

Lichen Planus

The etiology of this benign but annoying condition is unknown.

Diagnosis

The lesions are polygonal, red to violaceous, flat-topped, shiny papules, at times with fine scales (Fig. 6-9, *A*). The lesions may be annular, hyperpigmented, or erosive (Fig. 6-9, *B* and *C*). Histopathology is quite characteristic. The diagnosis is helped by the finding of typical lichen planus papules on other areas of the skin, particularly on the wrists and on the lower legs, and seeing whitish feathery patches in the oral mucosa. Differential diagnoses are with psoriasis, erosive fixed drug eruption, plasma cell balanitis, erythroplasia of Queyrat, erosive balanitis, and candidal balanitis.

Treatment

No cure is known for lichen planus. Erosive lichen planus may be more difficult to treat, as is the case when present in other mucosal areas. Improvement of the lesions may be achieved by the local application of steroid creams, such as 1% hydrocortisone cream once a day, or using a weak fluorinated steroid cream, such as 2% hydrocortisone valerate cream (Westcort cream). Prolonged use of stronger fluorinated steroid creams may cause irreversible skin atrophy.[11]

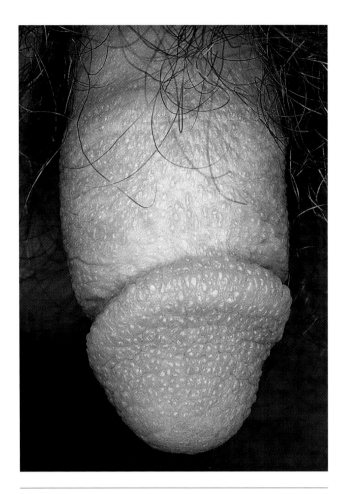

FIG. 6-10
Lichen Nitidus. Numerous tiny, skin-colored papules are observed on the glans and shaft of the penis.

Lichen Nitidus

Lichen nitidus is characterized by asymptomatic, tiny, shiny, pale, or skin-colored papules. These may be few or numerous (Fig. 6-10). The histology is characteristic. The etiology is unknown. The theory that it is a variant of lichen planus has not been proven yet. No adequate treatment for this benign condition is available. It may persist for an unpredictable duration.[12]

Psoriasis

Psoriatic lesions on the penis are fairly common and are quite similar to those encountered elsewhere on the skin, namely red, scaly patches, or papules (Fig. 6-11, *A* and *B*) On occasion, red patches may involve the glans with or without tiny pustules (Fig. 6-11, *C*). The condition may be confused with other papulosquamous diseases or with a nonspecific balanitis.

Diagnosis

The diagnosis of psoriasis may be facilitated if there is a family history of psoriasis and if a thorough examination of the patient is carried out. ▼ **In the examination look for red scaly patches, typical for psoriasis, located elsewhere on the skin, particularly in such typical areas as the elbows, knees, and scalp. Nails should be examined for onycholysis, pitting, or yellowish dystrophic changes; and the intergluteal fold should be examined for erythema and cracking.** ▲ The histology of psoriasis is fairly typical, so a biopsy may be very helpful to arrive at a correct diagnosis in atypical or doubtful cases.

Treatment

Currently there is no known cure for psoriasis. A satisfactory control may be achieved in many cases with nonfluorinated steroid creams, such as 1% hydrocortisone cream, rubbed into the lesions twice a day. A good preparation is 3% Liquor Carbonis Detergens (LCD, a tar solution) in 1% hydrocortisone cream used twice a day. When this treatment does not help, a weak fluorinated steroid cream or ointment, such as 2% hydrocortisone valerate with or without LCD, may be helpful. Although stronger steroid creams may cause temporary clearance, the prolonged use of fluorinated steroid creams may cause irreversible skin atrophy with or without erosions (Fig. 6-11, *D*).[13]

Balanitis Circinata

Balanitis circinata is part of Reiter's syndrome, which includes arthritis, conjunctivitis, urethritis, and stomatitis. The penile lesions consist of red, scaly, or scabby lesions around the urethra and anywhere else on the glans penis. Lesions are frequently but not necessarily annular or circinate (Fig. 6-12).[14]

FIG. 6-11

Psoriasis. **A,** Several dark-red, slightly scaly papules on the glans penis. **B,** Pink scaly patches on the glans penis, corona, and shaft of the penis. **C,** Red patches on the glans and mucosal aspect of the foreskin. Several small pustules on the glans, some in an arciform and annular pattern. **D,** Prolonged use of a fluorinated steroid cream on the glans penis has caused marked irreversible atrophy and erosions. Notice the psoriatic changes in the nails.

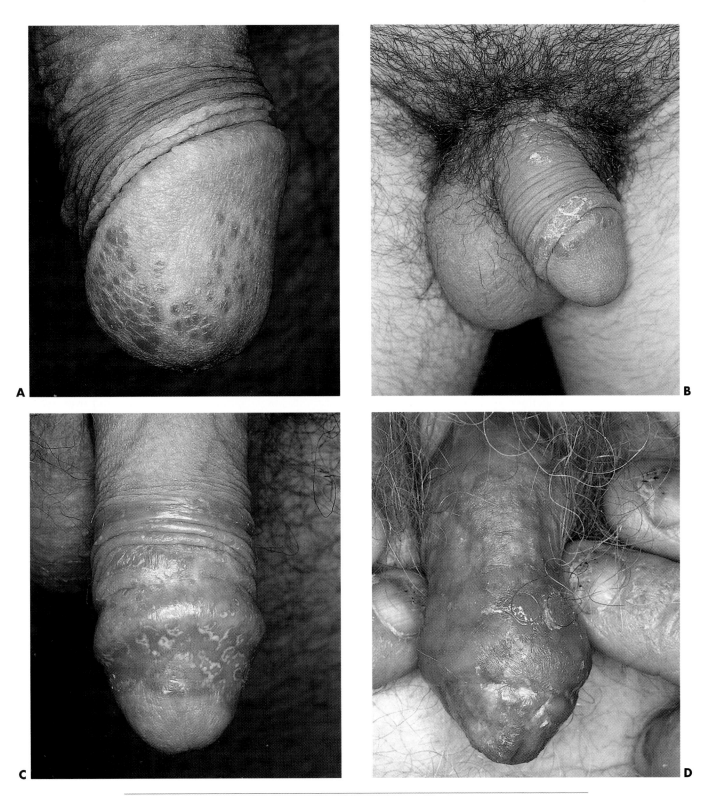

FIG. 6-11
For legend see opposite page.

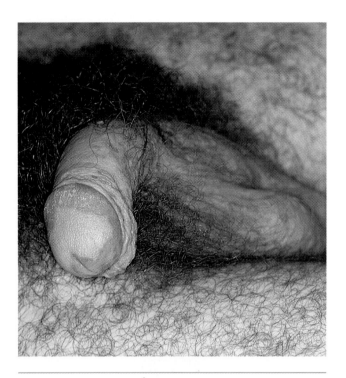

FIG. 6-12
Balanitis Circinata in Reiter's Syndrome. An annular lesion consisting of erythema and scaling is present on the periphery of the glans penis and around the urethral opening.

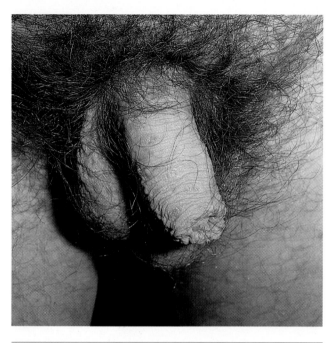

FIG. 6-13
Pityriasis Rosea. Salmon-colored, round and oval, scaly patches on the shaft of the penis.

Other Papulosquamous Conditions

Pityriasis Rosea

Pityriasis rosea shows the same lesions on the penis as are seen elsewhere on the body. The lesions on the penis are part of the general eruption. The lesions are round or oval, salmon-colored, scaly papules and patches that may or may not be itchy and usually disappear spontaneously after 6 to 8 weeks. A history of a preceding "herald patch" is very characteristic (Fig. 6-13).[15,16]

Pityriasis Lichenoides

Pityriasis lichenoides occurs in two forms that differ in severity. Transition between these two types occurs. Both are characterized by crops of pinkish-purplish, small, scaly papules that involve the trunk and to a lesser degree the extremities.

The milder form, pityriasis lichenoides chronica, is usually asymptomatic, and the lesions tend to involute spontaneously within several weeks or a few months. The more severe form, pityriasis lichenoides et varioliformis acuta ("PLEVA", Mucha-Haberman's disease), shows a more extensive eruption with many of the papules becoming hemorrhagic, necrotic, and scabby, which may end in scarring. The lesions may be quite itchy, and they may last for several months or years. The histology is fairly typical for both variants showing lymphocytic vasculitis as a common feature. The etiology is unknown.

Pityriasis lichenoides has the same type of typical scaly and scabby papules on the penis and scrotum as seen elsewhere on the body in this generalized eruption (Fig. 6-14). Treatment is usually unsatisfactory. Ultraviolet light treatment, oral tetracycline or erythromycin (500 mg four times a day), methotrexate, and short courses of prednisone have all been tried with variable, mostly temporary, success.[17]

The Red Scrotum Syndrome

Usually seen in individuals over 60 years of age, an occasional case of the red scrotum syndrome may be encountered in much younger patients. This entity has not been properly defined, although the rare description in the literature of cases that fit this diagnosis can be found. Most dermatologists have seen patients suffering from this condition. The patient seeks medical help because of a red and "burning" scrotum. The symptoms vary from the sensation of mild burning and discomfort in the scrotum and at times in the penis, to severe constant hypersensitivity, burning, itching, and pain, which may be aggravated by the mild pressure of a normal sitting position. Often the patient moves forward on the chair to have his scrotum hang down and not rest on the chair to prevent serious discomfort. This condition bothers the well-being of some patients to the extent that they even contemplate suicide. They give a typical history of going from doctor to doctor seeking help that is never found.

Diagnosis

The clinical picture is always the same. Bright red or dusky erythema of the anterior half of the scrotum, sometimes extending to the shaft of the penis (Fig. 6-15). Telangiectasia may be associated with the erythema, but oozing or scaling is not seen unless the patient develops an over-treatment contact dermatitis. The histology is usually nonspecific, showing a normal skin with a few dilated capillaries and a mild nonspecific inflammatory

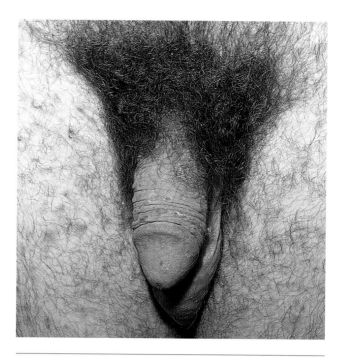

FIG. 6-14
Pityriasis Lichenoides et Varioliformis Acuta (PLEVA, Mucha-Haberman's Disease). Multiple pink, scaly, and scabby papules are present on the thighs and penis. Eruption was widespread.

infiltrate. The differential diagnoses include contact dermatitis and acute cellulitis.

Treatment

Numerous topical medications have been tried, including steroids, antibiotics, antifungals, metronidazole, and medications used for itching. Systemically used antibiotics, antifungals, antidepressants, and prednisone have also been tried. None of these has been found useful, although some of these medications may help anecdotally for a short while. The etiology of this condition is unknown, and its course seems to be protracted.[18]

Glucagonoma Syndrome (Necrolytic Migratory Erythema)

Glucagonoma syndrome is most commonly seen in association with a glucagon-secreting, alpha-cell tumor of the pancreas. In addition to skin and mucosal lesions, there is diabetes or an abnormal glucose tolerance test, elevation of serum glucagon (normal 100 to 200 pg/ml), weight loss, anemia, and hypoaminoacidemia. Skin lesions involve the face, mainly in a perioral distribution, groins, perineum, genitals, lower legs, ankles, and feet. Glossitis and angular cheilitis are commonly seen. Skin lesions are characterized by erythema, flaccid vesicles, and pustules that rupture easily and leave erosions, crusts, or superficial scales. Peripheral spreading causes circinate borders. A very typical finding is the presence of superficial scaling on an inflamed red background (Fig. 6-16).

The histology is typical with the lower half of the epidermis looking normal, whereas the upper half shows varying degrees of necrosis, depending on the stage of the lesion. If the condition is caused by an alpha-cell pancreatic tumor, its surgical excision is curative.[19]

Vasculitis

Vasculitis lesions are rarely seen on the penis as part of a widespread vasculitis on the body (Fig. 6-17). Lesions are typically those of palpable purpura, but may be macular or scabby. The histology is characteristic, showing a leukocytoclastic vasculitis with fibrinoid degeneration of small blood vessel walls.

Behçet's Syndrome

In this rare condition, the lesions are extremely painful and tender, presenting as small ulcers usually involving the scrotum, less often the penis (Fig. 6-18). These lesions are seen in association with oral aphthae, ocular disease (relapsing iridocyclitis, uveitis), various skin lesions (papules, pustules, folliculitis, erythema nodosum), and skin pathergy (the appearance of a pustule at the site of intrader-

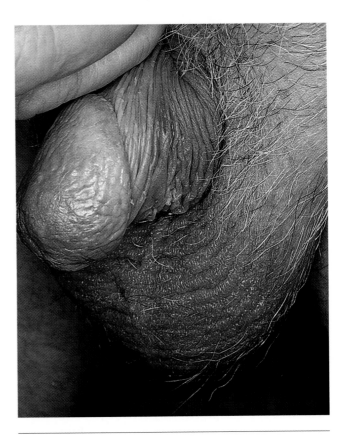

FIG. 6-15
The Red Scrotum Syndrome. Erythema of the anterior half of the scrotum, extending to the shaft of the penis.

mally injected saline). Other associations are gastrointestinal symptoms with diarrhea, arthritis, thrombophlebitis, generalized vasculitis, and various central nervous system manifestations.

Diagnosis
Differential diagnosis includes genital herpes, syphilis, chancroid, and ulcers associated with Crohn's disease.

Treatment
Systemic steroids, cytotoxic agents, or the combination of both is prescribed. Dapsone and colchicine may be beneficial for some patients.[20]

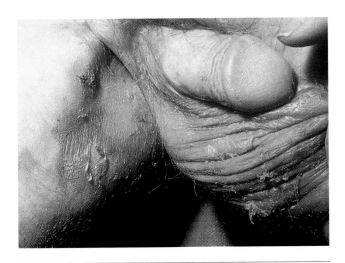

FIG. 6-16
Glucagonoma Syndrome (necrolytic migratory erythema). Erythema and superficial scaling on the scrotum, penis, and upper–inner thigh.
(Courtesy Dr. Colin A. Ramsey.)

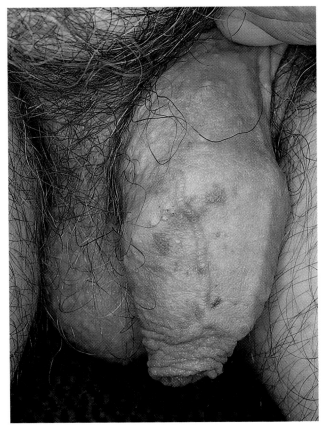

FIG. 6-17
Vasculitis. Palpable purpura observed on the shaft of the penis.

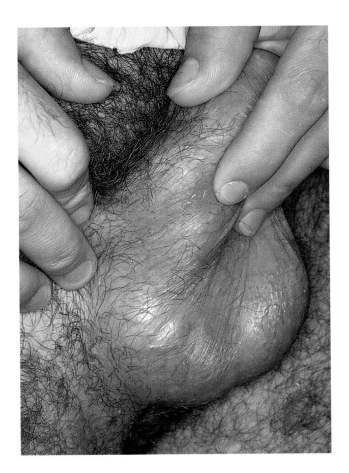

FIG. 6-18
Behçet's Syndrome. "Punched out" superficial ulcers are present on the base of the penis and scrotum.

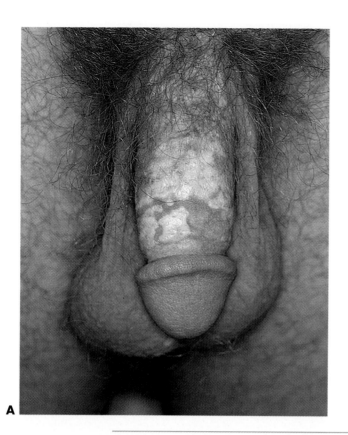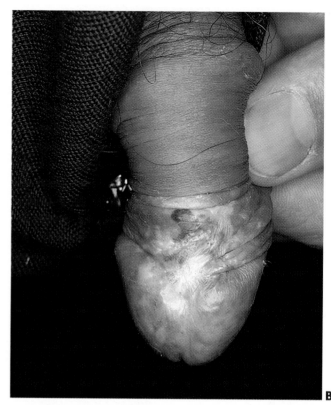

FIG. 6-19
Lichen Sclerosus et Atrophicus. **A,** White patches are present on the shaft of the penis. **B,** Whitish atrophic patches on the glans penis and on the mucosal aspect of the foreskin. The latter shows submucosal hemorrhages.

ATROPHIES

Lichen Sclerosus et Atrophicus

In this relatively rare condition, atrophic patches of unknown etiology involve the glans penis and at times the shaft of the penis (Fig. 6-19, *A*). They start as whitish atrophic papules that progress into small plaques. Most of the time the lesions are whitish, shiny, and atrophic, to the extent that any minor trauma causes submucosal or subepidermal hemorrhages with obvious bruising (Fig. 6-19, *B*). The atrophic process may cause shrinkage of tissue with narrowing of the meatal opening and phimosis of the foreskin. When these changes occur, the condition is called *balanitis xerotica obliterans* (Fig.

6-20, *A*). This is a precancerous lesion that requires periodic monitoring, at least twice a year.

Lichen sclerosus is one of the rare penile diseases that should be given a therapeutic trial with fluorinated steroid creams, such as 0.1% betamethasone cream, to try and control the condition. Shrinkage of the meatal opening may be helped greatly by treatment with the carbon dioxide laser (Fig. 6-20, *B*).[21,22,23]

Atrophoderma

The glans penis shows large areas of atrophy of the epidermis with smaller islands of normal epidermis. The condition is asymptomatic.

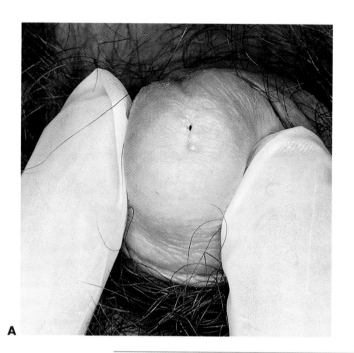
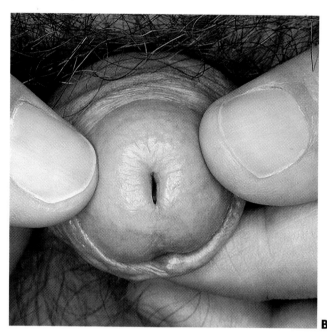

A

B

FIG. 6-20

Balanitis Xerotica Obliterans. **A,** A whitish, atrophic glans penis with scarring and almost complete closure of the meatal opening. **B,** Thirty-four days after treatment with the carbon dioxide laser. The laser was used after conventional surgery to open the meatus failed. The meatal opening remained patent and unchanged when patient was seen 2 years later.

ACNE AND ACNEIFORM ERUPTIONS

The penis has abundant sebaceous glands on the shaft, and it may present comedones and occasionally even pustules that are manifestations of low-grade acne (Fig. 6-21, *A*). Acneiform eruptions may also be caused by chronic exposure to machine oils (Fig. 6-21, *B*).

Hidradenitis Suppurativa

This severe acneiform eruption is a chronic, recurrent, deep-seated folliculitis, resulting in abscesses. This is followed by the formation of sinus tracts and various degrees of scarring. The groin's axillary and anogenital regions are the most commonly affected; less frequently lesions are seen on the buttocks, thighs, abdomen, and chest. Typical acne comedones, pustules, and small scars may precede the more severe lesions or may be seen concomitantly. Double and triple comedones that communicate under the skin surface are very typical for this condition. Sinus tracts may open into the penile shaft or scrotum and with time cause scarring and fibrosis (Fig. 6-22). When scarring and fibrosis occur in the groins, chronic lymphedema of the penis may develop. The condition starts after puberty, is more common in women and blacks, and is seen mainly in young adults.

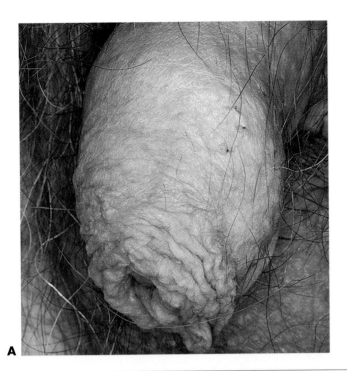

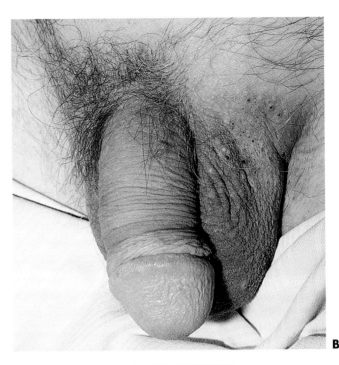

A

B

FIG. 6-21
A, Acne. Three grouped comedones are seen on the foreskin. **B,** Acneiform eruption on the scrotum, groin, and pubic area caused by exposure to machine oils ("chloracne"). Multiple open and closed comedones are observed.

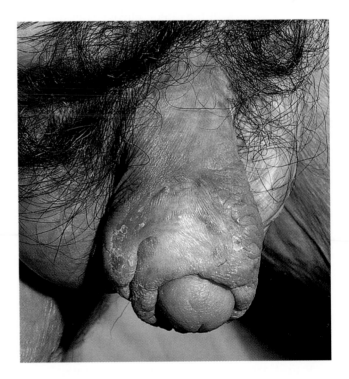

FIG. 6-22
Hidradenitis Suppurativa. Late stage is observed with scarring and fibrosis of the distal third of the shaft of the penis.

Treatment

Treatment is difficult and frustrating. Local anti-acne therapy may be useful for the very mild and early lesions. For the more advanced cases, systemic antibiotics, retinoids, and prednisone may help somewhat, but many of these patients will have to undergo radical excision of the diseased tissues with or without split-thickness skin grafting.[24]

Fordyce's Condition

Groups of minute, pin-point, yellowish papules are seen on the mucosal aspect of the foreskin. These are asymptomatic and may be discovered incidentally by the patient, who may worry about an infection. Histologically the lesions are ectopic, small, mature sebaceous glands. Fordyce's condition commonly occurs on the vermilion border of the lips. Lesions may be seen both on the mucosal aspect of the foreskin and on the lips in the same individual (Fig. 6-23). No treatment is necessary.

GRANULOMAS

Sarcoid of the Penis

Sarcoidal lesions confined to the penis and scrotum are rarely encountered. When this happens, the lesions are skin-colored, erythematous, hyperpigmented, or hypopigmented papules or small plaques, at times with slight scaling (Fig. 6-24). The histology is fairly characteristic, showing a sarcoidal granuloma. No satisfactory treatment is available.[25]

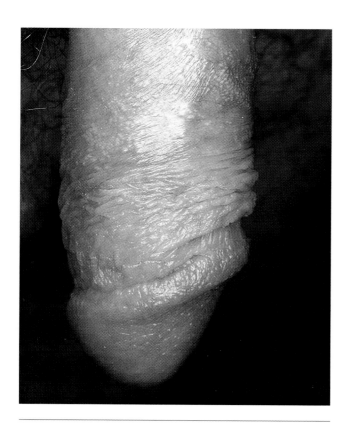

FIG. 6-23
Fordyce's Condition of the Mucosal Aspect of the Foreskin. Numerous yellowish, pin-point, submucosal papules are seen. These represent ectopic sebaceous glands. The patient had similar lesions on the vermilion border of his lips.

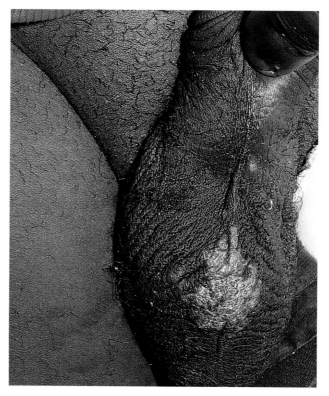

FIG. 6-24
Sarcoid of the Scrotum. Purplish, hypopigmented, slightly scaly papular plaque is located on the center of the scrotum.

Palisading Granulomas

The term *palisading granuloma* is a histologic one, describing lesions that show microscopically foci of collagen degeneration surrounded by an infiltrate composed largely of histiocytes in a palisading arrangement, intermingled with lymphocytes. Two clinical entities may be seen on the penis—granuloma annulare and necrobiosis lipoidica.[26]

Granuloma Annulare

The lesions present as asymptomatic skin-colored solitary or multiple papules that may be mistaken for warts. The histology of the lesion is quite typical, showing a "palisading granuloma," which establishes the benign nature of this condition. No effective treatment is available (Fig. 6-25). The patient should be reassured that this is an entirely benign condition of cosmetic significance only.

Necrobiosis Lipoidica (Diabeticorum)

The typical lesions usually involve the anterior tibial areas but may be seen anywhere. Lesions may or may not be associated with diabetes. They usually present as redish-yellowish, smooth or eroded, atrophic, well-circumscribed patches. Necrobiosis lipoidica lesions are rarely seen on the penis and usually are associated with diabetes (Fig. 6-26). Treatment with a fluorinated steroid cream may be helpful.

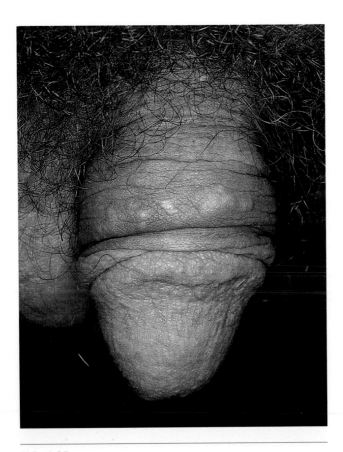

FIG. 6-25
Granuloma Annulare. Several pink dermal papules of various sizes are observed on the distal end of the shaft of the penis. The condition may be misdiagnosed as warts. Biopsy is typical.

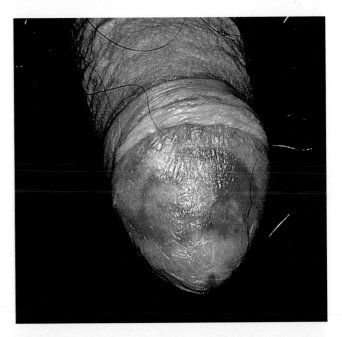

FIG. 6-26
Necrobiosis Lipoidica Diabeticorum. An eroded reddish-yellowish, well-circumscribed patch located on the glans penis in a patient with diabetes.
(Courtesy Dr. I. Braverman.)

Calcinosis Cutis

This may present as a solitary small ulcer secondary to a chronic irritation (Fig. 6-27, *A*) or as multiple small yellowish papules that mimic milia (Fig. 6-27, *B*).[27] The correct diagnosis is easily confirmed by biopsy.

Idiopathic calcinosis of the scrotum consists of multiple asymptomatic, skin-colored or slightly yellowish, small, smooth, round nodules on the scrotal skin. They first appear in childhood or early adult life and progressively increase in size and number. Some of the lesions break down and discharge a chalky material. Previously this condition was thought to be a specific entity,[28] but it is believed now that early lesions start out as epidermal or pilar cysts that with time become calcified and lose their cyst walls.[29]

REACTIONS TO DRUGS

Maculopapular drug eruptions may affect the penis as part of a generalized skin involvement. Hypersensitivity reactions to drugs may involve the penis and scrotum in a more specific and localized pattern. The most common is fixed drug eruption. Rarer types are localized angioedema, Foscarnet-induced erosions and ulcers, and drug-induced pressure lesions (coma bullae).

Fixed Drug Eruption

The penis is a frequent site for fixed drug eruptions that may be caused by several drugs, such as acetaminophen, long-acting sulfa drugs, antibiotics, phenolphthalein, and quinine. The lesions, which may be solitary or multiple, first start as

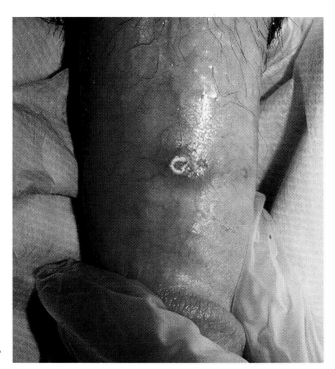

A

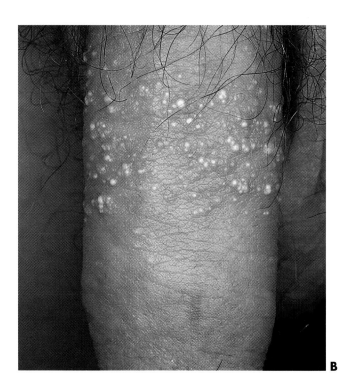

B

FIG. 6-27
Calcinosis Cutis. **A,** A large eroded yellowish papule located on the shaft of the penis, secondary to chronic irritation resulting from a condom catheter. **B,** Numerous milia-like small whitish papules observed on the shaft of the penis.
(**A,** Courtesy Dr. Kalman Watsky; **B,** courtesy Dr. Howard Harris.)

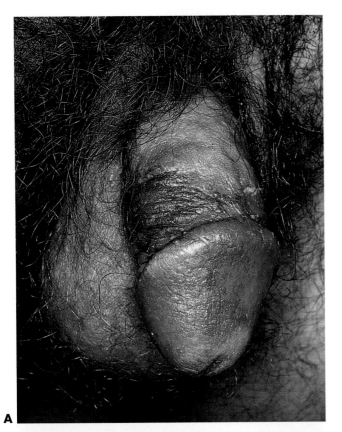

A

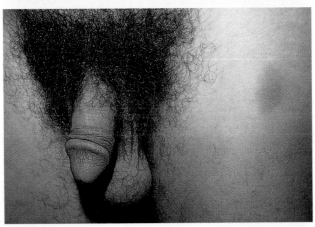

B

bright-red itchy patches that may blister (Fig. 6-28, *A*) and then heal with time, leaving a hyperpigmented patch (Fig. 6-28, *B*). When the offending medication is ingested again, the lesions tend to recur in the previously involved sites. The condition may become erosive (Fig. 6-28, *C*).[30,31]

Localized Angioedema

Sudden swelling of the penis and/or scrotum may be seen following the ingestion of certain medications, most commonly aspirin. This swelling, which subsides within a few days, may recur if the offending medication is taken again. A careful history helps to establish the correct diagnosis. Treatment is with antihistamines and avoidance of the causative drug.

Foscarnet-Induced Erosions and Ulcers

Foscarnet is an antiviral drug used primarily in AIDS patients with cytomegalovirus retinitis or in

FIG. 6-28
Fixed Drug Eruption. **A**, Eruption of the glans penis and shaft is caused by ingestion of trimethoprim-sulfamethoxazole (Bactrim, Septra). Acutely inflamed, dusky erythematous patches are seen. **B**, Healed lesions on the glans and distal end of the penile shaft have left dark-brown postinflammatory pigmentation. One active lesion is present on the left thigh. **C**, Erosive fixed drug eruption on the glans and shaft was caused by acetaminophen. Borders of red, eroded areas are hyperpigmented.

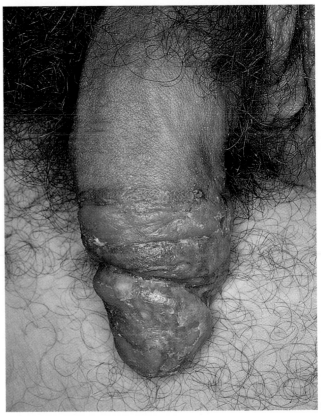

C

patients who have a herpes simplex virus infection that has become resistant to the commonly used drugs, such as acyclovir, famciclovir, or valacyclovir. Lesions in patients receiving foscarnet may appear 1 to 4 weeks after therapy has been started and often present as vesicles or bullae, which rapidly turn into bright-red painful erosions or ulcers, that usually involve the glans penis, foreskin and scrotum (Fig. 6-29). Rarely the oral mucosa and esophagus may be involved. The histology is nonspecific. The condition clears up rapidly when foscarnet is discontinued.[32,33]

Drug-Induced Pressure Lesions (Coma Bullae)

These lesions are commonly seen in individuals who have had prolonged coma secondary to carbon monoxide poisoning, prolonged surgery, or drug overdose, either accidentally or in a suicide attempt.

Lesions usually start as blisters in pressure areas on the extremities, mainly on bony prominences such as the knuckles, malleoli, or on the shins. Lesions on the penis are occasionally seen. The blisters, which may contain clear fluid or become hemorrhagic, show necrosis of the underlying eccrine sweat glands. The blisters dry up in several days leaving superficial scabs or erosions. Linear lesions, when seen, are very characteristic (Fig. 6-30). The lesions are usually superficial and heal within a couple of weeks without treatment.

Histology frequently shows necrosis of the epidermis and of the underlying eccrine sweat glands. Differential diagnoses include any of the blistering diseases (see Chapter 7), genital herpes, fixed drug eruption, and self-induced lesions.

Diagnosis is established by a history of prolonged coma, lesions at pressure sites (sometimes with a linear pattern), and a characteristic biopsy.[34]

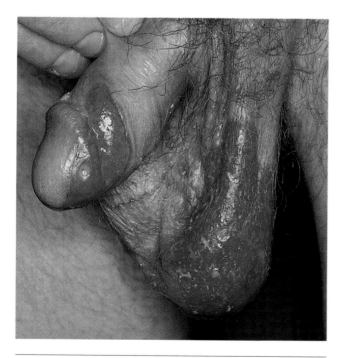

FIG. 6-29
Foscarnet-Induced Erosion and Ulcers. Large red erosions and rare small ulcers are observed on the penis and scrotum of a patient with AIDS being treated with foscarnet. When foscarnet was stopped, the lesions cleared up rapidly.
(Courtesy Dr. Lyn Guenther.)

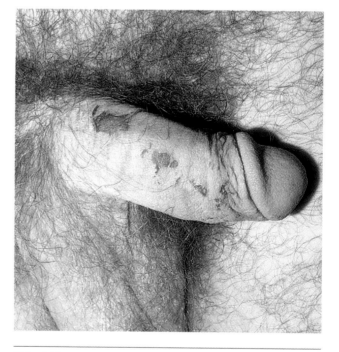

FIG. 6-30
Drug-Induced Pressure Lesions (coma bullae). Superficial scabs, some with linear borders, are present on the shaft of the penis. The patient tried to commit suicide with an overdose of diazepam.

REFERENCES

Acute Contact Dermatitis or Contact Balanitis

1. Fisher AA: Poison ivy/oak/sumac. Part II: specific features, *Cutis* 58:22-24, 1996.
2. Rietschel RL, Fowler JF, Jr: *Fisher's contact dermatitis*, ed 4, Baltimore, 1995, Williams & Wilkins, 59, 80-81.
3. Nödl F: Zur Klinick und Histologie der Balanoposthitis chronica circumscripta benigna plasmacellularis, *Arch Dermatol Syph* 198:557, 1954.
4. Souteyrand P, Wong E, MacDonald DM: Zoon's balanitis (balanitis circumscripta plasmacellularis), *Br J Dermatol* 105:195-199, 1981.
5. Davis DA, Cohen PR: Balanitis circumscripta plasmacellularis, *J Urol* 153:424-426, 1995.
6. Petersen CS, Thomsen K: Fusidic acid cream in the treatment of plasma cell balanitis, *J Am Acad Dermatol* 27:633-634, 1992.
7. Leventhal LC, Jaworsky C, Werth V: An asymptomatic penile lesion, *Arch Dermatol* 129:366-367, 369-370, 1993.

Gangrenous Lesions

8. Sanchez MH, Sanchez SR, del Cerro Herdero M, et al: Pyoderma gangrenosum of penile skin, *Int J Dermatol* 36:638-639, 1997.
9. Bour J, Steinhardt G: Penile necrosis in diabetes mellitus and end-stage renal disease, *J Urol* 132:560-562, 1984.

Papulosquamous Conditions

10. Horan DB, Redman JF, Jansen GT: Papulosquamous lesions of glans penis, *Urology* 33:1-4, 1984.
11. Boyd AS, Neldner KH: Lichen planus, *J Am Acad Dermatol* 25:593-619, 1991.
12. Aram H: Association of lichen planus and lichen nitidus: treatment with etretinate, *Int J Dermatol* 27:117, 1988.
13. Farber EM, Nall L: Genital psoriasis, *Cutis* 50:263-266, 1992.
14. Rothe MJ, Kerdel FA: Reiter syndrome, *Int J Dermatol* 30:173-180, 1991.
15. Parsons JM: Pityriasis rosea update: 1986, *J Am Acad Dermatol* 15:159-167, 1986.
16. Allen RA, Janniger CK, Schwartz RA: Pityriasis rosea, *Cutis* 56:198-202, 1995.
17. Gelmetti C, Rigoni C, et al: Pityriasis lichenoides in children: a long term follow-up of eighty-nine cases, *J Am Acad Dermatol* 23:473-478, 1990.
18. Fisher BK: The red scrotum syndrome, *Cutis* 60:139-141, 1997.
19. Kasper CS: Necrolytic migratory erythema: unresolved problems in diagnosis and pathogenesis. A case report and literature review, *Cutis* 49:120-122, 1992.
20. Mangelsdorf HC, White Wl, Jorizzo JL: Behçet's disease, *J Am Acad Dermatol* 34:745-750, 1996.

Atrophies

21. Meffert JJ, Davis BM, Grimwood RE: Lichen sclerosus, *J Am Acad Dermatol* 32:393-416, 1995.
22. Pride HB, Miller OF III, Tyler WB: Penile squamous cell carcinoma arising from balanitis xerotica obliterans, *J Am Acad Dermatol* 29:469-473, 1993.
23. Ratz JL: Carbon dioxide laser treatment of balanitits xerotica obliterans, *J Am Acad Dermatol* 10:925-928, 1984.

Acne and Acneiform Eruptions

24. Ebling FJG: Apocrine glands in health and disease, *Int J Dermatol* 28:508-511, 1989.

Granulomas

25. Vitenson JH, Wilson JM: Sarcoid of the glans penis, *Urology* 108:284-289, 1972.
26. Espana A, Sanchez-Yus E, Serna MJ, et al: Chronic balanitis with palisading granuloma: an atypical genital localization of necrobiosis lipoidica responsive to pentoxifylline, *Dermatology* 188:222-225, 1994.
27. Eng AM, Mandrea E: Perforating calcinosis cutis presenting as milia, *J Cutan Pathol* 8:247-250, 1981.
28. Fisher BK, Dvoretzky I: Idiopathic calcinosis of the scrotum, *Arch Dermatol* 114:957, 1978.
29. Song DH, Lee KH, Kang WH: Idiopathic calcinosis of the scrotum, *J Am Acad Dermatol* 19:1095-1101, 1988.

Reactions to Drugs

30. Sehgal VN, Gangarani OP: Genital fixed drug eruptions, *Genitourin Med* 62:56-58, 1986.
31. Sehgal VN, Gangarani OP: Fixed drug eruption: current concepts, *Int J Dermatol* 26:67-74, 1987.
32. Evans LM, Grossman ME: Foscarnet-induced penile ulcer, *J Am Acad Dermatol* 27:124-126, 1992.
33. Fitzgerald E, Goldman HM, Miller WG: A penile ulceration in a patient with the acquired immunodeficiency syndrome, *Arch Dermatol* 131:1447-1452, 1995.
34. Varma AJ, Fisher BK, Sarin MK: Diazepam-induced coma with bullae and eccrine sweat gland necrosis, *Arch Intern Med* 137:1207-1210, 1977.

CHAPTER 7

Blistering Diseases of the Penis

Blistering diseases usually involve the penis as part of a generalized eruption.

ERYTHEMA MULTIFORME

The "target" or "iris" type lesions, with or without blisters, frequently involve the mucosal surfaces (Fig. 7-1, *A*). When erythema multiforme is quite severe, with involvement of mouth, lips, conjuctiva, and genital mucosa, it is referred to as the Stevens-Johnson syndrome. It commonly involves the penis and scrotum and many of the lesions become bullous (Fig. 7-1, *B*). The most severe type of erythema multiforme, causing widespread erythema, vesiculation, and skin necrosis, is toxic epidermal necrolysis (TEN). Erythema multiforme may be secondary to an infection: viral (herpes simplex or Epstein-Barr virus), bacterial (streptococcal), mycobacterial (tuberculosis), mycoplasma, deep fungal infection (coccidioidomycosis, histoplasmosis); a manifestation of a drug eruption or of an occult lymphoma; or it may appear for no known reason.[1]

Herpetic DNA has been detected in skin lesions of recurrent erythema multiforme, using the polymerase chain reaction test.[2]

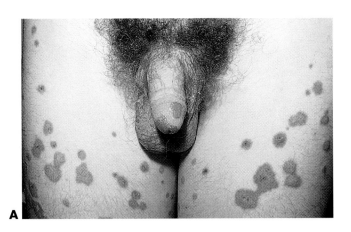
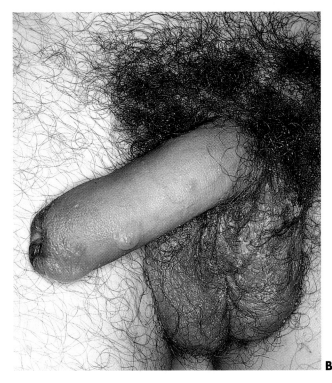

A B

FIG. 7-1
A, Erythema Multiforme. Multiple "target" or "iris" lesions are present on the thighs. Many of the lesions show flaccid blisters in their centers, some of which have become eroded. Two erosions are seen on the glans penis. **B**, Stevens-Johnson Syndrome. Several blisters are observed on the penis. The scrotal skin is red and inflamed, with several flaccid blisters and erosions.

TOXIC EPIDERMAL NECROLYSIS

Toxic epidermal necrolysis is usually secondary to an adverse drug reaction, for instance a long-acting sulfa, such as trimethoprim-sulfamethoxazole, allopurinol, or phenytoin.

Diagnosis

The skin is generally red and vesicular (Fig. 7-2, *A*). The penis is almost always involved, and the diseased necrotic epidermis sloughs off readily like wet tissue paper and leaves large denuded areas (Fig. 7-2, *B*). The penis is frequently the last area to heal in toxic epidermal necrolysis.

Treatment

The condition is life-threatening, and the patient should be treated as if he has been severely burned, preferably in a burn center if this facility is available.[3,4]

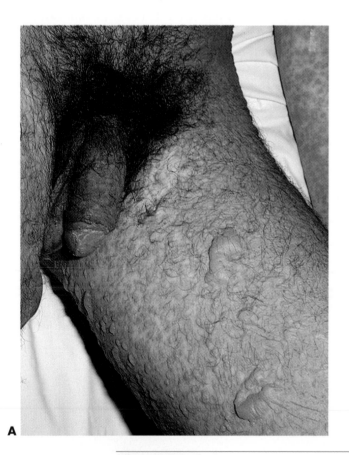

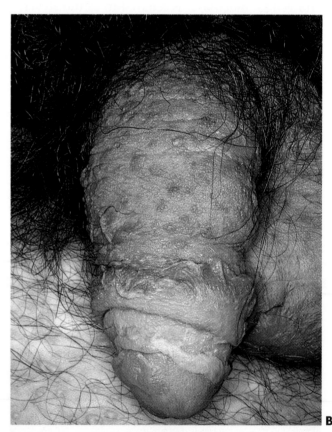

A   B

FIG. 7-2

A, Early phase of toxic epidermal necrolysis. The skin is red all over with numerous large and small blisters. The penis is involved. The disease was caused by trimethoprim-sulfamethoxazole prescribed to treat acne. **B,** Same patient as in *A*. The penis is red with several flaccid blisters. The grayish necrotic epidermis is ready to slough off.

PEMPHIGUS VULGARIS

Pemphigus is a severe autoimmune vesiculo-bullous disease that affects the skin and mucosa. It may start in the oral mucosa as a nonhealing erosion or erosions and may last for months or years before a biopsy identifies the true nature of the disease.

Diagnosis

Similar to lesions in the oral mucosa, penile lesions may linger for several months or even years before the condition is diagnosed correctly by a dermatologist (Fig. 7-3). Irritation and erosions on the penis may be the only signs, but a biopsy will show the characteristic intraepidermal, suprabasal acantholysis of pemphigus vulgaris. Small lesions may be confused with chronic recurrent herpes simplex. Like other blistering conditions of the penis, the blisters break off very easily and the diagnosis may have to be made by the presence of erosions or ulcers. A careful search may reveal occasional small vesicles at the borders of the lesions, as well as erosions in the mouth, or small blisters and scabs on the trunk and scalp. Positive immunofluorescence of histology sections confirms the diagnosis.

The differential diagnoses are with the other bullous diseases: Hailey-Hailey disease, bullous pemphigoid, cicatricial pemphigoid, erythema multiforme, as well as with erosive penile lesions such as erosive balanitis, erosive lichen planus, erosive fixed drug eruption, and genital herpes.

Treatment

Treatment is with systemic steroids. Preferably the treatment should be carried out by a dermatologist experienced in the management of this difficult condition.[5]

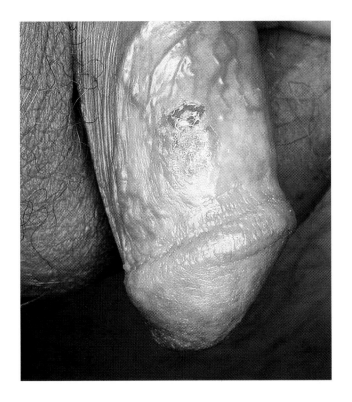

FIG. 7-3
Pemphigus Vulgaris. Recurrent erosions on the penis.

HAILEY-HAILEY DISEASE (FAMILIAL BENIGN CHRONIC PEMPHIGUS)

Hailey-Hailey is an autosomal dominant chronic blistering condition. It is manifested by plaques of small vesicles and erosions usually localized on the neck, trunk, armpits, and groins. The lesions may be annular or arciform and may be confused with a fungus infection.

Diagnosis

The condition may involve the penis, and then the eruption is similar to the one seen in the groins namely, red, eroded, cracked, and macerated plaques. (Fig. 7-4). The maceration and cracking are very typical for this condition. The biopsy is characteristic.

The differential diagnoses are with candidiasis, macerated dermatitis, pemphigus, and psoriasis.

Treatment

Treatment is unsatisfactory. Local and systemic antibiotics and steroids have been used with temporary relief. Currently there is no known cure for this condition.[6]

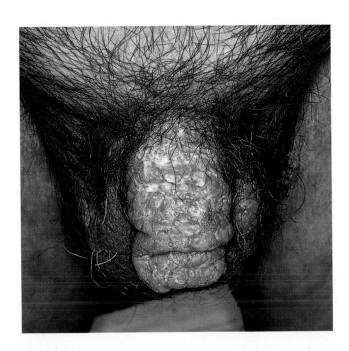

FIG. 7-4

Hailey-Hailey Disease. Erythema, maceration, and cracking of the shaft of the penis are observed. Identical lesions are usually seen in the groins.

BULLOUS PEMPHIGOID

Bullous pemphigoid is a rare autoimmune blistering disease seen mainly in the elderly. The individual lesion forms subepidermally, causing tense blisters that are less fragile than those of pemphigus vulgaris. The blisters may appear on normal skin or may be associated with areas of erythema, frequently showing an urticarial component. The penis is rarely involved as part of a generalized eruption (Fig. 7-5). The histology is quite typical, showing a subepidermal blister with many eosinophils in the blister cavity and in the underlying dermis.

Differential diagnosis is with the other vesiculobullous diseases such as pemphigus vulgaris and erythema multiforme.

Diagnosis

Diagnosis is made by the presence of tense blisters and a typical histology.

Treatment

Treatment of this condition is difficult. High doses of prednisone are needed initially (60 to 80 mg a day), which should be tapered off slowly. Immunosuppressive drugs (azathioprine, cyclophosphamide, methotrexate), dapsone, and tetracycline at the dose of 2 grams a day, have been used as steroid-sparing agents with various degrees of success. Treatment should be by a dermatologist experienced in managing this difficult condition.[7]

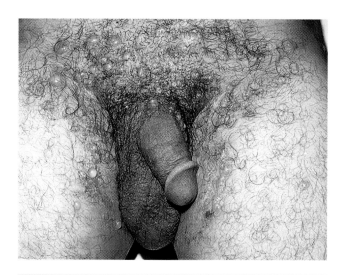

FIG. 7-5

Bullous Pemphigoid. Numerous tense blisters are observed on normal-looking skin. A few lesions are present on the base of the penis.

CICATRICIAL PEMPHIGOID (BENIGN MUCOUS MEMBRANE PEMPHIGOID)

Nothing is "benign" about this scarring, autoimmune, blistering disease that has a predilection to mucous membranes (oral, ocular, and genital) with scarring and irreversible tissue destruction. Lesions on the skin are rarely seen. Untreated ocular lesions frequently lead to blindness. Lesions of the penis are rare, showing vesicles, erosions, and scarring. The histology shows a picture identical to the one seen in bullous pemphigoid.

Diagnosis

Differential diagnosis is with the other blistering diseases and with various erosive penile lesions (see pemphigus vulgaris pp. 64-65). Diagnosis is made by the presence of blisters, erosions, and the obvious tendency to scarring in all mucosal areas, particularly the conjunctiva of the eyes. Histology and immunofluorescence are helpful.

Treatment

Treatment of the disease is difficult and unsatisfactory. Treatment should be aggressive, with high doses of steroids (60 to 80 mg a day), combined with cyclophosphamide or other steroid-sparing agents, such as azathioprine or dapsone. A consultation with an ophthalmologist should always be obtained.[8]

EPIDERMOLYSIS BULLOSA

This group of inherited bullous disorders is characterized by the appearance of noninflammatory blisters following minor trauma. Several variants of both dominant and recessive inheritance have been described, in addition to an acquired form (acquired epidermolysis bullosa, epidermolysis bullosa acquisita). Usually blisters first appear in infancy in friction areas and frequently involve the mucosal surfaces. The penis may be involved, with blisters, erosions, and scarring (Fig. 7-6).

Diagnosis

The diagnosis is made by a history of blisters appearing in early childhood, with other members of the family similarly inflicted. However, epidermolysis bullosa acquisita usually appears in middle-aged or older individuals. Electron microscopic examination of the skin is usually needed to accurately diagnose the specific type of the disease.

Treatment

Treatment is symptomatic.[9,10]

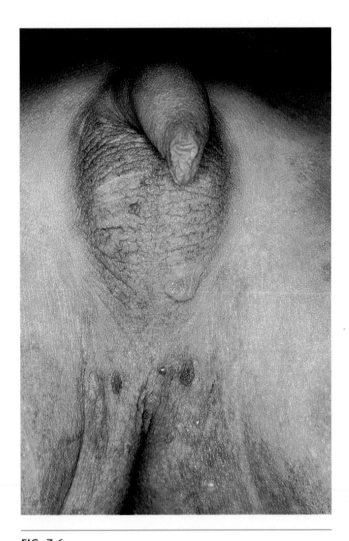

FIG. 7-6
Epidermolysis Bullosa in a Child. Blisters are present on the scrotum and upper inner thighs.

REFERENCES

Erythema Multiforme

1. Howland WW, Golitz LE, Weston WL, Huff JC: Erythema multiforme: clinical, histopathologic, and immunologic study, *J Am Acad Dermatol* 10:438-446, 1984.
2. Darragh TM, Egbert BM, Berger TB, Yen TS: Identification of herpes simplex virus DNA in lesions of erythema multiforme by the polymerase chain reaction, *J Am Acad Dermatol* 24:23-26, 1991.

Toxic Epidermal Necrolysis

3. Rohrer TE, Ahmed AR: Toxic epidermal necrolysis, *Int J Dermatol* 30:457-466,1991.
4. Bastuji-Garin S, Rzany B, Stern RS, et al: Clinical classification of cases of toxic epidermal necrolysis, Stevens-Johnson syndrome, and erythema multiforme, *Arch Dermatol* 129:92-96, 1993.

Pemphigus Vulgaris

5. Korman NJ: Pemphigus, *J Am Acad Dermatol* 18:1219-1238, 1988.

Hailey-Hailey Disease

6. Burge SM: Hailey-Hailey disease; the clinical features, response to treatment and prognosis, *Brit J Dermatol* 126:275-282, 1992.

Bullous Pemphigoid

7. Mutasim DF: Bullous pemphigoid: review and update, *J Ger Dermatol* 1:62, 1993.

Cicatricial Pemphigoid

8. Ahmed AR, Kurgis BS, Rogers RS III: Cicatricial pemphigoid, *J Am Acad Dermatol* 24:987-1001, 1991.

Epidermolysis Bullosa

9. Uitto J, Christiano AM: Inherited epidermolysis bullosa: clinical features, molecular genetics, and pathologic mechanisms, *Dermatol Clin* 11:549-563, 1993.
10. Woodley DT, Briggaman RA, Gammon WR: Acquired epidermolysis bullosa: a bullous disease associated with autoimmunity to type VII (anchoring fibril) collagen, *Dermatol Clin* 8:717-726, 1990.

HYPOPIGMENTED LESIONS
Vitiligo

Vitiligo of the penis is common. It may be seen on the shaft or glans. It may be part of a segmental vitiligo, involving larger skin areas (Fig. 8-1). Patients are usually unhappy about vitiligo of the penis, and they frequently do not find satisfactory the doctor's explanation that the condition is benign and of cosmetic significance only.

Treatment

No satisfactory treatment exsists for this condition of unknown etiology. Some lesions respond to fluorinated steroid creams or to ultraviolet light treatment, but these may cause more harm than good to the very thin skin of the penis. Generally it is better to leave the lesions alone.[1]

Chronic Contact Dermatitis of the Penis

Chronic contact dermatitis, particularly to antioxidants and rubber, may eventually cause hypopigmentation through destruction of the melanocytes in the involved areas (see Fig. 6-3, *D*).[2]

Lichen sclerosus et atrophicus also frequently causes hypopigmented lesions. (See Fig. 6-19.)

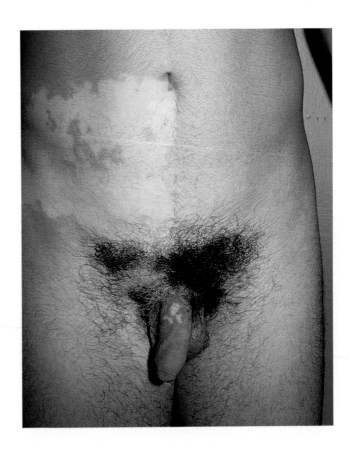

FIG. 8-1
Vitiligo. A patient with segmental vitiligo, showing whitish patches on the abdomen, groin, and penis, all localized to right side of body. Notice white hair as part of this condition.

HYPERPIGMENTED LESIONS
Lentigines

Lentigines (these are not freckles produced by exposure to sun) are commonly seen on the penis as anywhere else on the body and are entirely benign (Fig. 8-2).

Treatment

Treatment is unnecessary, although laser treatment, freezing with liquid nitrogen, or excision are options that could be used if the patient insists on treatment.[3]

Melanotic Macules

These lesions may present as hyperpigmented patches with irregular borders and may be indistinguishable clinically from a superficial spreading melanoma. Some of these lesions may persist for years without any change. (Fig. 8-3).

Diagnosis

A biopsy, nevertheless, is mandatory to establish the benign nature of this condition.[4]

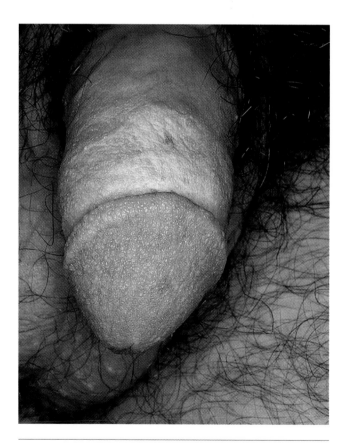

FIG. 8-2
Lentigines. Brown macules commonly seen on the penis. One lesion is seen here on the glans and another one is on the shaft. These are not sun-induced freckles.

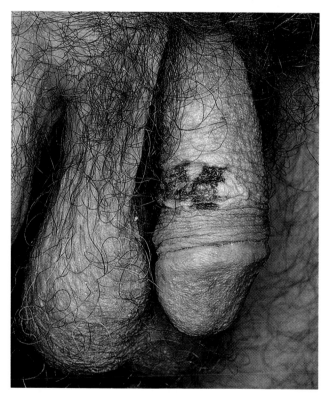

FIG. 8-3
Melanotic Macule. An irregularly pigmented, small patch with irregular borders. The lesion is indistinguishable clinically from a melanoma and must be biopsied.

Benign Melanocytic Nevi

These lesions are clinically the same as nevi elsewhere, light- or dark-brown in color (Fig. 8-4). They usually are flat junction nevi on the glans penis, but may be of the junctional, dermal, or compound type on the shaft of the penis. The location on the penis does not make nevi more susceptible to undergoing malignant changes. The patient, however, should be warned to look out for sudden changes, just as for nevi elsewhere on the skin.

Treatment

No prophylactic excision is warranted.

REFERENCES

Hypopigmented Lesions

1. Moss JR, Stevenson JC: Incidence of male genital vitiligo: report of a screening programme, *Br J Vener Dis* 57:145-146, 1981.
2. James O, Mayes RW, Stevenson CJ: Occupational vitiligo induced by a *p*-tert-butylphenol, a systemic disease? *Lancet* ii:1217-1219, 1977.

Hyperpigmented Lesions

3. Kopf AW, Bart RS: Tumor conference 43: Penile lentigo, *J Dermatol Surg Oncol* 8:637-639, 1982.
4. Revuez J, Clerici T: Penile melanosis, *J Am Acad Dermatol* 20:567-570, 1989.

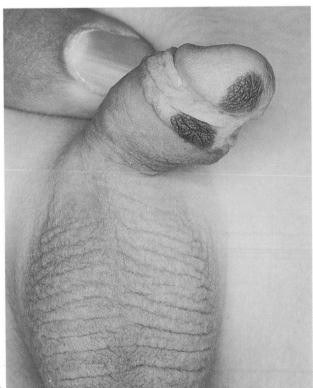

A

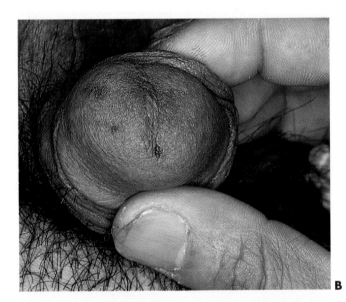

B

FIG. 8-4
A, Pigmented benign nevi present on the glans and shaft of the penis in a child. **B,** Pigmented junction nevi or melanotic macules on the glans penis of a dark-skinned individual. An exact diagnosis needs a histologic interpretation.

CHAPTER 9

Tumors of the Penis

BENIGN TUMORS

Sebaceous Hyperplasias

Sebaceous hyperplasias are small yellowish papules usually seen on the shaft and foreskin. They represent the benign enlargement of sebaceous glands normally found in these anatomic sites.

Treatment

No treatment except reassurance of the patient is necessary (Fig. 9-1).

Seborrheic Keratoses

Seborrheic keratoses are brown to gray, rough papules. Usually these lesions are seen on the shaft of the penis. Histologically typical, they show a basal cell papilloma (Fig. 9-2). Differential diagnoses are with pigmented nevi and warts.

Treatment

No treatment is necessary. In cases where the lesions are very bothersome, they could be removed by freezing with liquid nitrogen or by using electrodesiccation followed by gentle curettage.

Epidermal Inclusion Cysts

These cysts ("epidermal cysts", "sebaceous cysts") are rarely seen on the penis (Fig. 9-3, *A*), but they are fairly common on the scrotum (Fig. 9-3, *B*).

Physical Examination

They usually present as raised, round, skin-colored, yellowish or pink, smooth papules or nodules, at times with a centrally depressed black dot in their center (see Fig. 9-3, *A*).

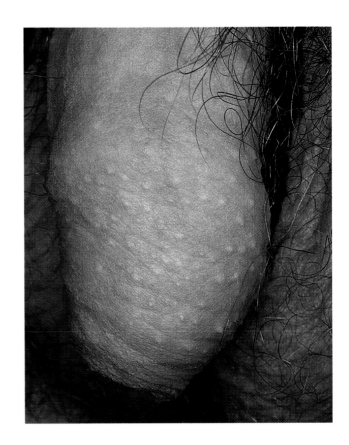

FIG. 9-1
Sebaceous Hyperplasia. Several small yellowish papules are present on the foreskin. These represent prominent sebaceous glands.

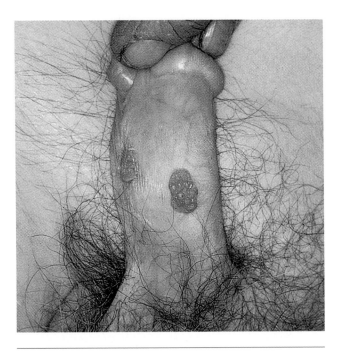

FIG. 9-2
Seborrheic Keratosis. A rough, raised brown papule is observed on the shaft of the penis. A similar, slightly more grayish lesion is seen nearby. The lesions are asymptomatic, and the histology is typical.

Diagnosis

When the small opening is present in the center and the lesion is squeezed, a threadlike yellowish material emerges, representing laminated keratin. This black depressed dot is usually not seen in scrotal cysts. The histology is very typical, showing a cyst containing laminated keratin surrounded by a true epidermal wall with all its layers.

Treatment

Usually no treatment is necessary for these asymptomatic lesions. In those rare instances in which the lesions become irritated or inflamed, or if they bother the patient cosmetically, surgical excision is curative. Old lesions may become calcified and with time lose their cyst walls, assuming the entity described as idiopathic calcinosis of the scrotum.[1]

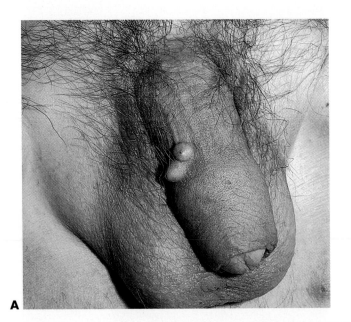

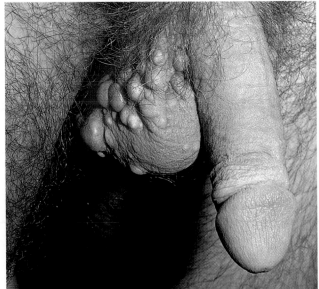

A   B

FIG. 9-3
Epidermal Inclusion Cysts. **A,** Two skin-colored, slightly yellowish smooth nodules are present on the shaft of the penis. Both lesions exhibit a centrally depressed black opening. **B,** Multiple skin-colored and yellowish nodules are located on the scrotum. Occasionally these lesions become calcified and lose their epithelial walls. The term *idiopathic calcinosis of the scrotum* was used to describe this occurrence.

BENIGN VASCULAR GROWTHS
Pearly Penile Papules

A very common, asymptomatic condition, pearly penile papules usually involve the coronal ring. The lesions appear as multiple pale, pink, or skin-colored, shiny, raised papules, arranged in one or a few rows (Fig. 9-4). The lesions may be few or numerous and may be seen occasionally on the base of the glans penis or on the sides of the frenulum. These lesions are histologically benign angiofibromas. They may be confused with penile warts, particularly if they are few in number.

Treatment

No treatment is necessary. Laser therapy is effective in removing these lesions if they bother the patient cosmetically.[2]

Varices

Varicose vein of the penis is an uncommon, soft, bluish, compressible, asymptomatic nodule, usually seen on the shaft of the penis (Fig. 9-5, *A*).

It is entirely benign and requires no treatment. Rarely it may become thrombosed and present a black or dark-brown papule that may arouse concern (Fig. 9-5, *B*).

Diagnosis

A biopsy establishes the benign nature of this condition.

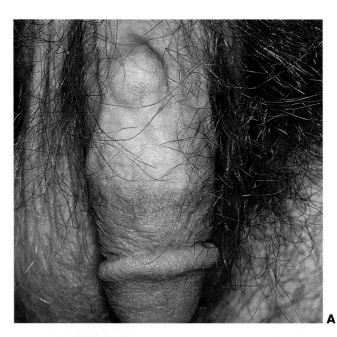

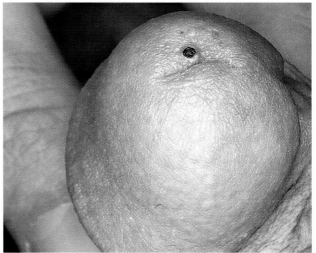

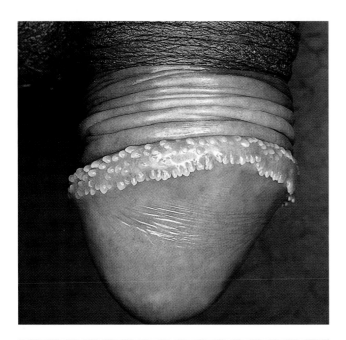

FIG. 9-4
Pearly Penile Papules. Rows of shiny, semi-transparent, "pearly" raised small papules are present on the corona. These are benign angiofibromas.

FIG. 9-5
A, Varicose vein of the penis is observed as a soft, bluish, compressible, asymptomatic nodule on the shaft. **B,** Thrombosed varix on tip of penis. Small, round, black scab is seen. Biopsy is typical.

Intravascular Papillary Endothelial Hyperplasia

Intravascular papillary endothelial hyperplasia (Masson's tumor) is a rare, benign lesion, presenting as a bluish, asymptomatic subcutaneous nodule on the shaft of the penis. The nodule may bleed spontaneously.

Diagnosis

The lesion is considered to represent a reactive response to trauma and venous thrombosis. The histology is very typical and shows some resemblance to angiosarcoma.

Treatment

Excision is curative.[3,4]

Angiokeratomas

Angiokeratomas of the penis are not rare. They may be angiokeratomas of Fordyce, identical to the lesions that commonly involve the scrotum (Fig. 9-6). The lesions are fairly characteristic. They are asymptomatic, violaceous, smooth, small papules that usually have no medical significance. If the lesions are present on the shaft of the penis, they may rarely bleed from intercourse. The histology is typical. They usually are of no significance except as a cosmetic problem to some individuals.

Treatment

They can easily be cured with laser treatment.[5]

Angiokeratoma Corporis Diffusum of Fabry

The penis is almost always involved in this x-linked systemic storage disease caused by the lack of the enzyme alpha-galactosidase-A. This causes an accumulation in the tissues of ceramide-trihexoside that eventually kills the patient from renal insufficiency, myocardial infarction, or cerebrovascular accident. The lesions consist of multiple angiokeratomas, indistinguishable clinically from other angiokeratomas (Fig. 9-7). Early lesions may mimic purpura.[6]

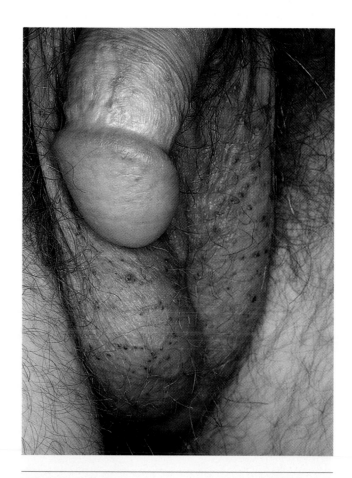

FIG. 9-6
Angiokeratoma of Fordyce is observed on the scrotum and penis. Numerous violaceous small papules are present on the scrotum, and three tiny lesions are on the glans penis.

Hemangiomas

These asymptomatic lesions may present as grouped, red or purplish, raised soft papules on the glans and shaft of the penis (Fig. 9-8, *A*); or as depressed, violaceous-grayish patches with or without a few angiokeratomas on the glans (Fig. 9-8, *B*).

Treatment

No treatment is necessary, unless symptoms such as bleeding precipitated by intercourse are present. Laser treatment is then indicated.

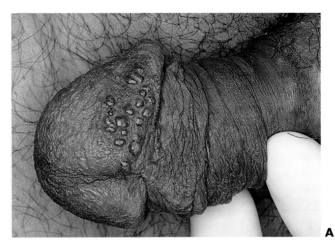

A

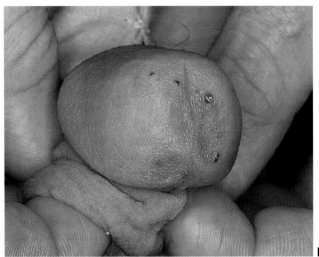

B

FIG. 9-8
Hemangiomas. **A,** Grouped, soft, red-purplish papules are present on the glans penis. **B,** Three grayish, depressed patches with a few angiokeratomas observed on the tip of the penis.

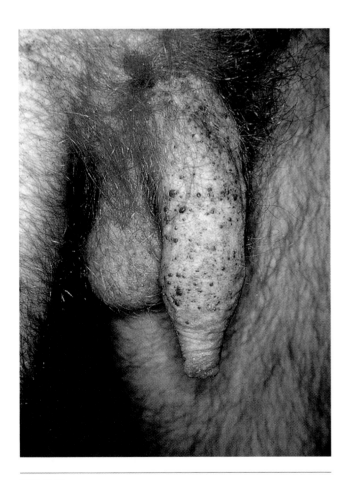

FIG. 9-7
Angiokeratoma Corporis Diffusum (Fabry's disease, Fabry-Anderson's disease). Numerous purplish and dark-red papules of various sizes are located on the shaft of the penis. The tiny lesions may mimic purpura.

BENIGN CYSTS

The most common variety of benign, fluid-containing cysts is the cyst of the median raphe of the penis (Fig. 9-9). This is an embryologic abnormality of the closure of the midline of the shaft (raphe). The lesion is asymptomatic and requires no treatment. It should be distinguished from apocrine hidrocystoma, which is seen less commonly in the same areas. Histologically the distinction is easy.[7]

Verruciform Xanthoma

This is a rare, benign, verrucous, yellowish growth usually seen on the glans penis, scrotum, and oral cavity. Lesions may present as solitary or multiple papules or as warty plaques that may mimic a giant condyloma or a squamous cell carcinoma (Fig. 9-10). The histology is very typical, showing acanthosis, papillomatosis, and densely packed, fat-filled foam cells in the papillary dermis. The nature of the fat has not been identified. The etiology is unknown. No malignant transformation has ever been reported.

Differential diagnoses are with warts, epidermal cysts, adnexal tumors, juvenile xanthogranuloma, giant condyloma, and squamous cell carcinoma.

Diagnosis

Diagnosis is established by the yellowish hue of this slow-growing lesion and by its characteristic histology.[8]

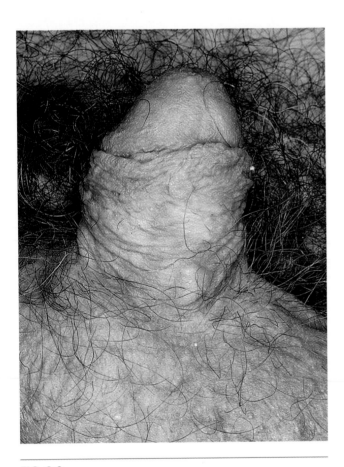

FIG. 9-9
Cyst of the median raphe of the penis. A soft, raised, compressible nodule is seen at the ventral aspect of the base of the penis in the midline (raphe).

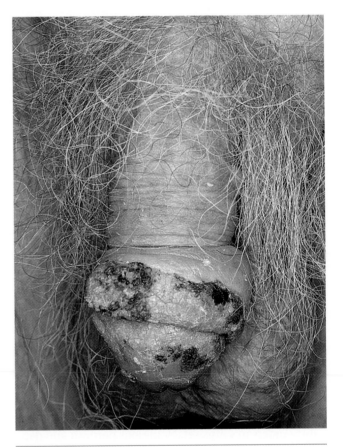

FIG. 9-10
Verruciform Xanthoma. A yellowish, verrucous, scabby plaque that involves the corona and glans penis. The lesion may mimic a giant condyloma or a squamous cell carcinoma. Biopsy is typical.

(Courtesy Dr. Sheetal Sapra and Dr. John B. Walter).

MALIGNANT TUMORS
Basal Cell Carcinoma

This condition is very uncommon on the penis. When seen, it is similar to basal cell carcinoma elsewhere on the skin; namely, a pearly, pink or skin-colored, often eroded, slow-growing, asymptomatic papule (Fig. 9-11). Most of the lesions are located on the shaft of the penis, but lesions on the prepuce and glans have been reported.[9] Lesions may be seen on black skin.[10]

Diagnosis

Lesions of basal cell carcinoma could be mistaken for molluscum contagiosum or for a syphilitic chancre. A biopsy establishes the definite diagnosis. No metastases have ever been reported from this locally invasive tumor.

Treatment

Treatment of choice is excision. There is no justification whatsoever for mutilating surgery, such as a penectomy, which has been occasionally used in the past.[11]

Squamous Cell Carcinoma

The most common malignant lesion of the penis is squamous cell carcinoma. It may be limited to the epidermal layer only (erythroplasia of Queyrat, Bowen's disease), or it may invade into the deeper layers (invasive squamous cell carcinoma).

Diagnosis and Treatment

Squamous cell carcinoma of the penis tends to metastasize early to the regional lymph nodes and should therefore be diagnosed and treated as soon as possible.[12]

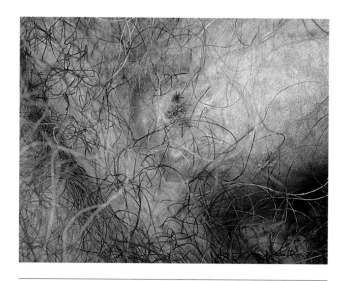

FIG. 9-11
Basal Cell Carcinoma. A large pearly, eroded papule at the base of the penis.
(From Goldminz D, Scott G, Klaus S: J Am Acad Dermatol 20:1094-1097, 1989.)

Erythroplasia of Queyrat

A carcinoma in situ, erythroplasia of Queyrat is confined mainly to the glans penis. The lesion is a smooth, shiny, velvety, red-colored patch (Fig. 9-12, *A*). In nonmucosal areas, carcinoma in situ is referred to as Bowen's disease.

Diagnosis

Bowen's disease on the shaft of the penis looks the same as Bowen's disease elsewhere; namely, a pink, well-demarcated, dry patch or flat papule that may be scaly (see Fig. 3-5), or a nonhealing, slowly growing, superficial red plaque (Fig. 9-12, *B*). With time these lesions invade the underlying tissues and become invasive squamous cell carcinomas.

Differential diagnoses are with any slow-healing erosive lesion such as chronic herpes simplex, erosive lichen planus, erosive drug reaction, pemphigus vulgaris, cicatricial bullous pemphigoid, and other malignant lesions such as extramammary Paget's disease.

Definite diagnosis is made by a biopsy showing the typical histologic picture of intraepidermal squamous cell carcinoma.

Treatment

Treatment should be carefully weighed for each individual case. Radiation, excision, carbon dioxide laser, topical 5% fluorouracil, and Mohs' surgery are all available options. Dermatologists, urologists, and surgeons are all competent to treat this cancer. Gynecologists, experienced with the use of the carbon dioxide laser in gynecologic cancers, can also be very helpful in treating penile cancers.[13,14]

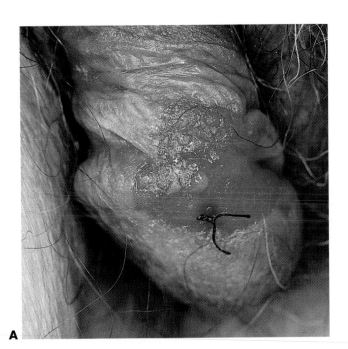
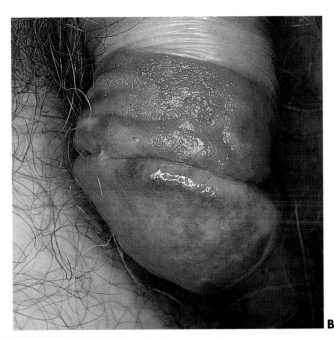

A **B**

FIG. 9-12

A, Erythroplasia of Queyrat. A red, shiny, smooth, well-demarcated patch located on the glans penis and extending to the shaft. The lesion is an intraepidermal squamous cell carcinoma (carcinoma in situ). **B,** Bowen's Disease. A large, red, superficial plaque present on the distal end of the shaft. The lesion represents a carcinoma in situ.

Invasive Squamous Cell Carcinoma

Invasive squamous cell carcinoma usually presents as a nonhealing ulcer of long duration (Fig. 9-13, *A*).

Diagnosis

One third of the cases metastasize early, so any suspicious lesion should be biopsied immediately and treatment instituted before metastasis or severe destruction of the penis occurs (Fig. 9-13, *B*). The primary lesion may be seen on the glans penis or may be hidden under the foreskin, where its presence may not be recognized until after regional lymph node metastases have already occurred (Fig. 9-13, *C*).

Treatment

Treatment options are surgery, radiation, carbon dioxide laser, or chemosurgery. Mutilating treatment is sometimes inevitable.[15,16,17,18,19]

Verrucous Carcinoma

This is a low-grade, locally aggressive, deeply invading squamous cell carcinoma, commonly termed *giant condyloma acuminatum of Buschke and Loewenstein.* It is usually seen on the glans penis in uncircumcised individuals. Clinically it is a slow-growing, cauliflower-like, compact verrucous nodule that looks like a large exophytic wart. The histology may be difficult to interpret because characteristic neoplastic features may be mild or absent. Aggressive treatment by surgery or laser is warranted (see p. 12 and Fig. 4-2, *E*).

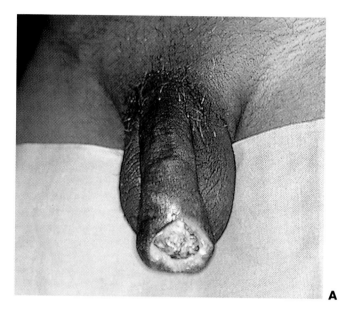

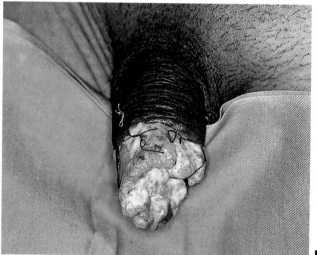

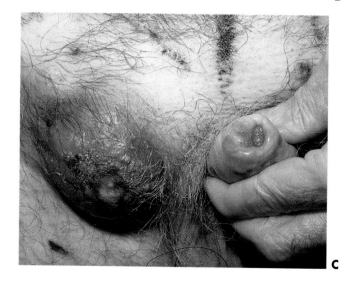

FIG. 9-13
Invasive Squamous Cell Carcinoma. **A,** A nonhealing, necrotic ulcer located on the tip of the penis. Metastases to regional lymph nodes have occurred. **B,** Severe destruction of the penis has occurred. **C,** A hidden carcinoma under the foreskin has caused large inguinal metastases.

Pseudoepitheliomatous Keratotic and Micaceous Balanitis of Civatte

This is a hyperkeratotic type of a low-grade squamous cell carcinoma. The lesion involves the glans penis and may be mistaken for a benign hyperkeratotic lesion. The term *micaceous* is used here because the hyperkeratotic lesion is composed of thin layers of scales that can be picked off like thin scales of mica, a mineral containing silicates of aluminum (Fig. 9-14).

Diagnosis

The differential diagnoses are with scaly plaques such as psoriasis, Reiter's disease, or Norwegian scabies. A biopsy establishes the true nature of this rare malignant condition.

Treatment

Treatment is the same as for invasive squamous cell carcinoma.[20]

Extramammary Paget's Disease

Extramammary Paget's disease of the penis presents as a red, sometimes moist, well-demarcated patch that usually starts in the groins and extends to the penis and scrotum (Fig. 9-15). It may be associated with underlying malignancy of the urethra, ureter, bladder, prostate, or lower gastrointestinal tract. The prognosis depends on the presence and type of the underlying malignancy, if any. A search for such a malignancy is mandatory.

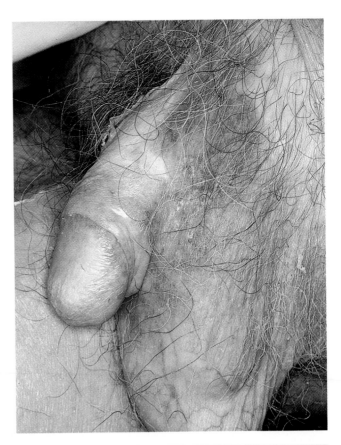

FIG. 9-15
Extramammary Paget's Disease. A large, red, ill-defined patch located on the scrotum and shaft of the penis.

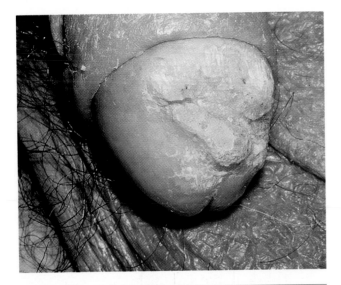

FIG. 9-14
Pseudoepitheliomatous Keratotic and Micaceous Balanitis of Civatte. Hyperkeratotic, scaly plaque present on the glans penis. This is a low-grade squamous cell carcinoma. (Courtesy Dr. Howard Bargman.)

Diagnosis

The differential diagnosis should include any long-standing red patch, such as a chronic contact dermatitis, psoriasis, yeast infection, Hailey-Hailey disease, and Bowen's Disease. The histology is quite typical.

Treatment

Treatment options are excision by surgery, carbon dioxide laser treatment, radiation, or Mohs' surgery.[21,22]

Kaposi's Sarcoma

Red, brown, or violaceous patches, papules or plaques, frequently with linear borders, may be seen either in the classic Kaposi's sarcoma type, or in the one associated with HIV infection (Fig. 9-16, *A*). The lesions are usually asymptomatic but cause great emotional distress to the patient because of their location. Rarely the lesion may enlarge and infiltrate the periurethral tissues, causing interference with urinary flow (Fig. 9-16, *B*).

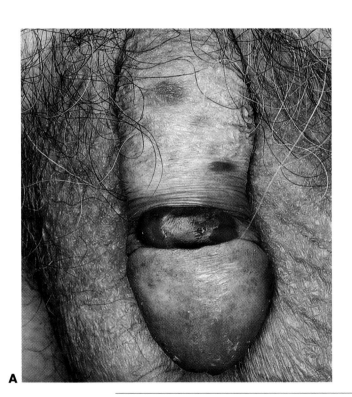
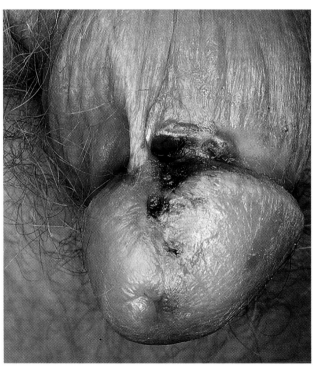

A　　　　　　　　　　　　　　　　　　　　　　　　　　**B**

FIG. 9-16
A, Kaposi's sarcoma in a non–HIV infected elderly individual. Bruise-like patches, one dark-red papule, and a similar plaque are present on the shaft of the penis. The latter two lesions have linear borders. **B,** Kaposi's sarcoma in an individual with AIDS. A dark-brown plaque is present on the ventral aspect of the penis. The tumor has infiltrated the periurethral area, causing obstruction to the urinary flow. Notice a purplish papule and distortion at the meatal opening.

Usually the clinical picture of Kaposi's sarcoma is fairly typical, but unsuspected lesions may be mistaken for hemangiomas, lichen planus, a bruise, or a melanocytic lesion. A biopsy will show the typical findings of Kaposi's sarcoma. Kaposi's sarcoma tumors respond temporarily to radiation therapy or to intralesional vinblastine injections.[23]

Recent work by Chang et al. strongly suggests that Kaposi's sarcoma is caused by a herpes virus (KSHV or HHV-8). Whether this virus alone can cause Kaposi's sarcoma or whether it needs additional cofactors remains to be elucidated.[24]

Hodgkin's Lymphoma

Lymphomas, such as Hodgkin's disease, are rarely seen on the penis. If the inguinal lymph nodes become involved, they may cause penile elephantiasis (Fig. 9-17).

Treatment

Treatment is for the underlying malignancy and is best carried out by an oncologist.

Mycosis Fungoides

This low-grade malignant cutaneous T cell lymphoma shows a typical three-stage evolution of skin lesions; starting usually with red scaly patches, frequently with a poikilodermatous component, progressing slowly into infiltrated plaques, and later into frank tumors. A rare variety of mycosis fungoides, seen as a solitary patch, showing the same typical histologic features of mycosis fungoides but behaving in an entirely benign way, is referred to as the Woringer-Kolopp disease or localized pagetoid reticulosis.[25]

Lesions of mycosis fungoides localized to the penis may be part of a generalized eruption or may be a solitary patch representing Woringer-Kolopp disease (Fig. 9-18). The histology is typical, showing atypical cells with hyperchromatic, irregularly shaped nuclei, with obvious tendency to invade the epidermis ("epidermotropism").

Treatment

Although treatment of mycosis fungoides is beyond the scope of this chapter, it should be noted that lesions of Woringer-Kolopp disease frequently disappear following local treatment with high-potency fluorinated steroid creams.

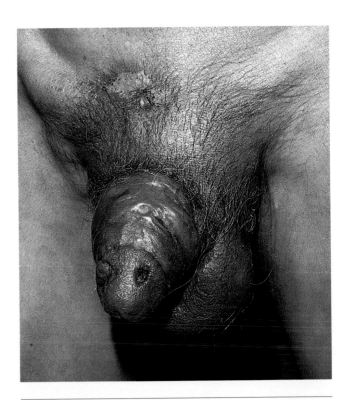

FIG. 9-17

Hodgkin's Lymphoma. Massive involvement of the inguinal and femoral lymph nodes has resulted in elephantiasis of the penis, with erosions and ulcerations.

Secondary Metastatic Lesions

Secondary metastatic lesions rarely involve the penis. The primary site in most cases is the bowel or the genitourinary tract.

Diagnosis and Treatment

The lesions may present as solitary nodules or may infiltrate the entire penis, causing induration and constant pain, necessitating amputation of the penis (Fig. 9-19).[26]

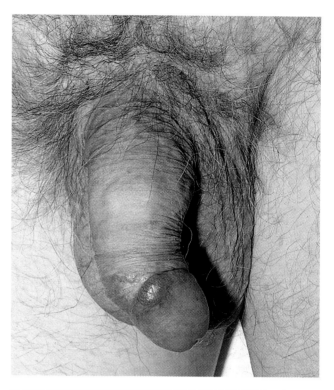

FIG. 9-19
Metastatic Lesions from Carcinoma of the Urethra. Metastatic nodules were seen on the glans and shaft of the penis, as well as on the lower lip. The malignant infiltrate caused painful induration and distortion of the shaft. The pain was so severe that the patient requested amputation of the penis.

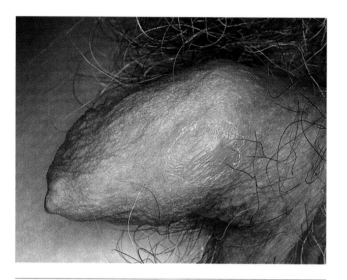

FIG. 9-18
Mycosis Fungoides. A solitary, superficial, pink patch, with slightly scaly borders is observed on the shaft of the penis. The lesion conforms to the Woringer-Kolopp variant of mycosis fungoides. A correct clinical diagnosis in this case was impossible. The lesion cleared up following treatment with a high-potency fluorinated steroid cream. (Courtesy Dr. Sheila Louisy.)

Melanoma

Rarely seen on the penis, melanoma occurs most commonly in the middle aged and elderly.

Physical Examination

Most lesions are seen on the glans penis. The lesion is usually an irregularly pigmented brown patch with or without a nodular component. It usually starts as a superficial spreading melanoma, which later may become nodular (Fig. 9-20).

Diagnosis and Treatment

The lesion has the same prognosis as melanoma elsewhere; the earlier the diagnosis, the better the prognosis. The prognosis also depends on the depth of the lesion at the time it is biopsied or removed. Wide surgical excision or amputation might be necessary, depending on the size and location of the lesion and how deeply it invades the underlying tissues.

It cannot be over-emphasized that an early diagnosis and treatment are necessary to save the patient's penis and life. Any suspicious lesion should be biopsied without delay.[27,28]

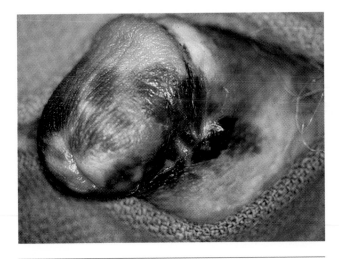

FIG. 9-20

Malignant Melanoma. Superficial spreading melanoma of the glans penis has extended to the shaft. An irregular brownish pigmentation with a black nodular component is located on the distal part of the shaft. The penis had to be amputated.

(Courtesy Dr. Leith Douglas.)

REFERENCES

Benign Tumors

1. Song DH, Lee KH, Kang WH: Idiopathic calcinosis of the scrotum, *J Am Acad Dermatol* 19:1095-1101, 1988.

Benign Vascular Growths

2. Ackerman AB, Kornberg R: Pearly penile papules: acral angiofibromas, *Arch Dermatol* 108:673-675, 1973.
3. Dekio S, Tsujino Y, Jidoi J: Intravascular papillary endothelial hyperplasia on the penis: report of a case, *J Dermatol* 20:657-659, 1993.
4. Paul AB, Johnston CAB, Nawroz I: Masson's tumor of the penis, *Br J Urol* 74:261-262, 1994.
5. Flores JT, Apfelberg DB, Maser MR, et al: Angiokeratoma of Fordyce: successful treatment with the argon laser, *Plast Reconstr Surg* 74:835-838, 1984.
6. Morgan SH, Crawford M d'A: Anderson-Fabry disease: a commonly missed diagnosis, *Br Med J* 297:872-873, 1988.

Benign Cysts

7. Dupre A, Lassere J, Christol B, et al: Canaux et kystes dysembryoplastiques du raphe genitoperineal, *Ann Dermatol Venereol* 109:81-84, 1982.
8. Geiss DF, Del Rosso JQ, Murphy J: Verruciform xanthoma of the glans penis: a benign clinical simulant of genital malignancy, *Cutis* 51:369-372, 1993

Malignant Tumors

9. Goldminz D, Scott G, Klaus S: Penile basal cell carcinoma, *J Am Acad Dermatol* 20:1094-1097, 1989.
10. Greenbaum SS, Krull EA, Simmons EB: Basal cell carcinoma at the base of the penis in a black patient, *J Am Acad Dermatol* 20:317-319, 1989.
11. Minami T, Chino I, Miki M, et al: Carcinoma of the penis: report of 2 cases and review of the record for the past ten years at the Jikei University Hospital, *Acta Urol Jpn* 11:321-328, 1965.
12. Norman RW, Millard OH, Mack FG, et al: Carcinoma of the penis: an 11 year review, *Can J Surg* 26:426-428, 1983.
13. Kaplan C, Kotah A: Erythroplasia of Queyrat (Bowen's disease of the penis), *J Surg Oncol* 5:281-290, 1973.
14. Bernstein G, Forgaard DM, Miller JE: Carcinoma in situ of the glans penis and distal urethra, *J Dermatol Surg Oncol* 12:450-455, 1986.
15. Narayana AS, Olney LE, Loening SA, et al: Carcinoma of the penis: analysis of 219 cases, *Cancer* 49:2185-2191, 1982.

16. Fraley EE, Zhang G, Sazama R, Lange PH: Cancer of the penis: prognosis and treatment plans, *Cancer* 55:1618-1623, 1985.
17. Micali G, Innocenzi D, Nasca MR, Musumeci ML, et al: Squamous cell carcinoma of the penis, *J Am Acad Dermatol* 35:432-451, 1996.
18. Burgers JK, Badalament RA, Drago JR: Penile cancer: clinical presentation, diagnosis, and staging, *Urol Clin North Am* 147:389-392, 1992.
19. Windhal T, Hellsten S: Laser treatment of localized squamous cell carcinoma of the penis, *J Urol* 154:1020-1023, 1995.
20. Tio TT, Blindeman L, van Ulsen J: Pseudoepitheliomatous, keratotic and micaceous balanitis of Lortat-Jacob and Civatte, *Brit J Dermatol* 123:265-266, 1990.
21. Perez MA, LaRossa DD, Tomaszewski JE: Paget's disease primarily involving the scrotum, *Cancer* 63:970-975, 1989.
22. Smith DJ, Hamdy FC, Evans JWH, et al: Paget's disease of the glans penis: an unusual urological malignancy, *Eur Urol* 25:316-319, 1994.
23. Schmidt ME, Yalisove B, Parenti DM, et al: Rapidly progressive penile ulcer: an unusual manifestation of Kaposi's sarcoma, *J Am Acad Dermatol* 27:267-268, 1992.
24. Chang Y, Cesarman E, Pessin MS, et al: Identification of herpes viruslike DNA sequences in AIDS-associated Kaposi's sarcoma, *Science* 266:1865-1869, 1994.
25. Burns MK, Chan LS, Cooper KD: Woringer-Kolopp disease (localized pagetoid reticulosis) or unilesional mycosis fungoides? an analysis of eight cases with benign disease, *Arch Dermatol* 131:325-329, 1995.
26. Robey El, Schellhammer PF: Four cases of metastases to the penis and a review of the literature, *J Urol* 132:992-994, 1984.
27. Oldbring J, Mikulowski P: Malignant melanoma of the penis and male urethra: report of nine cases and review of the literature, *Cancer* 59:581-587, 1987.
28. Rahid A-MH, Williams RM, Horten LWL: Malignant melanoma of penis and male urethra: is it a difficult tumor to diagnose? *Urology* 41:470-471, 1993.

CHAPTER 10

Miscellaneous Disorders of the Penis

HEREDITARY DISORDERS

Ichthyosis

The ichthyosiform dermatoses are a large group of hereditary keratinizing disorders characterized by the presence of abnormal scaling of the skin. Many types exist and most are quite rare. They may vary from being quite benign and manifesting dry skin (dominant ichthyosis vulgaris) to being extremely severe and life-threatening (harlequin ichthyosis). The four most common types are dominant ichthyosis vulgaris, X-linked ichthyosis, lamellar ichthyosis, and epidermolytic hyperkeratosis. Lesions on the penis may be seen in any of these conditions as part of the generalized skin condition (Fig. 10-1).[1]

Epidermal Nevi

Epidermal nevi are congenital, raised, linear, rough, usually hyperkeratotic plaques that most commonly involve an extremity or at times other areas. The penis may occasionally be involved (Fig. 10-2). The histology shows hyperkeratosis, acanthosis, and papillomatosis with elongation of the rete ridges, resembling a benign seborrheic keratosis.[2]

Treatment

Treatment is not recommended unless the lesion is very bothersome. If bothersome, excision or treatment with the carbon dioxide laser can be attempted.

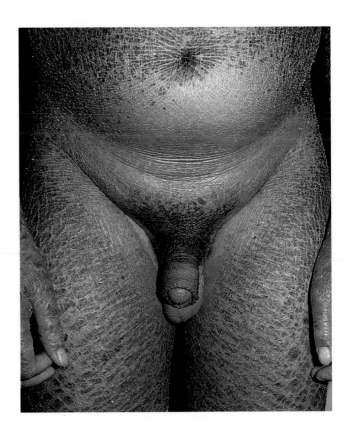

FIG. 10-1
Lamellar Ichthyosis. Large hyperpigmented scales are located on most of the body surface including the proximal half of the penis and pubic area.

Epidermolytic Hyperkeratosis

Localized epidermolytic hyperkeratosis (ichthyosis hystrix) looks clinically identical to epidermal nevus; but it manifests a totally different histologic picture of vacuolization of the mid and upper spinous layer of the epidermis, large keratohyaline granules in the vacuolated and thickened granular layer and hyperkeratosis. The lesions may be confined to the penis and scrotum (Fig. 10-3).[2]

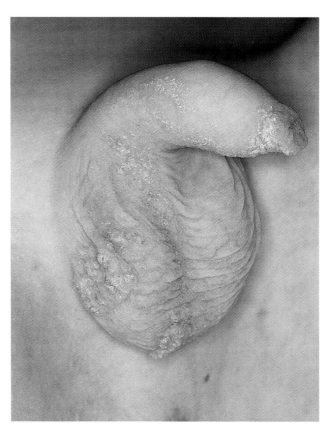

FIG. 10-3
Localized epidermolytic hyperkeratosis (ichthyosis hystrix) is observed with hyperkeratotic linear plaques limited to the penis and scrotum.

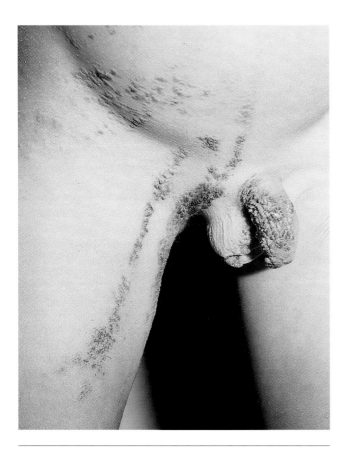

FIG. 10-2
Epidermal Nevi. Rough, hyperkeratotic and hyperpigmented linear streaks are observed on the right side of the body, penis, and scrotum.

SELF-INDUCED LESIONS
Neurotic and Psychotic Excoriations

These are rarely seen self-induced excoriations or ulcers, frequently with a linear border or a geometric pattern of the individual lesion (Fig. 10-4). Neurotic excoriations are commonly associated with depression.[3] Psychotic excoriations are associated with psychoses.

Treatment

Treatment of neurotic excoriation is with antidepressants. Patients with psychotic excoriations should be handled by a psychiatrist. Local supportive measure with topical antibiotics and protective dressings may be helpful.

Tattoos

Decorative tattoos are occasionally seen. Their design and appearance depend on the patient's ingenuity and the tattoo artist's skill (Fig. 10-5). Removal can be achieved with the neodymium-YAG laser; but it is a very rare occurrence indeed that the patient wants to part from this work of art.

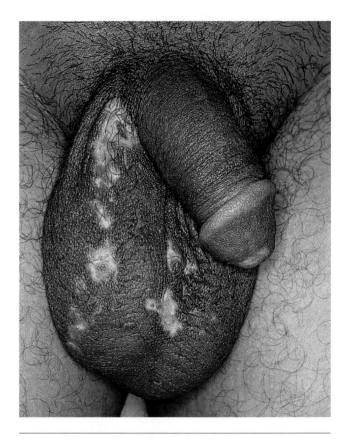

FIG. 10-4
Neurotic Excoriations. These self-induced erosions and ulcers are usually associated with depression.

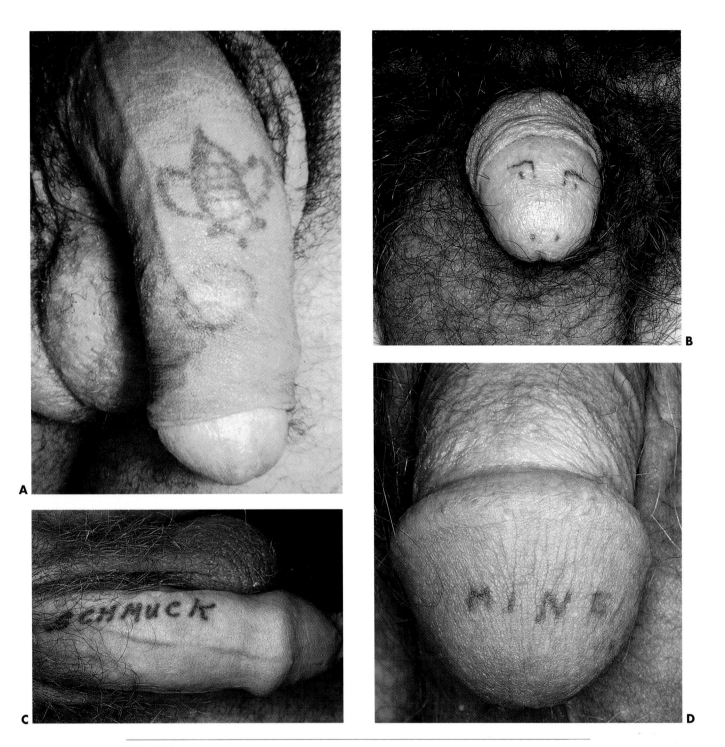

FIG. 10-5
Tattoos. **A,** "The Sting." **B,** "Snake-eyes." **C,** An individual's self-assessment. **D,** An individual's assertion of ownership.

Piercing of the Penis

Piercing and the wearing of decorative rings may be seen in individuals who enjoy piercing their skin and wearing rings and studs in the pierced areas. The ears, lips, tongue, nipples, and genitals are targeted. Rings in the penis are also used to promote sexual stimulation (Fig. 10-6).

Implantation of a Foreign Body

This may be done to promote sexual pleasure or for other more mundane purposes.[4] In one case, diamonds coated with paraffin were implanted under the skin of the penile shaft to carry the family jewels safely across hostile borders (Fig. 10-7).

THE PENIS AS A SYMBOL IN FOLKLORE

Phallic paintings, murals, and figurines have played a prominent part in many cultures mainly as a symbol of fertility (Fig. 10-8, *A*). Old murals and artifacts that display a prominent penis have been unearthed and can be seen in archaeologic sites (Fig. 10-8, *B*) and museums (Fig. 10-8, *C*).

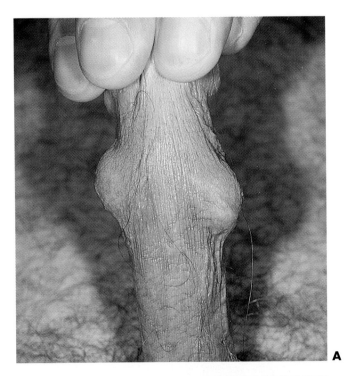

A

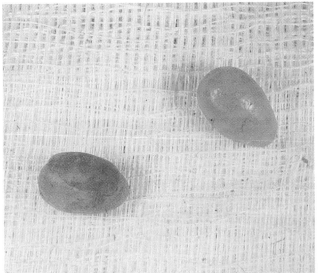

B

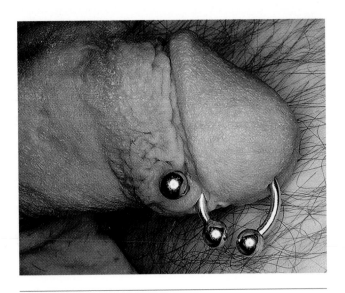

FIG. 10-6
A pierced penis with a golden ring and stud.

FIG. 10-7
Foreign Body Implantation. **A,** Diamonds coated with paraffin were implanted under the skin of the penile shaft to smuggle them safely across hostile borders. **B,** The paraffin-coated diamonds are seen following their surgical removal.
(Courtesy Dr. Jay Herbst.)

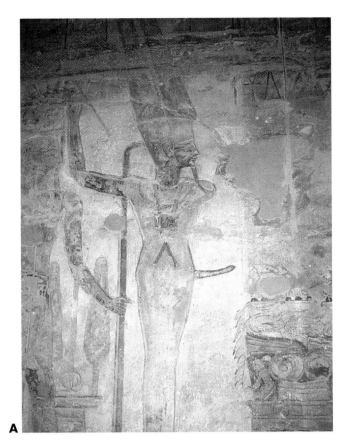

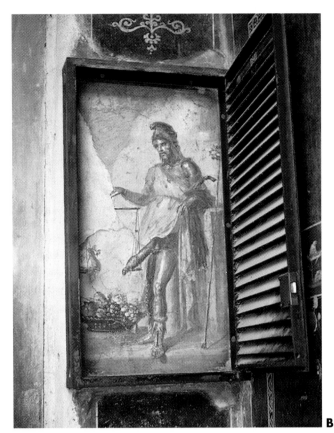

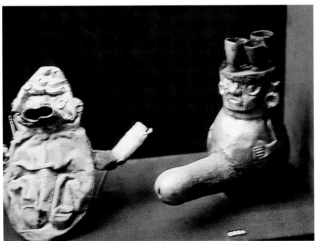

FIG. 10-8

A, A mural in Abou-Simbel, Egypt, depicting King Ramses the Second. The prominent phallus is a symbol of fertility. **B**, A mural in ancient Pompeii, Italy. A Roman gentleman is shown holding a scale. On one side is his large penis, on the other is a purse, presumably full of gold coins. The message: a healthy penis is literally worth its weight in gold. **C**, A golden archeologic artifact that exhibits a prominent penis. Part of an exhibit at the Gold Museum, Lima, Peru.

ANATOMIC ABERRATION
Double Penis

Approximately 100 cases of double penis (diphallia, diphallus) have been recorded in the medical literature up to 1997. Many of these show one normal penis and one rudimentary penis. Frequently they are associated with multiple congenital anomalies, mainly of the genitourinary tract.[5] Rarely two penises of normal size may be seen (Fig 10-9). In this particular case one penis was perfectly normal and the other one was an imperforate penis. The proud owner could use only one penis for voiding or ejaculating, but one or both together for sexual intercourse. He thus could manipulate the situation for "procreation" or for "recreation."[6]

REFERENCES

Hereditary Diseases
1. Rand RE, Baden HP: The ichthyoses: a review, *J Am Acad Dermatol* 8:285, 1983.
2. Su WPD: Histopathologic varieties of epidermal nevus, *Am J Dermatopathol* 4:161-170, 1982.

Self-Induced Lesions
3. Fisher BK, Pearce KI: Neurotic excoriations: a personality evaluation, *Cutis* 14:251-254, 1974.
4. Cohen EL, Kim S-W: Subcutaneous artificial penile nodules, *J Urol* 127;135, 1982.

Anatomic Abberation
5. Johnson CF, Carlton CE Jr, Powell NB: Duplication of penis (review), *Urology* 4:722-725, 1974.
6. Pendino JA: Diphallus (double penis), *J Urol* 64:156-157, 1950.

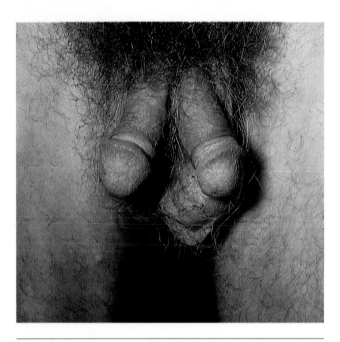

FIG. 10-9
Double Penis (diphallia, diphallus).
(Courtesy Dr. Morris Waisman.)

LYNETTE J. MARGESSON

INTRODUCTION

Women with genital cutaneous problems find it very difficult to locate experienced caregivers. They sometimes find themselves being shuttled from their general practitioner to gynecology, urology, dermatology, venereology, and even neurology experts. Some practitioners have had little or no training in the area and are unsure how to approach diagnosis and management. I was one of these physicians over 20 years ago when I first started to see vulvar patients in my private practice. With the encouragement of my patients and with the selfless help of the excellent dermatologic mentors who pioneered in vulvar disease, I have acquired some modest expertise. There has been a Multidisciplinary Regional Vulvar Clinic at Queen's University for almost a decade, staffed by me and an excellent group of gynecologists and a gynecologic oncologist, Dr. Peter Bryson. I strongly encourage a multidisciplinary approach to vulvar disease when possible. ▲

CHAPTER 11

Normal Anatomy of the Vulva

Understanding the anatomy of the vulva is vital to managing the wide array of vulvar disorders. This anatomy is often not understood by healthcare professionals, nor by women themselves. Healthcare professionals are at a disadvantage because they have never been taught the anatomic variations. Women also have little education about this area. Therefore it is difficult, if not impossible, for them to visualize this area and recognize what they can see. Furthermore, their culture may have taught them to consider the area "dirty" or even repulsive. Their caregivers labor under the burden of legal, social, and moral restrictions that further complicate history taking, physical examination, and effective care.

This chapter provides only an overview. The reader is encouraged to look at the list of suggested readings for in-depth descriptions.

PERINEUM

The vulva is located in the perineum. The perineum is diamond shaped and is bounded anteriorly by the symphysis pubis, posteriorly by the tip of the coccyx, and bilaterally by the ischial tuberosities. It is divided into two distinct parts that are roughly triangular and are defined by drawing a line between the ischial tuberosities. The anterior triangle is referred to as the urogenital triangle; the posterior is the anal triangle. The vulva lies principally within the urogenital triangle but does extend up onto the pubic symphysis.

VULVA

The vulva is defined as the female anatomy bound laterally by the genitocrural folds, anteriorly by the mons pubis, and posteriorly by the anus. The main anatomic structures are the mons pubis, labia majora, labia minora, clitoris, vestibule, urethral meatus, hymen, vestibular glands, and Bartholin's glands. There is considerable anatomic variation here as anywhere else on the body. The pattern of hair growth, pigmentation, structural size, and shape all vary according to genetic background, hormonal status, and age (Fig. 11-1).

MONS PUBIS

The mons pubis is the subcutaneous fat pad over the symphysis pubis. It becomes progressively thicker and is covered with pubic hair at puberty.

LABIA MAJORA

The labia majora form the lateral borders of the vulva. They are made up of folds of adipose and fibrous tissue fusing anteriorly with the mons pubis and posteriorly to form the posterior commissure . They are covered with a varying amount of hair and contain sebaceous, sweat, and apocrine glands. The small cavity between the posterior commisure and the vaginal opening is called the posterior vestibule. The fold between the labia majora and labia minora is called the interlabial sulcus.

LABIA MINORA

The labia minora are the two thin pigmented folds of the vulva. They are medial to the labia majora and are made up of loose connective tissue and blood vessels but devoid of subcutaneous fat. They are quite small in childhood, grow at puberty, and then atrophy again after menopause. Each labium divides anteriorly into two parts: the lateral parts join anteriorly to form the prepuce of the clitoris, the medial parts pass posterior to the clitoris, and then join to form its sling or frenulum. The labia

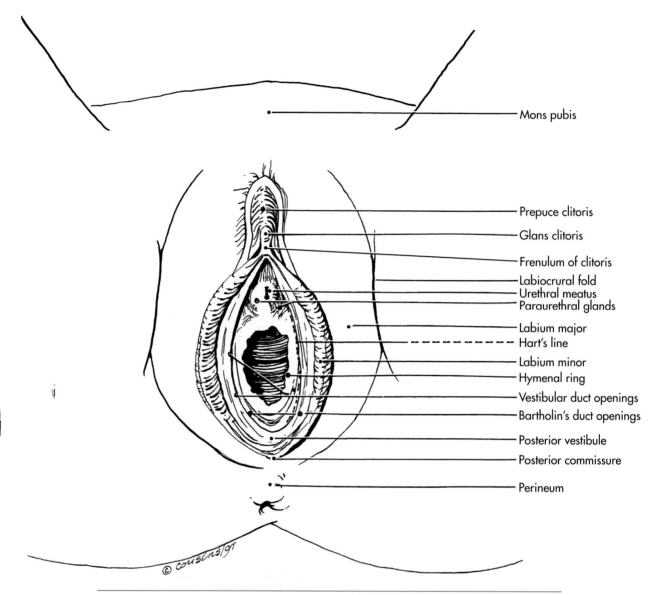

Mons pubis

Prepuce clitoris

Glans clitoris

Frenulum of clitoris

Labiocrural fold

Urethral meatus

Paraurethral glands

Labium major

Hart's line

Labium minor

Hymenal ring

Vestibular duct openings

Bartholin's duct openings

Posterior vestibule

Posterior commissure

Perineum

FIG. 11-1
Normal Anatomy of the Vulva.

minora have abundant sebaceous glands on their outer one third. Their inner aspects blend into the vulvar vestibule, and the junction of squamous epithelium (labial) and the transitional epithelium (vestibular) forms Hart's line.

CLITORIS

The clitoris is the erectile body of the vulva. It corresponds to the penis in the male. It is situated posterior to the pubic symphysis at the apex of the vulvar vestibule. It is composed of a body and a glans. The body consists of two corpora cavernosa covered by their ischiocavernosus muscles. The glans is a small mass of erectile tissue that caps the body of the clitoris and is hidden by the prepuce.

VULVAR VESTIBULE

The vulvar vestibule is the part of the vulva that extends from the clitoral frenulum posteriorly to the posterior commissure and laterally to Hart's line, where the nonkeratinized transitional epithelium of the vestibule joins the keratinized squamous epithelium at the base of the medial aspects of the labia minora. This vulvar mucosa is responsive to estrogen, which is responsible for thickening the mucosa at puberty. Within the vestibule are the urethral meatus, the openings of Skene's paraurethral glands, the minor vestibular glands, the Bartholin's gland duct openings, and the lateral hymenal surface. Central to the hymenal ring is the vaginal orifice. The similarity of the vulvar, oral, and conjunctival mucosae may explain their coinvolvement in some of the inflammatory and bullous diseases.

URETHRAL MEATUS

The urethra opens just anterior to the vaginal introitus within the vestibule. It may have two or three small over-hanging lips. The opening may be either star-shaped or slit-like. On either side are the Skene's glands with their small openings.

HYMEN

The hymen is a thin membrane of connective tissue separating the vestibule and the vagina. The shape of the prepubertal and/or virginal hymen varies, but most commonly it is annular or crescentic (Fig. 11-2). It is very prominent in a newborn child as a result of antenatal exposure to maternal estrogen, but it regresses to its thin prepubertal state during childhood. The normal hymen changes with puberty. Sexual intercourse and childbirth cause the disappearance of its larger part, leaving only remnants.

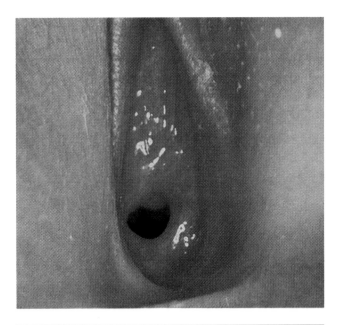

FIG. 11-2
A Normal Crescentic Hymen in a Child.
(Courtesy Dr. G.D. Oliver.)

VESTIBULAR GLANDS

Around the hymenal ring and extending in two arcs up to and beside the urethra are the openings of the mucus-secreting minor vestibular glands. The largest of these are the Bartholin's glands, one on each side, opening at the 5 and 7 o'clock positions just outside the hymenal ring. These glands are located deep in the musculature with ducts that are up to 2.5 cm long.

NEUROVASCULAR SUPPLY

The arterial blood supply is from branches of the external and internal pudendal arteries. Lymph drains from the vulva into the medial group of superficial inguinal nodes on both ipsilateral and contralateral sides. The sensory nerve supply to the anterior vulva is via the genitofemoral nerve (L1 and L2) and the cutaneous branch of the ilioinguinal nerve (L1). The posterior part of the vulva and the clitoris are supplied by the pudendal nerve (S2 through S4). It courses through the lower pelvis where it is subject to trauma in many forms. A small area of the posterior vulva is also served by the perineal branch of the posterior cutaneous nerve of the thigh. Motor innervation of the perineal muscles is by the pudendal nerve.

PERIANAL AND PELVIC MUSCLES

The perineum can be considered a diamond-shaped area. Two triangles in apposition comprise this area. Anteriorly is the urogenital triangle, and posteriorly is the anal triangle. A line between the ischial tuberosities represents this division. The urogenital triangle is divided into a superficial space and a deeper space, each with its own muscles, vessels, and nerves.

The superficial perineal space contains the bulbospongiosus muscle, the ischiocavernosus muscle, the superficial transverse perineal muscle, and the urogenital diaphragm. The superficial transverse perineal muscle runs between the ischial tuberosities and inserts into the central tendon/perineal body that is interposed between the anal canal and the vagina to form a vital support system (Fig. 11-3). To this perineal body also attaches the deeper levator ani muscle that supports the posterior wall of the vagina. The ischiocavernosus muscles arise from the ischial tuberosities, insert into the medial parts of the pubic arch, and form the crus of the clitoris. Medially, in the same plane, is the bulbospongiosus muscle (sometimes called the bulbocavernosus). It serves as the vaginal sphincter. Both the ischiocavernosus and bulbospongiosus muscles are responsible for clitoral erection. Deep to the bulbospongiosus muscle is the vestibular bulb, equivalent to the penile bulb in the male, which also aids in erection.

The deep perineal space is also called the perineal membrane or triangular ligament. It contains the muscles of the urethral sphincter and the deep transverse perineal muscle, plus parts of the urethra and vagina. Thus the muscles of the urogenital triangle/diaphragm are also involved with micturition.

The main pelvic organs, plus the urethra, vagina, and rectum, are all held in place by the deeper pelvic floor muscles of the pelvic diaphragm. Often referred to as the levator ani, this is a three-part muscle that not only supports the pelvic viscera but also provides the elasticity of the pelvic floor. Through it pass the urinary, vaginal, and rectal canals. Unlike the muscles of the urogenital triangle mentioned above, these muscles occupy much of the anal triangle but are not confined to it (also extending anteriorly). The posterior (first) part of the muscle is the ileococcygeus, a fan-shaped muscle passing from the ischial spines to the anococcygeal ligament. The anococcygeal ligament traverses the space between the coccyx and the posterior external anal sphincter in an anterior-posterior direction. The anterior (second) part is the pubococcygeus muscle that sweeps from the pubis around the urethra and vagina and inserts into the perineal body and the anococcygeal ligament. It envelops and is attached to the urethra, vagina, and rectum. The third part, the puborectalis muscle, forms half of a heavy muscular sling from the pubic bone to the anococcygeal ligament behind the rectum. This area is supplied by L1 and L2 and S1 through S4 nerve roots.

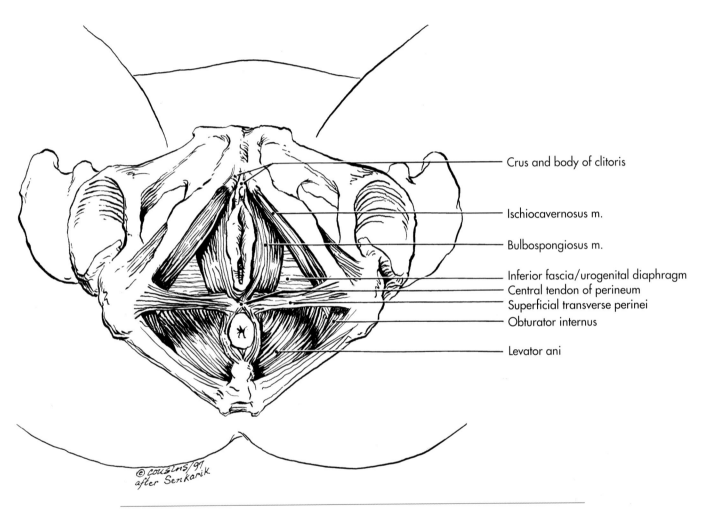

Crus and body of clitoris

Ischiocavernosus m.

Bulbospongiosus m.

Inferior fascia/urogenital diaphragm
Central tendon of perineum
Superficial transverse perinei
Obturator internus

Levator ani

© cousins/91
after Senkarik

FIG. 11-3
Normal Anatomy of the Pelvic Floor.

ANATOMIC VARIATIONS
Sebaceous Hyperplasia

The sebaceous glands on the inner aspect of the labia minora can become quite prominent. This is referred to as sebaceous hyperplasia and is completely harmless (Fig. 11-4, *A*). The clinician unfamiliar with this change may be concerned about missing an unusual rash or neoplasm.

Vulvar Papillomatosis

The vulvar vestibular area may have prominent vestibular papillae in about half of premenopausal women (Fig. 11-4, *B*). These are small tubular or slightly filiform projections along the vulvar vestibule. They are soft and completely asymptomatic. They can be confused with condylomata. Condylomata are firm and can be differentiated with palpation, colposcopy, or biopsy.

AGE-RELATED CHANGES

Significant age-related changes occur in the vulva.

Childhood

At birth the vulvar tissue has been stimulated by placental estrogen. The hymen is somewhat plump and pale, and the vulvar vestibule is swollen and pink. This can last for weeks. The loss of maternal estrogen leaves the vestibule and vagina somewhat thinned and susceptible to minor trauma. In childhood the labia majora are plump fat pads, but the labia minora are quite tiny (Fig. 11-5, *A*). The whole area is hairless and lacking nonethnic pigmentation. The hymen has a smooth edge ("intact"), but in almost all girls is patent. There may be a build-up of greasy secretion called smegma in the interlabial sulcus, depending on hygiene practices.

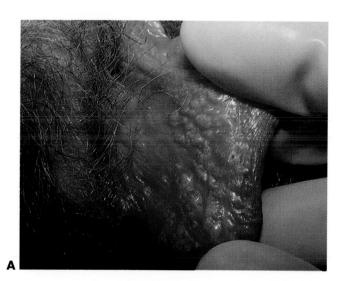

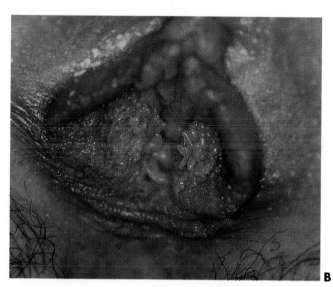

A   B

FIG. 11-4
Papules. **A,** On the inner edge of the labia minora are variably sized yellow papules. These are normal sebaceous glands—sebaceous hyperplasia. **B,** On either side of the hymenal ring are obvious filiform papules filling the whole area. This is vulvar papillomatosis.
(**A,** Courtesy Dr. M. Moyal-Barracco.)

Adult Reproductive Age Group

The vulva shows a varying degree of hair growth over the mons pubis, labia majora, and perineum, with a variable amount of pigmentation (Fig. 11-5, *B*).

The labia majora are fully developed and vary in size. The labia minora may have some slight notching along the edges and are definitely more prominent than before puberty.

Post-Menopausal Age Group

With the gradual loss of estrogen the vulva atrophies. The vestibular mucosa pales (Fig. 11-5, *C*).

The pubic hair thins and gradually the hairs themselves whiten. Pigmentation fades. The labia majora atrophy and in thin women can become floppy. The labia minora can atrophy and almost disappear. The clitoris may appear somewhat larger as a result of a relative increase in androgens and decrease in prepuce covering. Aging and multiple deliveries produce a weakening of the muscular structures, resulting in a tendency toward prolapses of urethra, bladder, uterus, vagina, and rectum.

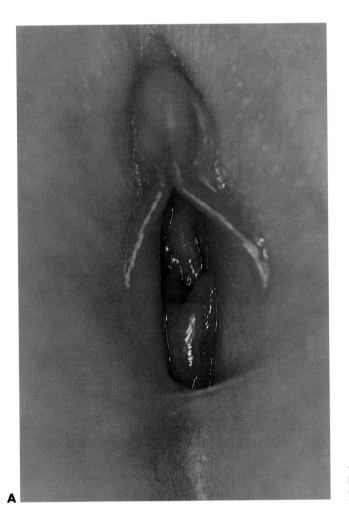

A

FIG. 11-5

Normal Vulvas. **A**, A normal vulva in 20-month-old child.

continued

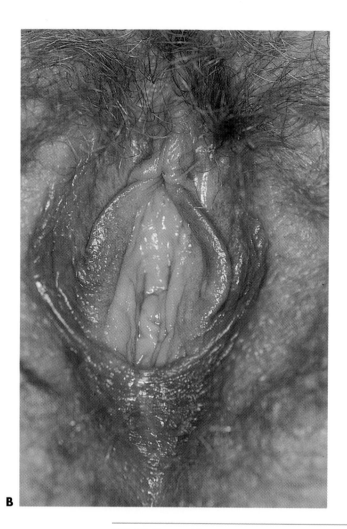

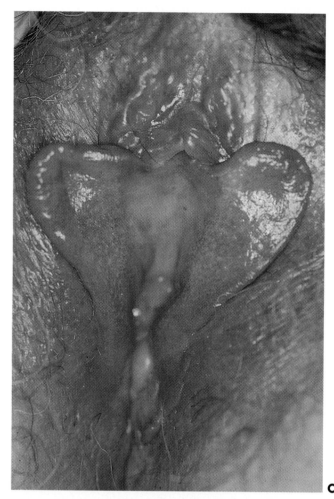

FIG. 11-5, cont'd
B, An adult vulva with a normal pattern of hair, etc. Note the normal pigmentation in this olive-skinned woman. **C**, In this 60-year-old woman, a pale vulvar vestibule and thinning pubic hair is consistent with her age.

ATROPHIC VULVOVAGINITIS

Without adequate estrogen, the epithelium of the vagina and vulvar vestibule atrophy. This thinned surface is friable, very easily irritated, and susceptible to secondary infection.

The cause of atrophic vulvovaginitis is loss of estrogen resulting from menopause, castration, antiestrogens (tamoxifen), or ovarian destruction. Natural menopause is the most common cause. With a thin atrophic vaginal epithelium there is a shift in pH and the growth of normally commensal organisms may occur, with resulting infection.

Note: *There is a relative estrogen deficiency before menarche, post-partum, and during breast-feeding.*

Patient history includes complaints of vulvar burning, dysuria, pruritus, tenderness, and dyspareunia. A watery, scalding discharge may occur. There may be exquisitely painful fissures, with slight bleeding around the introitus.

Physical Examination

The labia majora are lax, and the labia minora may shrink and even disappear. The vulvar trigone and vagina are paler, the vaginal walls are smoother, and the tissues thinner. There may be introital stenosis. Petechiae and fissures may be seen. The discharge may be heavy, malodorous, gray, or even green in color, with a pH of 6 to 7.

Diagnosis

Diagnosis is made clinically.

Treatment

Treatment is nonspecific (see Appendix C for details). The patient can be instructed to do the following:

- Avoid irritating soaps and hygiene products
- Cleanse gently with Cetaphil (cleanser)
- Use lubricants and emollients
- Treat intercurrent infections

Specific treatment is estrogen replacement therapy (ERT):

Topical

Conjugated estrogen cream: 0.625 mg/g, 2g intravaginally qhs for 2 to 3 weeks, then 1g qhs given 2 to 3 times per week as required

Dienestrol cream: 5g intravaginally qhs as above, then 2.5g given 2 to 3 times per week as required

Systemic

Oral conjugated estrogens: estradiol-17-ß patches, with or without medroxyprogesterone acetate, and other preparations are used in a wide variety of regimens. ▲ **If patients do not tolerate estrogens, suggest a vaginal lubricant such as Replens or K-Y Long Lasting.** ▼

SUGGESTED READINGS

DiSaia DJ: Clinical anatomy of the female genital tract. In Scott JR, editor: *Danforth's obstetrics and gynecology,* ed 7, Philadelphia, 1994, Lippincott, 1-8.

Ridley CM: *The vulva,* Edinburgh, 1988, Churchill Livingstone, 39-65.

Snell RS: *Clinical anatomy for medical students,* ed 5, Boston, 1992, Little, Brown, 320-325, 348-366.

CHAPTER 12

Congenital Malformations of the Vulva

Developmental abnormalities of the female genital tract are rare. They inevitably cause anxiety and upset in the family. The abnormality may involve parts of the vulva or the whole vulva. There may be abnormalities of the openings of the urinary or digestive tract and malformation of the external genitalia, resulting in sexual ambiguity. In-depth discussion of these conditions is beyond the scope of this text.

AMBIGUOUS EXTERNAL GENITALIA

At birth, if the external genital organs are not clearly female or male then there is sexual ambiguity. The majority of these cases are due to excessive androgenization of a female fetus. Such infants usually present with an enlarged phallus alone or associated with some degree of labioscrotal fusion. These cases represent female pseudohermaphroditism. The two other main etiologic categories are male pseudohermaphroditism and disorders of differentiation.

Female Pseudohermaphroditism

Accounting for 80% of ambiguous genitalia, female pseudohermaphroditism is usually due to a recessive congenital enzymatic defect of adrenal steroid biosynthesis. These infants are 46XX with normal ovaries. The most common defect is 21-hydroxylase deficiency, resulting in underproduction of cortisol and overproduction of androgens that virilize the

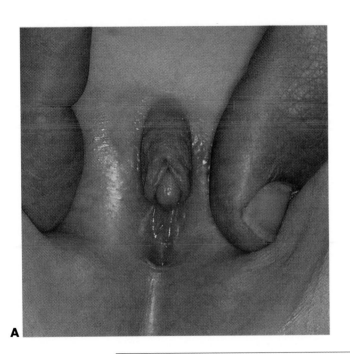

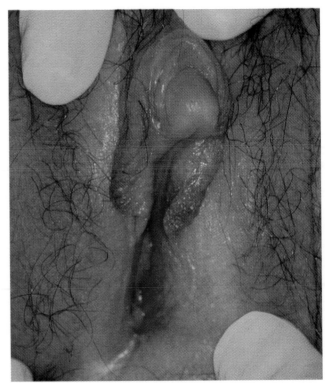

A

B

FIG. 12-1
For legend see opposite page.

fetal female external genitalia (Fig. 12-1). Rarely it is associated with sodium depletion, which can be life-threatening in the neonate. Less common is the 11-hydroxylase deficiency, which produces the same clinical picture.

Although rare, maternal factors can also virilize a female fetus. If a mother has an ovarian or adrenal androgen-producing tumor or ingests androgens during fetal development, pseudohermaphroditism can develop.

Male Pseudohermaphroditism

Male pseudohermaphroditism occurs in about 15% of cases of ambiguous genitalia. These infants are normal 46XY but have had a partial or complete block in the masculinization process during development. This results in the underdevelopment of male genitalia and in the most extreme cases can yield a female phenotype (Fig. 12-2). The mechanism can be a lack of gonadotrophin, an enzyme defect in testosterone biosynthesis, or a defect in androgen-dependent target tissue response (e.g., androgen receptor defect or 5-α-reductase deficiency).

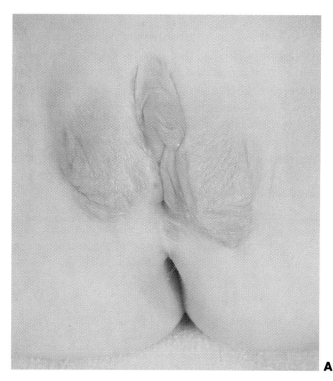

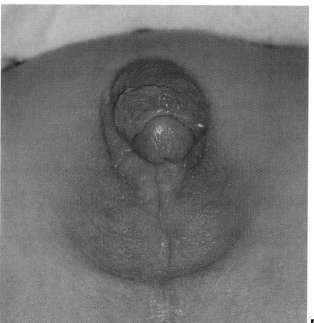

FIG. 12-1

A, Clitoromegaly with posterior labial fusion in congenital adrenal hyperplasia. An example of female pseudohermaphroditism. **B,** An 11-year-old girl with increasing facial hirsutism, thick genital hair, normal vagina, and clitoromegaly as a result of a 21-hydroxylase deficiency. (**B,** Courtesy Dr. G.D. Oliver.)

FIG. 12-2

A, Male pseudohermaphroditism resulting from a partial androgen sensitivity. Ambiguous genitalia in an XY child raised as a girl. **B,** Ambiguous genitalia in an XY child with partial androgen insensitivity. (Courtesy Dr. G.D. Oliver.)

Disorders of Gonadal Differentiation

In these three conditions there is an abnormality of the number or structure of the X and Y chromosomes or of a male-specific transplant antigen (H-Y antigen) that interacts with the Y chromosome to induce testicular differentiation.

Ovarian dysgenesis can occur in several chromosomal abnormalities, but the most common is Turner's syndrome (45X) or a Turner's mosaic (45X/46XX). The phenotype at birth is appropriately female, but pubertal development fails.

True hermaphroditism is the presence of both ovarian and testicular tissue in the same patient (Fig. 12-3). External and internal genital development varies, with multiple possible permutations and combinations of features.

Dysgenesis of seminiferous tubules can occur in Klinefelter's syndrome.

Treatment

Infants with ambiguous genitalia must be assessed immediately by the appropriate pediatric gynecologist, geneticist, and/or endocrinologist. The salt-losing form of congenital adrenal hyperplasia must be ruled out, and other hormonal and chromosomal studies must be undertaken to assign an appropriate sex to the infant.

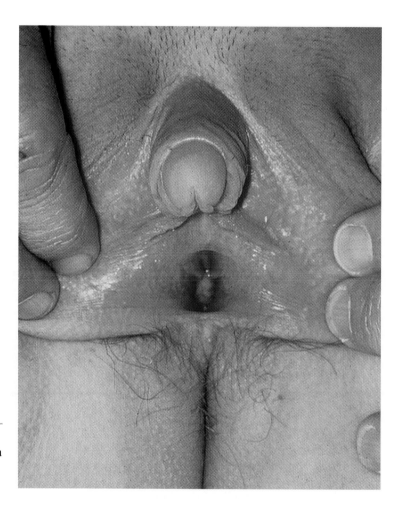

FIG. 12-3
A vulva in a true hermaphrodite XY/XX with a penis, vagina, testes, ovary, and hemiuterus.
(Courtesy Dr. G.D. Oliver.)

Androgen-Producing Tumors

Note: *Rapid clitoral enlargement in a young girl with a sudden onset of hirsutism and virilization should trigger an investigation for underlying androgen-producing tumors. Congenital adrenal hyperplasia can also present late (at puberty) but is usually more gradual.*

CONGENITAL LABIAL HYPERTROPHY

Hypertrophy of the labia minora is not an uncommon developmental abnormality. The etiology is usually an anatomic variant rather than a malformation. It is noted at puberty. Rarely it occurs because of lymphostasis or chronic physical pulling on the labia. The patient history is asymptomatic except as a nuisance with hygiene, physical activity, or sexual intercourse. The large labia may be unilateral or bilateral (Fig. 12-4). If there is difficulty with hygiene, there may be erythema and irritation.

Treatment

If the hypertrophy is asymptomatic, no treatment is needed. Surgical reduction can be considered when the condition is problematic.

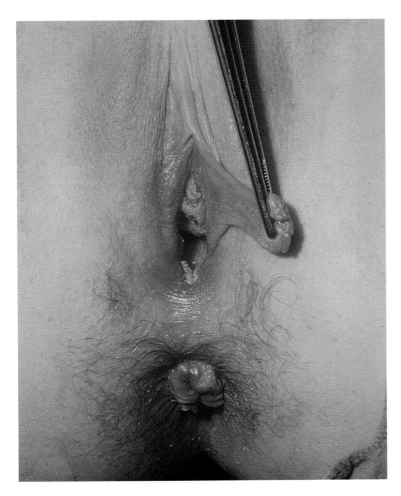

FIG. 12-4
An elongated left labium minor.
(Courtesy Dr. P. Bryson.)

LABIAL ADHESIONS

Labial adhesions result from fusion of the labia minora. This occurs in 1.4% of prepubertal girls. The etiology is unknown. Contributing factors can be local irritation, poor hygiene, and lack of estrogen, resulting in a mild inflammatory reaction. The patient is prepubertal and often asymptomatic. Often the parent or medical caregiver notices a reduction in vaginal opening. Other presentations include dysuria, urinary retention, urinary tract infection, or genital irritation and burning.

The extent of fusion varies. Sometimes only a pinhole opening is seen, with the vaginal introitus and urethral meatus trapped behind (Fig. 12-5, *A*).

The natural history is of spontaneous resolution with pubertal estrogenization.

Treatment

A topical conjugated estrogen (Premarin) cream applied in a thin layer twice a day for two to three weeks, along with gentle traction, often leads to separation (Fig. 12-5, *B*). Long-term application of a bland ointment (e.g., petrolatum) after a daily warm water soak and gentle traction is recommended to reduce the risk of recurrence. Reassurance is important. Manual separation with some form of anesthesia may be necessary, especially when urinary sequelae are present. Rarely carbon dioxide laser surgery is useful here.

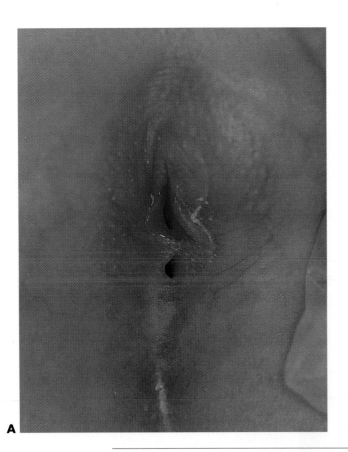
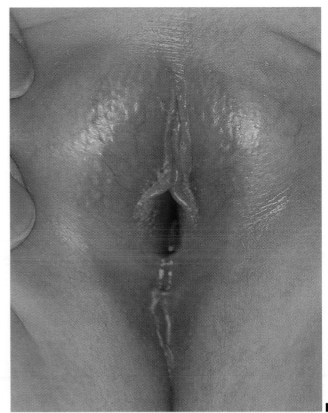

A
B

FIG. 12-5

A, Labial adhesions in a 3-year-old girl with a tiny opening before treatment. **B**, One month later after treatment with a topical estrogen cream.

HYMENAL ABNORMALITIES

The hymen is a thin membrane of connective tissue in the vestibule, over the entrance of the vagina. It normally has a round or crescentic opening. Different patterns occur, including several microperforations (cribriform/fenestrated hymen) or no opening at all (imperforate hymen) (Fig. 12-6). The etiology involves failure of complete or uniform embryonic canalization. Partial canalization may lead to recurrent vaginal infection in the premenarchal years as a result of trapped secretions, urine, and bacteria. An imperforate hymen may present with primary amenorrhea and complaints of lower abdominal discomfort, usually noticed cyclically for 1 to 3 months or more.[1] There is progressive severe cyclical lower abdominal pain. Occasionally an imperforate hymen is noted at birth with a microcolpos from maternal estrogen exposure.

With an imperforate hymen, the hymen is completely intact (Fig. 12-7, *A*). The vagina is distended, may be large and sausage-shaped, and causes the hymen to protrude out the "introitus," sometimes with a blue discoloration. Examination may be difficult because of the pain. An abdominal examination may demonstrate lower abdominal swelling (Fig. 12-7, *B*) resulting from the blood accumulation in the vagina (hematocolpos) and even in the uterus (hematometra). As mentioned earlier, a bulging imperforate hymen may be noted in the neonate as a result of trapped vaginal secretions. In all cases a rectal examination may be helpful.

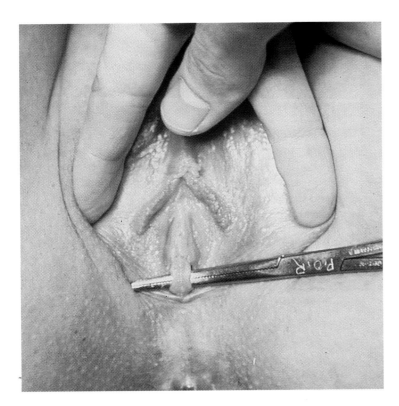

FIG. 12-6
A Septate Hymen.
(Courtesy Dr. G.D. Oliver.)

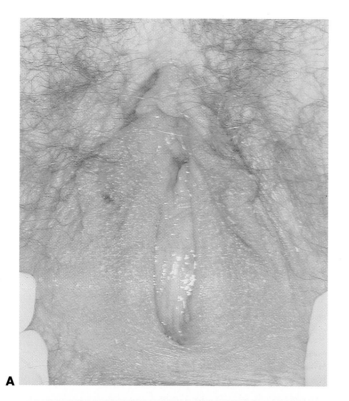

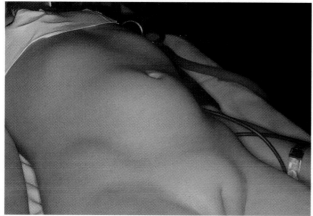

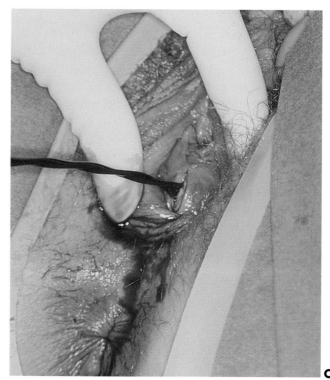

FIG. 12-7
A, An imperforate hymen in a 13-year-old adolescent who presented with an acute abdomen. **B**, In the same patient, abdominal swelling resulting from hematocolpos is present. **C**, The patient's imperforate hymen is incised, and the old blood is released.
(Courtesy Dr. G.D. Oliver.)

Diagnosis

Clinical diagnosis includes taking the patient history, performing a physical examination, and occasionally using ultrasound to determine the appropriate diagnosis.

Treatment

For an imperforate hymen a surgical hymenotomy by a surgeon or gynecologist should be performed (Fig. 12-7, *C*). This involves a cruciate incision and adequate drainage of the hematocolpos.

REFERENCES

Hymenal Abnormalities

1. Wilkinson EJ, Stone IK: *Atlas of vulvar disease,* Baltimore, 1995, Williams & Wilkins, 201-202.

SUGGESTED READINGS

Congenital Malformation

Hewitt J, Pelisse M, Paniel BJ: *Diseases of the vulva,* London, 1991, McGraw-Hill, 64-71.
Ridley CM: *The vulva,* Edinburgh, 1988, Churchill Livingstone, 1-38.

CHAPTER 13

Trauma to the Vulva

ACCIDENTAL TRAUMA

Accidental trauma to the vulvar area is uncommon. The vulva can be injured only when the thighs are open or are flexed on the trunk.

Vulvar trauma is most common in children. Risks include falling astride a bicycle bar, fence, or barrier with blunt or sharp edges; being kicked; falling violently while water skiing or surf boarding; becoming impaled with a stake, etc. (Fig. 13-1).

Bruise

The most common physical finding is bruising, especially where there are torn muscles, and it is most noticeable over bony attachments (Fig. 13-2). The vulva itself can form one large hematoma, and a thrombosis involving the perineum may generate intense pain.

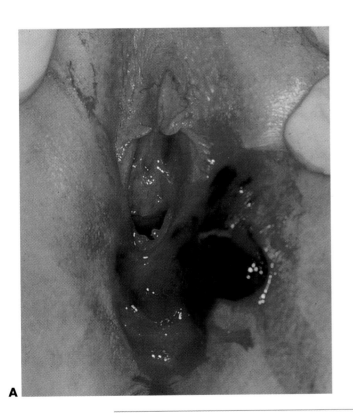
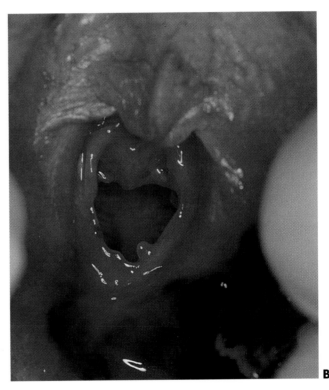

A

B

FIG. 13-1
A, Straddle injury showing perineal lateral laceration on the left side with bleeding and swelling. **B,** Close up of *A* showing an intact hymen and swelling and bleeding at the site of the laceration.
(Courtesy Dr. G.D. Oliver.)

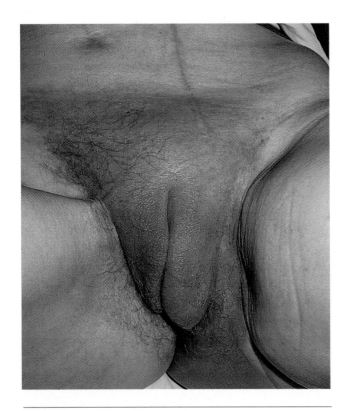

FIG. 13-2
A hematoma extending from the mons pubis and vulva to the left buttock area.
(Courtesy Dr. P. Bryson.)

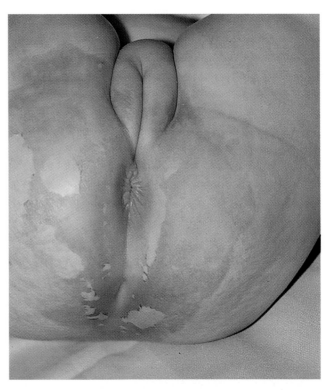

FIG. 13-3
A resolving burn caused by hot water in a physically abused 3 year old.

Lacerations

The extent of lacerations depends entirely on the force involved in the injury and the sharpness of the offending object. If the penetrating wound is deep, it can involve the vagina, urinary tract, rectum, or even the abdomen.

Burns

Burns can result from any one of several sources of heat—hot water (Fig. 13-3), cooking fluids, and most commonly, fire. The degree of injury often depends on the type of clothing being worn by the victim.

TATTOOS

A tattoo results from the introduction of exogenous pigments into the skin. Decorative tattooing has been practiced since ancient times. It has become much more popular in the last decade in both sexes. Although still rare, it is becoming more common in the genital area (Fig. 13-4, *A*).

Technique and Materials

Tattoos may be administered by a professional or an amateur. The professional uses an electric motor-driven multi-headed needle for introducing the pigment particles into the dermis, whereas the amateur usually uses any pointed object with ink or soot. The most common pigment colors are black (carbon), red (cinnabar), green (chromic oxide), yellow (cadmium sulfide), and blue (cobaltous aluminate).

Complications

Complications include an introduction of infections (e.g., pyoderma, hepatitis, AIDS) and allergic reactions to the pigment (e.g., chromate).

Dissatisfaction and embarrassment may also be problems and are further complicated by the difficult and sometimes costly removal. A Q-switched ruby laser can be used for blue and black ink. Other lasers are used for other colors with variable success. It may not be possible to completely destroy a green, yellow, or amateur tattoo without scarring.

BODY PIERCING

Like tattoos, body rings are also very popular these days. The genital area is the third most common area after the head (ears, nose, lips) and the umbilical area (Fig. 13-4, *B*).

Body piercing involves passing a sharp instrument through the skin. This is followed by the placement of a ring or stud through the opening. The jewelry is left in place and the wound heals, leaving a permanent sinus.

This procedure may result in a local inoculated infection (as in tattoos), contact dermatitis (usually to nickel), or keloidal scarring. Rings may be traumatically pulled and the sinus partially or completely torn, with pain and scarring.

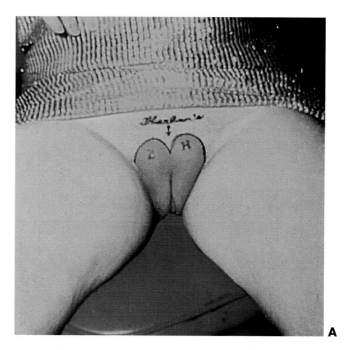

A

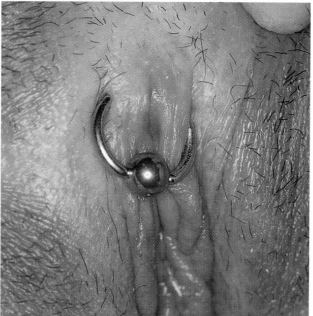

B

FIG. 13-4
A, Tattoo of the vulva: outline is in black and the mons pubis and labia are colored red. **B**, Ring inserted through the clitoral area.
(**A**, Courtesy Dr. Howard Bierman and Dr. Norman Goldstein.)

FEMALE GENITAL MUTILATION

Female genital mutilation is an ancient cultural practice encompassing a variety of female genital operations. These include the following:

Simple incision of the clitoral prepuce

Circumcision—removal of the prepuce

Excision—removal of the clitoris and labia minora

Infibulation—removal of the clitoris, labia minora, and two thirds of the labia majora followed by almost complete oversewing of the vaginal introitus

A synonym for female genital mutilation is female circumcision. It is a standard practice and commonly occurs in 26 African countries.

In Somalia alone 80,000 procedures are done yearly. It is estimated that 85 to 115 million girls have been subjected to this procedure at a rate of 6000 per day worldwide.

The purpose of the genital mutilation is both religious and cultural, often for purity and cleanliness, and to curb female sexual desire. The membership of a girl in her community is based on this procedure. In Somalia and Sudan infibulation has "always" been done. In the countries where this is common, to change the tradition would upset and destroy the basis of the culture.

Procedure

The operations are performed by the older women of the community. Surgery is usually crude, using a variety of sharp instruments, and anesthetic use is rare. In infibulation, after the tissue is removed the vulva is held together with sutures or herbal mixtures and pressure. The child is then immobilized for 7 to 40 days until healing occurs.

Complications

The occurrence of complications depends on the degree of trauma, sanitation, personnel training, and type of circumcision. Serious complications occur in 50% of infibulations. Acute complications include hemorrhage (18%), infection (15%), and urinary retention and dysuria (4%). Chronic com-

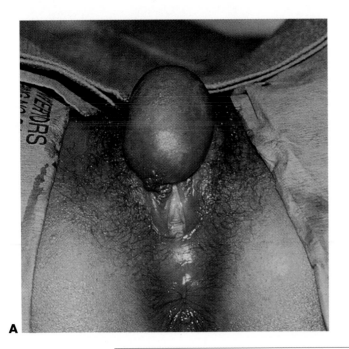

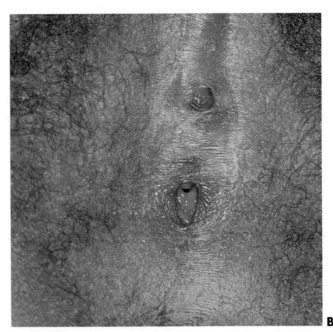

A

B

FIG. 13-5
Female Genital Mutilation. **A,** A large sebaceous cyst that developed after circumcision. **B,** Scarring in an African woman with two small openings remaining after infibulation.
(**A,** Courtesy Dr. T.L. MacLeod; **B,** courtesy Dr. G.D. Oliver.)

plications include genitourinary infection, dysmenorrhea, cysts (Fig. 13-5, *A*), and dyspareunia (Fig. 13-5, *B*).

Note: *Consummation of marriage necessitates opening this scar with fingers or a sharp instrument.*

Treatment

A knowledgeable gynecologist is needed for the management of the scarring from infibulation (Fig. 13-6).

Ethical Questions

Major ethical questions have been raised in the West about this procedure, and in fact it is banned in many parts of the world. Understanding this tradition is important, particularly with the increase in travel and immigration from Third World countries. Professionals dealing with these patients need sensitivity and access to the appropriate technical skills.

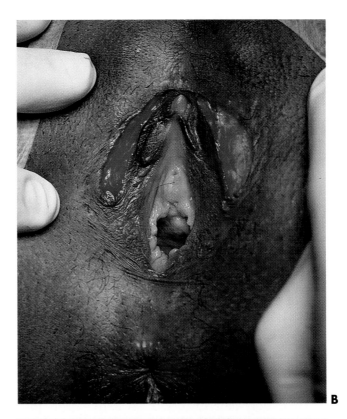

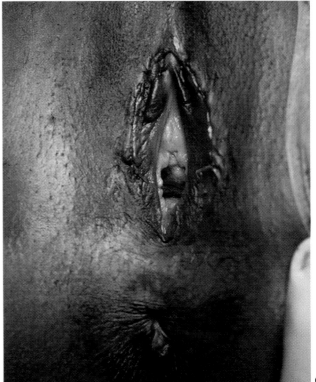

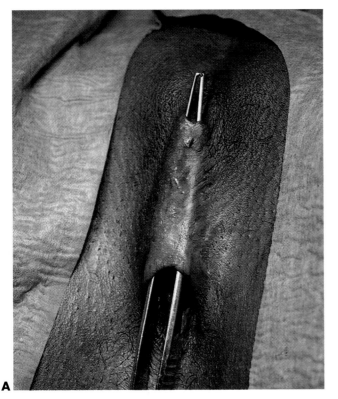

FIG. 13-6
Repair of the Vulva After Female Circumcision. **A**, Scar over introitus. **B**, Results of the removal of the scarred tissue. **C**, Result with final sutures in place after the repair.
(Courtesy Prof. B.J. Paniel.)

FISSURES OF THE VULVA

Painful splits or fissures can occur anywhere on the vulva. The etiology of fissures involves the following:

1. Infections are the most common cause, *Candida* most frequently. Beta hemolytic *Streptococcus* and, infrequently, *Staphylococcus aureus* are also implicated.
2. Dermatoses can result in a dry scaly surface. Scratching produces painful fissures in psoriasis, lichen sclerosus, lichen simplex chronicus, tinea cruris, contact dermatitis, etc.
3. Estrogen deficiency predisposes to thinning of the tissue in the posterior vestibule and commissure. This is usually post-menopausal but can occur post-partum and with some birth control pills.

The patient complains of recurrent or persistent painful splits in the vulva.

▼ These tiny insignificant fissures cause a disproportionate amount of pain (like paper cuts) and are often missed if not carefully sought. ▲

There may be a history of an itchy "rash" preceding this problem. Clothing, sanitary napkins, and sexual intercourse may be very uncomfortable. Cyclic flaring of the problem before the woman's menstrual period may occur (as with cyclic *Candida* infections). Intercourse may aggravate an area that is dermatitic, causing splitting and possibly precipitating both a *Candida* infection and further splitting.

If the condition is due to hormonal change, then the history includes onset post-partum or after the initiation of birth control pills.

Physical Examination

The splits are tiny and shallow and rarely longer than 1 cm. In the infections and dermatoses they are most commonly found in the interlabial sulcus. In the atrophic conditions the splits are in the area of the posterior commissure (Fig. 13-7, *A*). These splits may be accompanied by changes typical of other concurrent conditions such as lichen sclerosus (Fig. 13-7, *B*) or psoriasis.

Diagnosis

The diagnosis is made clinically with the appropriate cultures for infection when indicated.

Treatment

Diagnose the underlying cause of the dermatosis, infection, or atrophy and treat appropriately. The patient should gently cleanse the area with Cetaphil (cleanser). Instruct the patient to avoid harsh irritating soaps, detergents, sanitary pads, or vulvar lubricants.

In the case of *Candida* prescribe a ketoconazole or clotrimazole cream 2 to 3 times a day and after sexual intercourse.

Mupirocin ointment 2 to 3 times a day should be used for bacterial infections.

Estrogen deficiency should be treated with a topical conjugated estrogen (Premarin) 0.625 mg/g or estradiol (Estrace) 0.01% cream nightly for 2 to 3 weeks then twice a week as needed.

Sometimes simple petroleum jelly applied after cleansing is all that is needed. If it is not possible to correct the fissuring in the posterior commissure, then perineoplasty may need to be considered.

FOREIGN BODIES

Foreign bodies inserted into the vagina more commonly cause troubles in children than in adults. These children develop a chronic vaginal discharge and an irritant dermatitis in the vulva. At times the whole vulvovaginal area may be swollen. The child may complain of itching, burning, or soreness. One of the most common foreign bodies is toilet tissue (Fig. 13-8) but toys, peanuts, and other small items may be found.

In adults foreign bodies such as forgotten tampons can cause copious malodorous discharge and an irritated vulvovaginitis with itching and burning. Other foreign bodies, medical (e.g., pessary) or nonmedical (e.g., molded phallus) may cause vulvovaginitis and nonspecific vulvar problems.

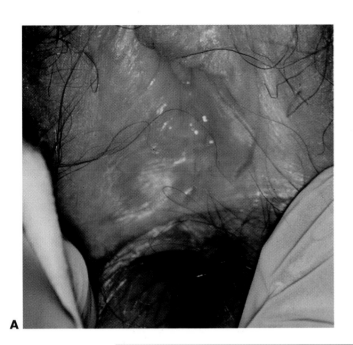

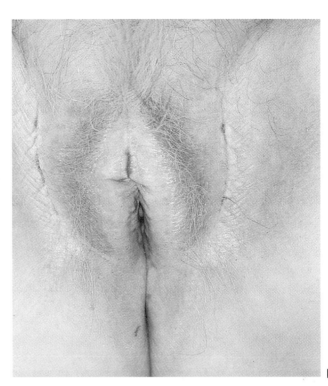

FIG. 13-7
Fissures. **A**, Small fissures in the area of the posterior commissure. These are tiny but exquisitely tender. **B**, Large fissures in the scarred clitoral area and in the genitocrural folds in extensive lichen sclerosus.
(**A**, Courtesy Dr. M. Steben.)

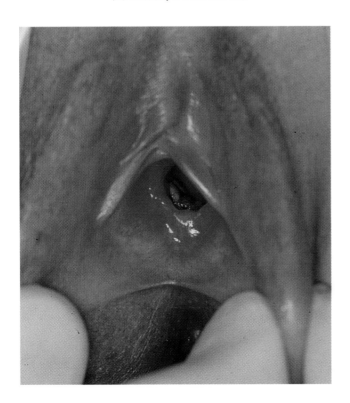

FIG. 13-8
A 6-year-old girl who presented with scratching, pain, bleeding, and vaginal discharge showing intact red hymenal ring with tissue paper just inside opening.
(Courtesy Dr. G.D. Oliver.)

OBSTETRIC/SURGICAL TRAUMA

With precipitous delivery and/or a very large baby, stretching, bruising, or frank tearing of the vulva can occur, resulting in laceration and variably sized hematoma formation. Rarely a perineal tear can extend anterior to the meatus or posterior to the rectum.

Obstetric trauma is frequent and involves vulvoperineal tears and genital thrombosis. Vulvar tears may be anterior around the meatus or clitoris and are usually unilateral with bleeding.

The lateral tears in the labia minora are usually minor. Occasionally part of the labia minora can be torn away or perforated.

Perineal tears can be partial, complete, or complicated. Partial tears range from a simple split to a complete tear of the perineal body down to the anal sphincter. The complicated tear (third degree) involves the whole perineal body, anal sphincter, and the anterior wall of the rectum.

Gynecologic surgery may also produce significant hematoma formation (Fig. 13-9, *A*) Scarring can occur anywhere in the vulva following such surgery, particularly the extensive surgery needed for hidradenitis suppurativa, squamous cell carcinoma, Paget's disease, or melanoma. The resulting scarring can result in significant vulvar or vaginal stenosis (Fig. 13-9, *B*).

Vulvectomy may be necessary for some of these patients, and there may be resulting numbness, urinary difficulties, and sexual dysfunction. These patients may be depressed, with loss of self-confidence.

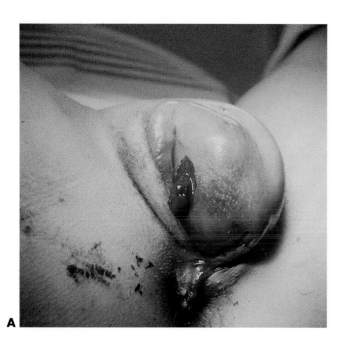

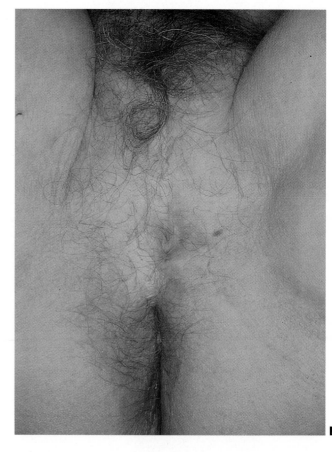

FIG. 13-9
Vulvar Surgery. **A**, Vulvar hematoma and bleeding following surgery. **B**, Vaginal stenosis and loss of vulva after radical vulvectomy for cancer.
(Courtesy Dr. P. Bryson.)

RADIODERMATITIS

Radiotherapy of malignant vulvar or pelvic tumors usually results in a degree of secondary cutaneous reaction, either acutely or chronically.

Acute radiation vulvitis occurs at the end of the course of irradiation. Clinically there is edema with violaceous discoloration, pain, burning, and occasionally frank bullae and necrosis.

In late radiodermatitis the changes are seen years after radiation therapy. The vulvar skin is thinned, whitish, scarred, and shows extensive telangiectasia (Fig. 13-10). This is relatively asymptomatic.

Treatment

See Appendix D for the recommended treatment for acute vulvar ulcerative disease.

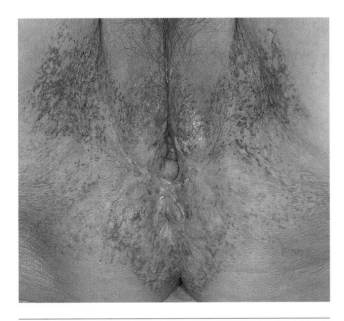

FIG. 13-10
Chronic radiodermatitis of the vulva with extensive telangiectasia and marked scarring of the perineum.

SELF-MUTILATION

Psychiatrically ill patients and patients with mental handicaps may uncommonly mutilate their own genitalia. This may occur during masturbation, as the result of a delusion or as an act of self-destruction. The causes of trauma vary. Recognizing the causes may be difficult. Chronic excoriation and picking are fairly easily recognized. Cigarette burns may be difficult to diagnose.

It may take strong suspicion by the physician and very careful questioning to diagnose the cause of problems in the patient who appears normal. These individuals often present as honest and straightforward. Only with time do the underlying psychologic problems start to appear. Treatment requires a nonconfrontational approach and a lot of patience.

The synonym for self-mutilation is factitial vulvitis. The classification of such destruction includes the following:
1. Secondary trauma inflicted on underlying dermatoses (e.g., psoriasis, lichen sclerosus).
2. Lesions in individuals who neurotically manipulate, overtreat, or pick at minor, insignificant, or imagined vulvar lesions.
3. Factitial ulcers resulting from self-mutilation by psychotic individuals.

Investigating a patient's history may not be helpful. There may be no complaints, and the patient is often unable to explain the lesions. There may be major symptoms of incapacitating itch, crawling sensations, burning, etc. Other parts of the body may also be a problem. The patient usually denies a self-induced component. In factitial ulcers the history may be very bizarre.

Physical Examination

Scattered ulcers of variable size with crusts and surrounding erythema may be seen (Fig. 13-11, *A*). Old lesions may show hyperpigmentation with central scarring. Similar lesions may be found elsewhere on the body. Usually there is no primary lesion or dermatosis in the vulva.

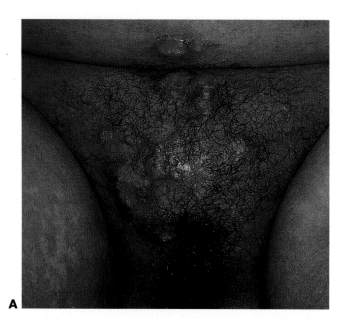

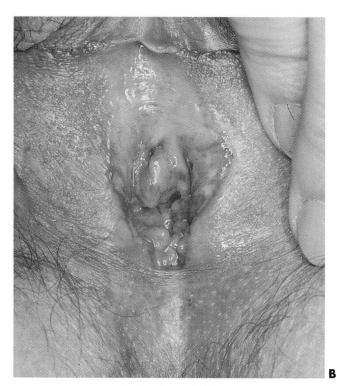

FIG. 13-11

Self-Mutilation. **A**, Extensive deep and open self-inflicted ulcers with surrounding hyperpigmentation in a patient with molluscum contagiosum. Note molluscum on right thigh. **B**, Self-inflicted erosions and ulcers in perihymenal area resulting from an alkali burn.

(Courtesy Dr. M. McKay.)

In factitial ulcers, the presentation depends on the agent or instrument used—cigarette, alkali (Fig. 13-11, *B*), or sharp instrument.

Diagnosis

Clinical suspicion leads to a diagnosis. The physician must rule out other possible underlying causes.

Treatment

If the trauma inflicted on the vulva is secondary to a dermatosis, treat that underlying condition. In the other cases, treatment is often difficult. Confrontation is often counterproductive. Support, but not sympathy, is important. Although psychiatric help is needed, patients often refuse to see a psychiatrist. The Selective Serotonin Reuptake Inhibitor (SSRI) medications fluoxetine, fluvoxamine, and sertraline can be helpful.

SEXUAL TRAUMA

Rape

Rape is defined as sexual intercourse with a woman without her consent. This includes sex by fraud, threat, and situations in which the woman is mentally handicapped, impaired, unconscious, or so young she is unable to understand the nature of the act.[1]

Sexual assault is the fastest growing violent crime in the United States.

The degree of vulvovaginal injury is variable. Lacerations are common and very extensive in the young child or virgin. Considerable hemorrhage and hematoma formation can also occur (Fig. 13-12). The laceration can involve the hymenal ring and extend into the vagina with profuse bleeding. In a child the lacerations can be much deeper even into the rectum and bladder. Other types of injury may be present on the body and include scratches, abrasions, bruises, and hematoma depending on the degree of force.

Treatment

Treatment is best provided by a specially trained team involving gynecology and emergency medicine with psychologic support. Major attention has to be given not only to the physical wounds but also to the psychologic ones. In each jurisdiction there are medicolegal issues that must be addressed. Details are beyond the scope of this book.

Sexual Abuse in Children

Sexual abuse refers to the involvement of a dependent, developmentally immature child, or adolescent in sexual activities by an older person for their own sexual stimulation or for gratification of others as in pornography or prostitution. Activities involve oral-genital, genital-genital, and anal-genital contact, including exhibitionism, sexualized kissing, fondling, masturbation, and digital or object penetration of the vagina and anus.

Sexual abuse is a complex medical and social problem.[2] It involves the misuse of power and the betrayal of the child's trust by an older person. It is estimated that 40% to 50% of women are sexu-

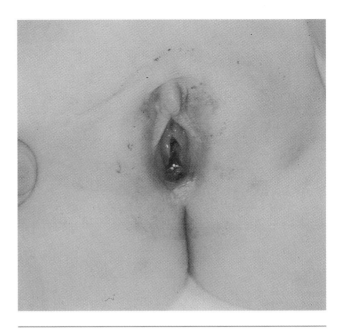

FIG. 13-12
Perineal laceration through the hymen and posterior fossa with hematoma formation and surrounding bruising in a raped child.
(Courtesy Dr. G.D. Oliver.)

ally abused during their lifetime. In-depth discussion of this complicated problem is beyond the scope of this book.

Major long-term problems occur with sexually abused children and their families. Being aware that sexual abuse is such a common problem should alert the physician to consider it when examining children who present with an infection (condyloma acuminata, herpes simplex, gonorrhea, and other sexually transmitted diseases [STDs]) or with trauma that includes scratches, bruising or hematoma, lacerations or fissures, scars, and gaping of the anus or introitus.

Obtaining an appropriate history requires interview techniques used by specially trained personnel. These children often have poor self-esteem. They may have withdrawn or be acting out. Sometimes they are very anxious to please.

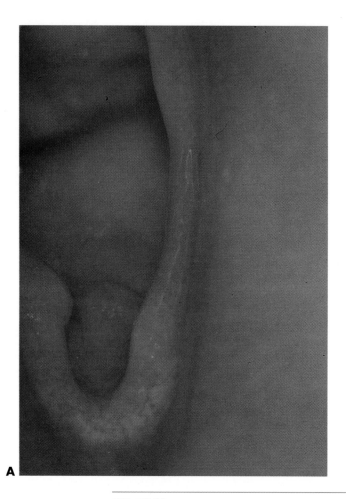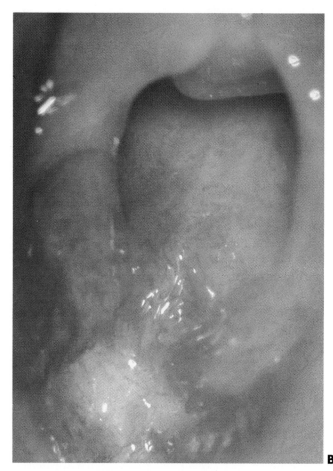

A

B

FIG. 13-13

A, A 5-year-old girl with a typical keyhole deformity of the hymenal ring at the 6 o'clock position resulting from penetration, laceration, and scarring—sexual abuse. **B**, Same child (supine position) 2 years later with a healed scar at the 6 o'clock position. (Courtesy Dr. G.D. Oliver.)

Physical examination often involves following special local protocols. Total physical examination is necessary plus cultures for all of the STDs where indicated. Understanding the normal anatomy is important (see Chapter 11). The hymen is usually annular or crescentic in children. A variety of notches and bumps are quite normal. Changes are usually chronic, showing healed transections of the hymen between the 4 and 8 o'clock positions and sometimes partial hymenal loss (Fig. 13-13). The majority of sexual abuse does not show changes of painful or forced trauma. In some cases there may be abrasions, lacerations, or bruising, but the area heals very quickly (Fig. 13-14).

Any question of child abuse must be referred to the proper authorities.[2]

Diagnosis
Differential diagnosis includes lichen sclerosus. It can present as bruising in children (Fig. 13-15). Scratches and odd scarring can also be mistaken for signs of abuse.

Treatment
Like rape, abuse is best managed by a specialized team.

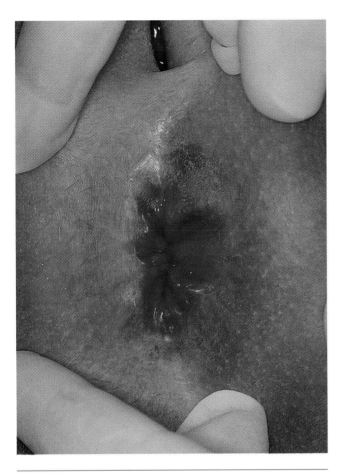

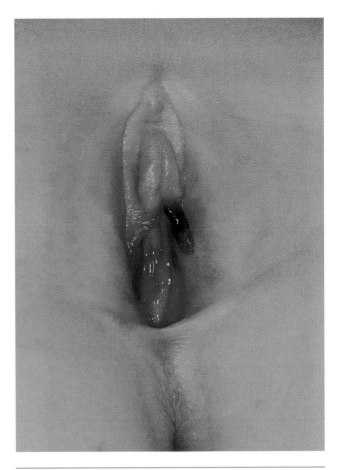

FIG. 13-14
Anus of a sexually abused little girl showing tears, bruising and laxity with normal hymen above.
(Courtesy Dr. G.D. Oliver.)

FIG. 13-15
A 4-year-old girl with hematoma formation and questionable sexual abuse. No abuse in this case, just typical changes of lichen sclerosus with the white figure of eight extending from the vulva to perianal area, plus purpura and a normal hymenal ring.

REFERENCES

Sexual Trauma

1. Kaufman RH, Faro S: *Benign diseases of the vulva and vagina,* ed 4, St Louis, 1994, Mosby, 391-396.
2. Heger A, Emans SJ: *Evaluation of the sexually abused child,* New York, 1995, Oxford University Press, 79-145.

ADDITIONAL READINGS

Female Genital Mutilation

Daya S: Female genital mutilation: a call to abandon this traditional custom, *J SOGC* 17(4):315-318, 1995.
MacLeod TL: Female genital mutilation, *J SOGC* 17(4):333-342, 1995.
Toubia N: Female circumcision as a public health issue, *N Eng J Med* 331(11):712-716, 1994.

Obstetric/Surgical Trauma

Ridley CM: *The vulva,* Edinburgh, 1988, Churchill Livingstone, 222-223.
Tovell HMM, Young AW: *Diseases of the vulva in clinical practice,* New York, 1991, Elsevier, 62-63.

VIRAL DISEASES

Human Papillomavirus—Warts

Genital warts are caused by the human papillomavirus (HPV). They are among the most common sexually transmitted infectious diseases. Synonyms for HPV include venereal warts, condylomata acuminata, and HPV infection. A DNA papovavirus, HPV has 70 subtypes; the most common infections (90% of cases) are caused by types 6 and 11 (Table 14-1).

Transmission of the virus can be sexual or nonsexual. The majority of cases in adults are sexual. Children may acquire genital warts from infected caregivers or by autoinoculation from hand warts. ▼ **Of children with anogenital warts, 30% to 40% have been abused and this must always be ruled out.** ▲ HPV infects mostly young adults between the ages of 16 and 25 years.

Table 14-1   Human Papillomavirus Type and Clinical Disease

Clinical Disease	HPV Type
Common warts	1,2,4,7
Anogenital warts	6,11,16,18 Less common 31,33,35,51,52
Genital intraepithelial neoplasia	16,18,31,33,35,51,52*

Vulvar + Penile intraepithelial neoplasia
  Bowen's disease
  Bowenoid papulosis	

Carcinoma Squamous cell carcinoma (cervix)	16,18

*Only 3 to 10% of anogenital warts are caused by these types. Only 0.1% of population develops anogenital malignancy. Types 16 and 18 are strongly associated with squamous cell carcinoma of the cervix.

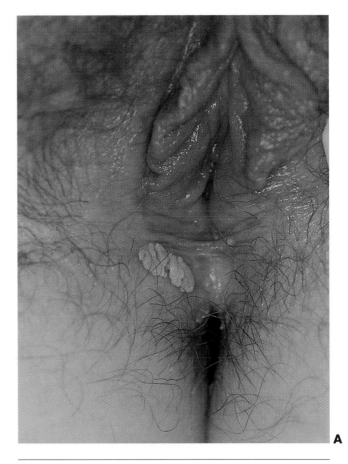

A

FIG. 14-1

Condyloma. **A,** Solitary condyloma just below the posterior commissure.

Note: *Incidence of HPV has risen dramatically in the last twenty years.*

Usually there is a history of exposure, weeks to months previously, to a sexual partner who has venereal warts. The incubation period is 2 to 3 months. There may be a history of prior warts. Some patients are immunosuppressed. The lesions are usually asymptomatic. If very large and exophytic, they can be traumatized, fissured, and sore.

Physical Examination

Initial pin-head papules develop into filiform papules that are often symmetric and on apposing skin surfaces. The lesions of condylomata acuminata can be small or large, skin-colored to reddish, and may grow into cauliflower-like clusters (Fig. 14-1). Their surfaces can be smooth or velvety. They are located around the vaginal introitus and perianal area most commonly. A less common clinical pattern is that of papules or plaques, single or multiple, skin-colored or hyperpigmented.

Note: *Fifty percent of women with genital warts will have associated HPV of the cervix.*

Diagnosis

Diagnosis is clinical but can be confirmed by biopsy. Vinegar (acetic acid 5%) applied for 5 to 10 minutes to keratinized skin and for 1 minute to

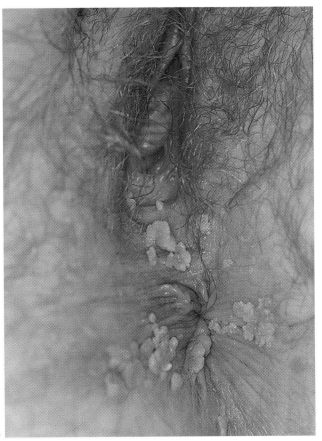

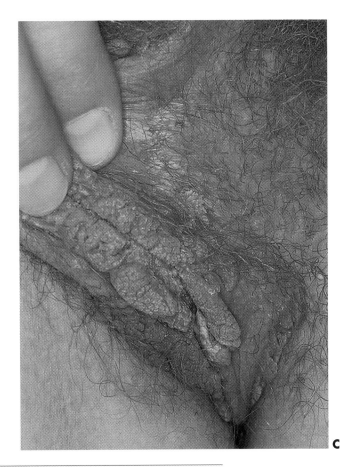

FIG. 14-1, cont'd
Condyloma. **B,** Multiple condylomata in the perineum and perianal area. **C,** Solid plaque of condylomata along labia minora edges and in linear thin plaques in the labiocrural folds.

nonkeratinized mucous membrane highlights the HPV lesions (acetowhitening). ▼ **Rule out neoplasia in patients with HPV using colposcopy and biopsy if indicated.** ▲ Also it is important to rule out other associated sexually transmitted diseases. Differential diagnoses include molluscum contagiosum, lichen planus, enlarged sebaceous glands, condylomata, and vulvar intraepithelial neoplasia.

Treatment

No treatment is guaranteed to cure genital warts, and patients should understand and must accept the unpredictability of response to treatment. Up to 30% of cases spontaneously regress. Most treatment modalities are destructive in nature.

Indications for treatment of genital warts include the following:

To manage symptoms of itching or burning

To prevent spread

To treat disfiguring lesions

To return or preserve normal function (e.g., stop postcoital bleeding or dyspareunia)

The following treatments are listed in order of preference.

Cryotherapy—A cotton-tipped applicator or spray is used on a weekly basis. This is best for small warts but can be very painful. It is safe for pregnant women.

Trichloroacetic acid (TCA)—A 25% to 50% solution is applied with a toothpick or cotton-tipped applicator to warts weekly. The warts turn white, and the area is neutralized immediately with water. Although this can burn, it is safe during pregnancy.

Podofilox—A 5% solution is used at home by the patient. It is applied to the warts twice a day on three consecutive days a week for 4 weeks. If there is no improvement, another therapy is chosen.

Electrodesiccation—Small warts can be electrodesiccated after local anesthesia. For exophytic masses in localized areas scissor excision can be used to remove the mass and the base is then electrodesiccated. If the wart mass is significant, general anesthesia should be considered. Scarring can occur.

Carbon dioxide laser—This can be an ideal method of treatment. The wounds usually heal quite well without scarring. There may be considerable post-operative pain. It can be used for pregnant women.

Also it is important to rule out other associated sexually transmitted diseases.

Note: *Viruses can be transmitted in the smoke plume.*

5-Fluorouracil—A 5% cream is applied over the warty areas nightly on two consecutive nights a week. This can be used intravaginally by applying about 3 mL at bedtime weekly for 8 to 10 weeks. It is not to be used in pregnant women.

Imiquimod 5% cream (Aldara)—An immune response modifier applied 3 times a week (Monday, Wednesday, Friday) for 6 to 10 hours, for up to 16 weeks with 50% clearing (up to 73% clearing at 20 weeks reported). Side effects are mainly itching and burning.

Interferon alpha 2b recombinant (Intron-A)— This is injected into the warts three times a week for 3 weeks using 3 million units/treatment. This often results in a flulike reaction after treatment.

Podophyllin Resin—25% to 50% in tincture of benzoin is applied with a cotton-tipped applicator or a small wooden stick to cover the wart surface. After 1 to 2 minutes the whole area is dusted with a fine powder to keep the resin from smearing and irritating the surrounding skin. The resin is washed off after 4 hours. This is repeated weekly and works best for less keratinized warts. *It is not to be used during pregnancy.* It has recently been reported to contain mutagens; therefore podofilox is preferred (see the preceeding discussion).

Follow-Up

Because of the association between HPV and Vulvar Intraepithelial Neoplasia (VIN), follow-up with Papanicolaou smears on a once yearly basis is recommended. Suspicious areas should be culposcopically examined and biopsied. Sexual partners should be notified as treatment may be necessary.

Herpes Simplex

Herpes simplex virus (HSV) of the vulvar area is usually sexually transmitted. It is characterized by recurrent outbreaks of pain, grouped vesicles, and erosions. Synonyms for HSV include herpes genitalis, herpes progenitalis, and cold sore. It is most common in sexually active adults. The etiology of genital herpes is usually HSV type 2, less commonly type 1. HSV1 is found in 50% to 70% of the population with genital HSV but recurs in about 25% of cases. HSV2 is found in 20% of the population but recurs in about 89% of cases. Individuals with Human Immunodeficiency Virus (HIV) and genital HSV have both HSV1 and HSV2. Transmission is by person-to-person contact, usually sexual, with an incubation period of 2 to 20 days (with an average of 7 days).

There may be a history of recent exposure, usually sexual, to a person with cold sores. Most HSV infections are transmitted during periods of asymptomatic viral shedding. Most infected individuals do not know they are infected or infectious. Classic primary herpes vulvitis is not commonly seen.

An initial paresthesia for 2 to 3 days is followed by fever, malaise, headache, and myalgia for another 2 to 3 days. Discomfort may vary from irritation to deep boring pain that is moderate to severe. When the pain is severe there is difficulty with urination. Catheterization may be necessary.

In recurrent infections (much more common than primary infections) tingling, itching, and burning usually occur before the onset of vesiculation, and the symptoms are usually less severe and of shorter duration.

Physical Examination

Primary Herpes Simplex. The vulva becomes very red and swollen. Extensive groups of vesicles appear, rapidly become pustular, and break open, leaving very tender erosions that last for 14 to 16 days. Primary herpes simplex is usually on the labia, perineum, vagina, and cervix and may involve the urethra, bladder, and anus (Fig. 14-2, *A*).

Recurrent Herpes Simplex. The lesions are much less extensive and of shorter duration than those of primary herpes simplex. There may be only mild swelling and a few vesicles that become pustules and erosions (Fig. 14-2, *B*). They recur in about the same area each time and may be *sine eruptione* (without blisters). These patients complain of cyclic episodes of burning pain and discomfort but no "rash." Recurrent infection is usually labial.

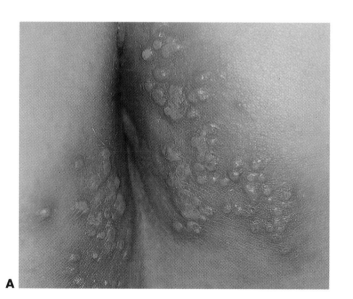

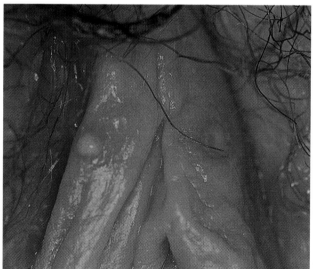

A   B

FIG. 14-2

Herpes Simplex. **A**, Primary herpes simplex on the perineum and buttock with groups of vesicles on a red base. **B**, Recurrent herpes simplex with periclitoral pustule and erosion.

continued

Immunosuppressed Herpes Simplex. These patients often develop areas of ulceration, papules, verrucous lesions, or vegetating plaques that extend peripherally and may be necrotic, painful, and indolent (Fig. 14-2, *C*).

Note: *With any of these HSV infections the inguinal nodes can be swollen and tender.*

Diagnosis

Although usually clinical, the diagnosis is confirmed with a viral culture, Tzanck's smear (showing viral acantholytic giant cells), monoclonal antibody test, or histopathology. Tzanck's smear consists of scraping the base of a vesicle with a #15 scalpel blade, smearing the material on a microscopic glass slide, and staining with Giemsa or Wright's stain. The test confirms the presence of HSV in 75% of cases by showing multinucleated syncytial epithelial giant cells.

Differential diagnoses are chancroid, syphilis, trauma, pemphigus, aphthous ulcers, herpes zoster, Behcet's disease, granuloma inguinale, and lymphogranuloma venereum. ▼ **The pattern of HSV most often missed is the recurrent episodes of vulvar burning with cyclic episodes of itching and burning but no skin eruption.** ▲

Course and Prognosis. Herpes Simplex Virus 2 recurs six times more commonly than HSV 1. About 95% of primary HSV 2 will recur in 1½ to 2 months. Women experience recurrences less commonly than men. The more severe the primary infection, the more recurrences.

Treatment

Nonspecific care for the acute swollen vulva consists of the following (see Appendix C):

Burow's solution 1:40 (mix 1 packet or tablet of Domeboro or Bluboro in 500 mL of water) in a sitz bath or as a cool compress 2 to 3 times a day to decrease the swelling and heal the erosions. A bland barrier ointment—petrolatum, zinc oxide, or Ihle's paste (see Appendix D)—can also be used to promote healing.

For pain use lidocaine-prilocaine cream (EMLA) applied in a thick layer under plastic wrap for 20 minutes for local anesthesia as needed.

Catheterization and sedation may be necessary.

Specific treatment for primary HSV includes the following:

Valacyclovir (Valtrex) 1g po bid × 7 days
Famciclovir (Famvir) 500 mg po tid × 7 days
Acyclovir (Zovirax) 400 mg po at 7 and 11 AM and 3, 7, and 11 PM × 7 days.

Specific treatment for severe mucocutaneous HSV includes the following:

Valacyclovir (Valtrex) 1g po bid × 5 days
Famciclovir (Famvir) 500 mg bid × 5 days
Acyclovir (Zovirax) 400 mg po at 7 and 11 AM and 3, 7, and 11 PM × 7 days.

If systemic involvement is suspected, acyclovir (Zovirax) 5 mg/kg IV every 8 hours for 5 to 7 days (assuming normal renal function).

Specific treatment for recurrent HSV includes the following:

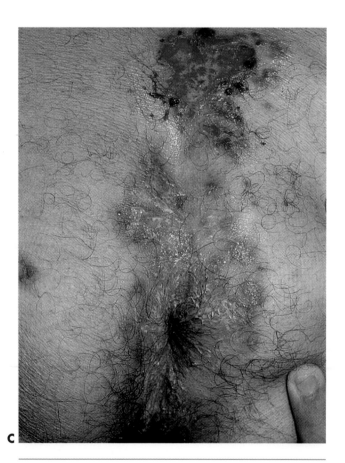

C

FIG. 14-2, cont'd
C, Extensive nonhealing perianal ulcers and erosions resulting from herpes simplex in a patient with lymphoma.

Valacyclovir (Valtrex) 500 mg po bid × 5 days

Famciclovir (Famvir) 125 mg bid × 5 days

Acyclovir (Zovirax) 200 mg po as above × 5 days

Specific treatment for immunocompromised HSV includes the following:

Acyclovir (Zovirax) 5 mg/kg IV every 8 hours × 5 to 7 days

Foscarnet (Foscavir) 40 mg/kg IV every 8 hours until resolution. Foscarnet is used only if there is intolerance to acyclovir, famciclovir, or valacyclovir and the safety of this drug in pregnancy is not established.

Specific treatment for asymptomatic viral shedding is given indefinitely.

Valacyclovir (Valtrex) 1g daily

Acyclovir (Zovirax) 400 mg bid

Famciclovir (Famvir) 250 mg bid

These reduce viral shedding by 92%.

No treatment for HSV is a "cure" or prevents asymptomatic shedding completely. The response to treatment depends on the patient's individual immunity.

In primary herpes simplex, rule out other STDs. Herpes patients often need a lot of support and counseling. Education with up-to-date information is very important.

Herpes Zoster

Herpes zoster is an acute vesiculobullous infection caused by the varicella-zoster virus (VZV) and usually involves the skin of a single dermatome. A synonym for herpes zoster is shingles. The virus is deposited in cutaneous nerves during an earlier episode of chickenpox and remains latent in dorsal root ganglia. It becomes active as a result of impaired immune surveillance caused by old age, AIDS, neoplasia, etc.

The first symptom of herpes zoster is that of pain or paresthesia—itching, burning, or tingling—in the involved dermatome. This lasts for several days before the eruption. There may be headache, fever, and malaise.

Physical Examination

Red swollen plaques arise in a dermatomal distribution, develop groups of vesicles on the surface, and over about 7 to 10 days these go on to form pustules and crusts with increasing pain in the area, particularly in older patients (Fig. 14-3, *A*). Involvement of the vulvar area is uncommon, and can be difficult, with associated urination and defecation problems (Fig. 14-3, *B* and *C*).

Diagnosis

Diagnosis is clinical, supported by a Tzanck's smear and/or biopsy. Electron microscopy shows the virus, and monoclonal antibody confirms the diagnosis.

Differential diagnoses include herpes simplex, cellulitis, contact dermatitis, and pemphigoid.

Treatment

Nonspecific care for the acute swollen vulva is covered in Appendix I and consists of the following:

Burow's solution 1:40 (mix 1 packet or tablet of Domeboro or Bluboro in 500 mL of water) in a sitz bath or as a cool compress 2 to 3 times a day to decrease the swelling and to heal the blisters.

For pain use lidocaine-prilocaine cream (EMLA) applied in a thick layer under plastic wrap for 20 minutes for local anesthesia as needed.

Catheterization and sedation may be necessary.

Specific treatment includes the following:

Acyclovir (Zovirax) 800 mg po at 7 and 11 AM and 3, 7, and 11 PM × 7 days

Famciclovir (Famvir) 500 mg tid × 7 days

Valacyclovir (Valtrex) 1g po tid × 7 days if renal function is normal

For severe disease note the following:

Acyclovir (Zovirax) 10 mg/kg IV q8h × 7 days

For immunosuppressed patients: Foscarnet (Foscavir) 40 mg/kg IV q8h × 7 to 10 days (only if intolerant to acyclovir)

For pain control the following is recommended:

Acetaminophen and codeine 15 to 30 mg q 3-4 h

Pentazocine 25 to 100 mg q 4-6 h

Herpes zoster of the vulva and the dermatomes S1 through S4 can be very incapacitating and ultimately depressing. Early institution of a low to moderate dose (10 to 50 mg/day) of amitriptyline may reduce the zoster-associated pain complex. Usually the lesions settle in three to four weeks with some degree of scarring and, in the elderly, postherpetic neuralgia may result. The use of prednisone to prevent the neuralgia is controversial.

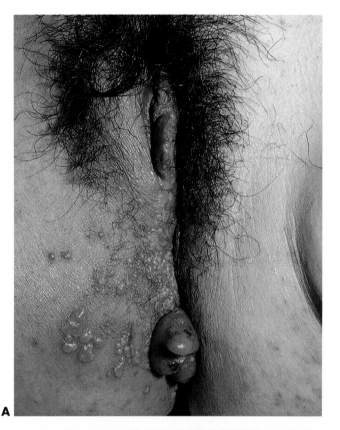

A

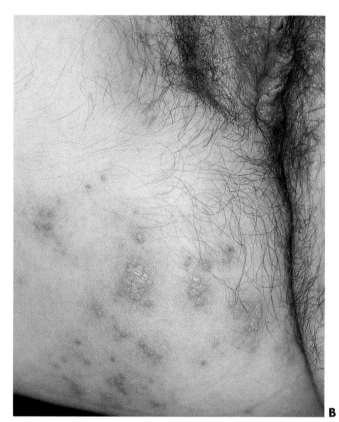

B

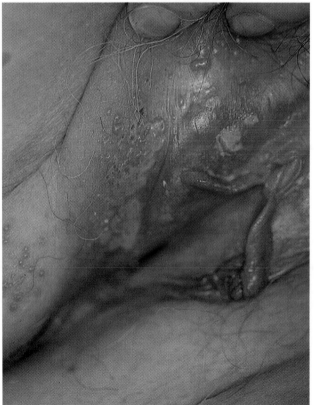

C

FIG. 14-3

Herpes Zoster. **A**, Extensive vesicles, erosions, and pustules in S3 to S4 (and hemorrhoid) from the varicella-zoster virus (VZV). **B**, Swelling of the right labium minor with vesicles and pustules on buttocks in herpes zoster. **C**, Groups of vesicles and confluent pustules with swelling on the vulva.

Molluscum Contagiosum

A poxvirus infection of the skin, molluscum contagiosum presents with discrete, firm, flesh-colored, umbilicated papules, affecting children and young adults. Caused by a DNA poxvirus, it is normally acquired innocently by children; but when seen in adults, it is usually acquired sexually. Often these lesions are completely asymptomatic but they can be mildly itchy. They start few in number and then spread. In a patient with HIV they can be very extensive.

Physical Examination

These discrete little dome-shaped, umbilicated, skin-colored papules can be scattered or in groups. They are usually in the suprapubic area or inner thighs (See Figs. 13-11, *A* and 14-4).

Diagnosis

Direct examination with Giemsa stain of material extruded from lesions shows the typical molluscum bodies. They are easier diagnosed by their clinical presentation.

Differential diagnoses include warts, basal-cell carcinoma, and, in the immunocompromised, the deep fungi *Cryptococcus neoformans* and *Histoplasma capsulatum.*

Treatment

Molluscum treatment involves destructive techniques. Liquid nitrogen is most commonly used, every 1 to 2 weeks. Each lesion is individually treated with a white frosted 1 mm border. Alternatives include the following:

Topical cantharidin 0.7% (Cantharone) is applied in *a thin film* to the lesions and dried. The lesions are taped for two to four hours, then washed off. This is repeated as needed every 2 to 3 weeks. Using *one drop* can make a nasty blister.

Curettage with or without local anesthesia. In children consider the use of lidocaine-prilocaine (EMLA) cream under occlusion for 1 to 1½ hours before treatment.

Light electrodesiccation with or without local anesthesia.

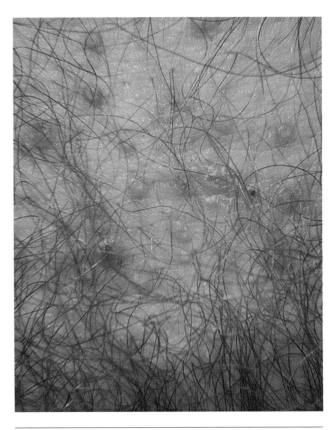

FIG. 14-4
Multiple dome-shaped pink papules of molluscum contagiosum in the suprapubic area.

FUNGAL
Candidiasis

This is a mucocutaneous yeast infection that is very common in women, giving a variety of anogenital manifestations, particularly in those with impaired immunity. Its synonym is moniliasis. Occurrence can take place at any age.

The majority of yeast infections are a result of *Candida albicans*. Less common are the non-albicans species (in 25% of cases *C. tropicalis* and *C. glabrata*). Women have this organism in their vaginal and gastrointestinal tracts and, under the influence of a number of factors, the organism becomes pathogenic. The factors include medications, particularly antibiotics, corticosteroids, chemotherapeutic agents, and diseases such as diabetes and immunodeficiency. Even the hormonal changes of pregnancy and birth control pills can predispose to vulvovaginal candidiasis. The sexual partner may be a source of infection.

Conceptually, it is best to consider that these patients are not only infected with yeast but are allergic to their yeasts. Some have large populations of the organism with relatively minor symptoms other than the discharge. Others have severe symptoms with relatively small populations of the organisms. It is this variable reaction to the organism that produces the spectrum of clinical presentations described in the following discussion.

History and Physical Examination

The history and physical findings of vulvovaginal candidiasis depend on the clinical pattern, and each is quite different. The most common presentations are pruritus and vulvitis.

Acute Vulvovaginal Candidiasis. The classic type of candidiasis, it presents with a sudden onset of itching, burning, curdy discharge, and dyspareunia, even dysuria in some cases. On examination, the vulva can be swollen around the vestibule and labia minora with some degree of erosion and typical satellite pustules. If the condition is very extensive, it can extend up into the crural folds and down onto the thighs. There may even be scratch marks (Fig. 14-5, *A*).

Recurrent and Chronic Vulvovaginal Candidiasis. The patient may complain of recurrent itching and curdy white discharge that will clear when it has been treated but continues to recur. In some patients, despite treatment, these symptoms persist, with chronic itching, irritation, and a varying degree of discharge (Fig. 14-5, *B*). ▼ **Treatment of recurrent candidiasis for at least six months is advised.** ▲

Eczematous Candidiasis. These patients are so persistently itchy that they develop thickening of the skin (lichenification) of the vulva, with excoriations, redness, and chronic swelling. This looks clinically like lichen simplex chronicus or chronic contact dermatitis, showing persistent erythema and swelling around the interlabial sulcus and labia minora with some degree of involvement of the labia majora. The discharge may be scant or absent (Fig. 14-5, *C*).

Recurrent Fissuring Candidiasis. Small tiny fissures are located in the interlabial sulcus and peri-

clitorally with pin-point areas of pain, worse with urination or wiping. There may be a degree of erythema and little to no discharge (Fig. 14-5, *D*).

Cyclic Vulvovaginitis. Patients have episodes of burning, itching, and irritation that last for 5 to 10 days or more at a specific time each month, typically just before or after the menstrual cycle. They also complain of dyspareunia with burning after sex. They sometimes have fissuring but show minimal to no discharge.

Note: *There are symptom-free times.*

Diagnosis

Diagnosis is clinical, with an attention to pattern. Confirmation is by culture and wet smear using potassium hydroxide 10% to lyse the epithelial cells and reveal the budding yeast organisms. The vaginal pH will be 4.5 or less.

Differential diagnoses include intertrigo, seborrheic dermatitis, psoriasis, eczema, contact dermatitis, lichen simplex chronicus, and vestibulitis (with which this complex may coexist). ▼ **The diagnosis is most often missed in cyclic vulvar candidiasis with recurrent episodes of itching and burning, fissuring, or eczematous vulvar change.** ▲

Treatment

The management of candidiasis really depends on recognition of the pattern and identification of the organism. The first aim of treatment is to control whatever contributing factors may be playing a role—antibiotic use, diabetes, etc.

Note: *The non-albicans yeasts can be resistant to the common imidazoles.*

Nonspecific care for the acute swollen vulva (see Appendix C) includes the following:

Burow's solution 1:40 (mix 1 packet or tablet of Domeboro or Bluboro in 500 mL of water) in a sitz bath or as a cool compress 2 to 3 times a day to decrease swelling.

Cold packs

Topical treatments for an acute infection are covered in Table 14-2. Note that patients should have a culture-positive diagnosis. The shorter imidazole treatments for 1 to 3 days have a lower cure rate than the 7 to 14 day regimens. The one- and three-

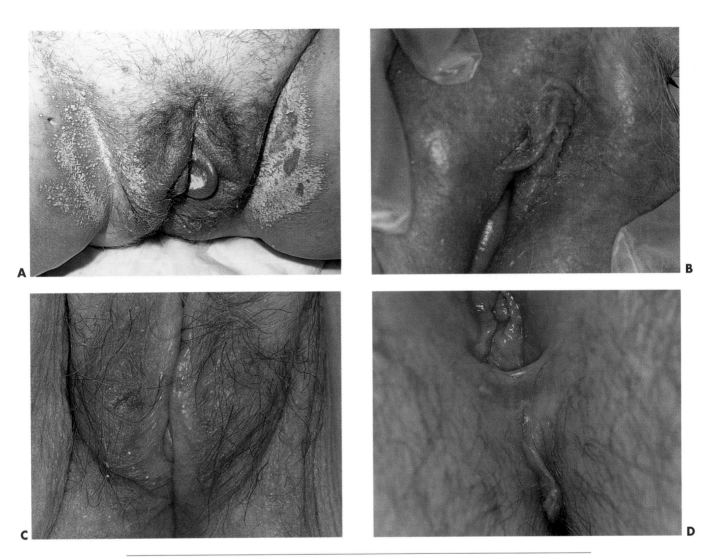

FIG. 14-5

Candidiasis. **A**, Diffuse edema and erythema with sheets of pustules and white curdy discharge in acute candidiasis. **B**, Red, irritated vulva in recurrent candidiasis. **C**, Red swollen excoriated labia majora in eczematous candidiasis. **D**, Painful fissures on perineum in fissuring candidiasis.

day products can be very irritating if the vulva is raw and causing a lot of burning. This may be avoided with the seven-day formulations. As the non-albicans yeasts are becoming more common, consider terconazole.

Systemic antifungal treatments are listed in Table 14-3. These medications are best reserved for those patients with difficult recurrent or persistent disease, appreciating that these systemic medications have a variety of side effects. For patients with chronic or recurrent infection or cyclic candidiasis the following are recommended:

Fluconazole (Diflucan) 100 mg daily × 5 days, then 150 mg before each monthly flare or 150 mg once a week × 2 months, then every 2 weeks × 2 months, then monthly

Table 14-2   Topical Treatment for Vulvovaginal Candidiasis

Name	Formula	Dose
Nystatin	100,000 IU vaginal tablet	100,000 IU × 14 days
Miconazole	2% cream	5 g × 7 days
	100 mg vaginal tablet	100 mg × 7 days
		200 mg x 3 days
Clotrimazole	1% cream	5 g × 7 to 14 days
	100 mg vaginal tablet	100 mg × 7 days
		200 mg × 3 days
	500 mg vaginal tablet	500 mg × 1 dose
Econazole	150 mg vaginal ovule	150 mg × 3 days
	2% cream	5 g × 3 days
Terconazole	6.5% cream	5 g × 1 dose
	0.4% cream	5 g × 7 days
	0.8% cream	5 g × 3 days
	80 mg vaginal insert	80 mg × 3 days

Table 14-3   Systemic Treatment for Acute Vulvovaginal Candidiasis

Name	Formula	Dose
Fluconazole	150 mg capsule	150 mg once
	100 mg capsule	100 mg × 5 days
Itraconazole	100 mg capsule	200 mg × 3 days
Ketoconazole	200 mg tablet	400 mg × 5 days

Ketoconazole (Nizoral) 400 mg a day × 2 weeks, then 100 mg daily for 6 months

Itraconazole (Sporanox) 200 mg a day × 3 days, then 200 mg once a month

A topical choice for chronic or recurrent infection or cyclic candidiasis is terconazole (Terazol) 0.4% cream nightly for 2 weeks, then half an applicator full (2.5g) Monday, Wednesday, and Friday for 3 to 6 months. In the cyclic cases, one applicator full can be used for the 3 to 5 days just before symptoms occur each month.

If suppressive anticandidal therapy is not effective, remove copper-bearing intrauterine devices (IUDs) and consider contraception with medroxy-progesterone acetate 150 mg IM q3months.

For pregnant patients, only topical treatments are used.

Dermatophytosis

Dermatophyte infections are superficial fungal infections. In the groin they present as a typical erythematous skin eruption with annular scaling margins. Synonyms for dermatophytosis are tinea cruris and ringworm. The organisms include *Epidermophyton floccosum*, *Trichophyton rubrum*, or *Trichophyton mentagrophytes*. This condition is more common in men than in women and is usually found in young adults. It can be spread from a sexual partner or via autoinoculation from tinea pedis by shaving infected toes, then the bikini line. An itchy irritated rash in the groin develops and spreads slowly over a number of weeks. It is worse in those wearing tight synthetic clothing.

Physical Examination

The eruption is a well-defined, sharply margin-ated pale red rash with a scaly border. It spreads peripherally with a typical annular pattern. In women it is usually in the hair-bearing portion of the vulva, extends out into the inguinal creases and around the buttock area, and is often bilaterally symmetric (Fig. 14-6).

Diagnosis

The clinical pattern alone can be diagnostic. Scale from the periphery is put on a glass slide, followed by a drop of 10% potassium hydroxide

(KOH), and then a cover slip. The typical hyphae then can be seen as the skin cells are cleared by the KOH. A scraping for culture on Sabouraud medium defines the exact organism.

Differential diagnosis includes erythrasma, candidiasis, psoriasis, and contact dermatitis.

Treatment

Local treatment for the infection involves keeping the area cool and dry. Wash the area with a triclosan solution (Tersaseptic), rinse well, and pat dry.

Topical treatment is with the following creams bid for 14 days:

Clotrimazole 1%	Ciclopirox olamine 1%
Miconazole 2%	Ketoconazole 2%
Econazole 2%	Terbinafine 1%

Systemic treatment for the infection includes the following:

Terbinafine (Lamisil) 250 mg daily × 2 weeks

Itraconazole (Sporanox) 100 or 200 mg bid × 1 week

Ketoconazole (Nizoral) 200 to 400 mg daily × 2 weeks

Griseofulvin 500 mg a day for 2 to 6 weeks

Fluconazole (Diflucan) 150 mg once a week × 3 to 4 weeks

BACTERIAL DISEASES

Abscess

An abscess is a deep bacterial infection of hair follicles forming a walled-off collection of pus in a painful, firm, or fluctuant mass. The synonyms for an abscess are boil and furuncle. Coalescing abscesses form a carbuncle. Abscesses are most common in adolescents and young adults.

Staphylococcus aureus and much less commonly *Escherichia coli* or *Pseudomonas aeruginosa* are the cause of abscesses. This problem is found in those who are chronic carriers of *Staphylococcus* in the nares or perineum, and their infections are typically around areas of friction. Although more frequently present under the abdominal pannus in the obese, an abscess may appear in the vulvar area or the inner thigh or buttock. An exquisitely tender localized lesion forms, throbbing with pain, sometimes accompanied by malaise and a low-grade fever.

Physical Examination

In the groin, inner thighs, or perianal area a hard, red nodule develops that may progress to a fluctuant mass with a central necrotic plug. The surface may show exuding pus (Fig. 14-7).

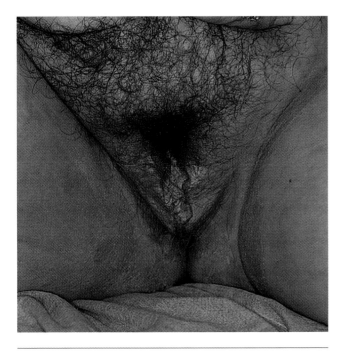

FIG. 14-6
Tinea Cruris. Annular, symmetric, red rash with a scaly border present on the inner thighs.

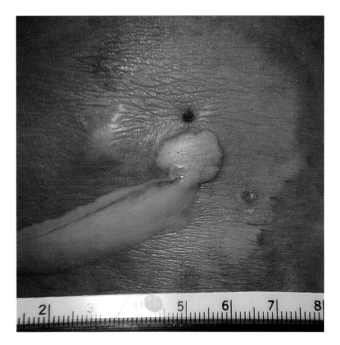

FIG. 14-7
A draining abscess located on the thigh.

Diagnosis

The clinical picture plus a culture of the purulent drainage determines the diagnosis. A Gram stain of the drainage confirms the organisms. Differential diagnoses include hidradenitis suppurativa, severe herpes simplex, and ruptured epidermal cyst.

Treatment

With a simple lesion, local application of heat and drainage may be all that is necessary. Deeper lesions may need packing after drainage.

Antibiotics are used for recurrent disease. The choice depends on the culture and sensitivity. For *Staphylococcus aureus,* cloxacillin 500 mg qid, cephalexin 250 mg qid, erythromycin 250 mg qid are prescribed (adjust doses depending on the patient's size).

For those with nasal or gluteal cleft carriage, use mupirocin (Bactroban) or fusidic acid (Fucidin) ointment applied qid for one week.

For continued recurrences, a combination of cloxacillin and rifampin is used.

Cellulitis/Erysipelas

Cellulitis is an acute, spreading subcutaneous bacterial infection causing areas of hot, red, tender skin. Group A ß-hemolytic *Streptococci* (GABHS) and *Staphylococcus aureus* are primarily found. The organism enters through a small abrasion or split in the skin and then spreads. It is more common in patients with diabetes or chronic lymphedema. This is not a common vulvar problem.

The infection can be quite subtle when it involves the vulva, with only slight tenderness and soreness and a mild fever. If involvement is extensive, there may be intense tenderness, fever, and malaise.

Physical Examination

The labia may be red and warm or hot. In the perineum, sharply demarcated red indurated plaques may occur and gradually spread (Fig. 14-8). In severe cases there are sometimes bullae and erosions.

"Erysipelas" is caused by group A streptococci and is a very superficial type of cellulitis involving the lymphatics. It has a very obvious margin that

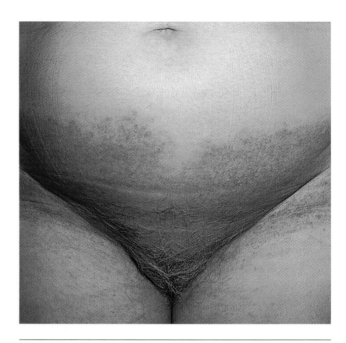

FIG. 14-8
Diffuse painful cellulitis present on the lower abdomen, groin, and thigh.

is raised and demarcated from normal skin. It is painful. If there has been any significant alteration in local lymphatic drainage caused by a prior infection, hidradenitis suppurativa, Crohn's disease, or repeatedly infected lichen simplex chronicus, then recurrent cellulitis/erysipelas can be a problem. There is always a degree of residual lymphedema predisposing to recurrent episodes of erythema and swelling of the area. With time, the labia can become permanently lymphedematous.

Diagnosis

The diagnosis is clinical. Culture helps in only 25% of the cases. Differential diagnoses include contact dermatitis, urticaria, fixed drug eruption, and herpes zoster.

Treatment

The following drugs are recommended:
Cloxacillin 0.5 to 1g po q6h × 7 to 10 days
Erythromycin 500g po q6h × 7 to 10 days

For chronic recurrent disease, long-term penicillin (penicillin V potassium 300 to 500 mg po qid for weeks, tapering to one dose daily over 3 to 6 months) is prescribed. For associated lymphedema, see the section on vulvar lymphedema.

Folliculitis

Small follicular papules and pustules result from this bacterial or yeast infection of the hair follicles. *Staphylococcus aureus, Candida albicans,* and *Pseudomonas aeruginosa* are the most common infectors. This may be seen in the vulvar area associated with shaving and waxing. Patient history involves slightly tender to itchy lesions developing in pubic hair or anywhere in the shaved vulvar area. *Pseudomonas* infection is associated with exposure to hot tubs.

Physical Examination

Isolated (Fig. 14-9) or scattered follicular pustules with surrounding erythema are seen. In the late stages of the infection, crusting occurs.

Diagnosis

Gram stain and culture confirm the offending organism. Differential diagnosis includes scabies, insect bites, herpes simplex, and tinea.

Treatment

Eliminate the point of entry of the causative organism. This may involve changing techniques for shaving and hair removal.

For *Pseudomonas* infection, the patient's exposure to hot tubs must be stopped. Use Cipro 250 to 500 mg or trimethoprim-sulfamethoxazole, double strength bid × 5 to 7 days.

For *Staphylococcus* infection use the following:
Erythromycin 250 mg qid × 10 to 14 days
Cloxacillin 500 mg qid × 10 to 14 days
Cephalexin 500 mg qid × 10 to 14 days

For yeast folliculitis resulting from *Candida,* use topical imidazole cream twice a day for 7 to 14 days (e.g., miconazole 2% cream, ketoconazole 2% cream, econazole 1% cream).

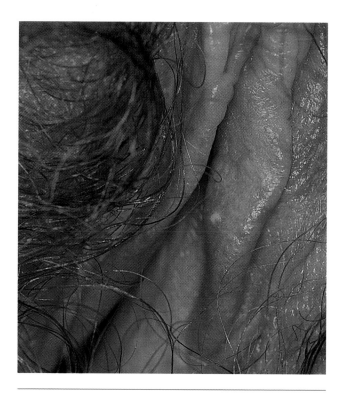

FIG. 14-9
A small, isolated, very tender pustule of folliculitis is observed.

Erythrasma

This is a chronic, reddish-brown, scaling, bacterial infection of adult intertriginous areas, caused by *Corynebacterium minutissimum.* This organism prefers the warm intertriginous areas of the groin, toes, and axilla. Patient history includes mild irritation, particularly in warm humid climates.

Physical Examination

Sharply marginated reddish-brown patches and bilaterally symmetric plaques extending from the edge of the labia majora through the crural folds out onto the inner thighs (Fig. 14-10, *A*).

Diagnosis

The clinical pattern is highly suggestive. Wood's light examination shows the typical coral red fluorescence (Fig. 14-14, *B*).

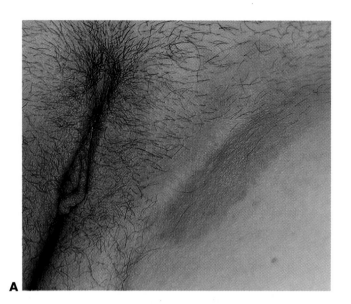
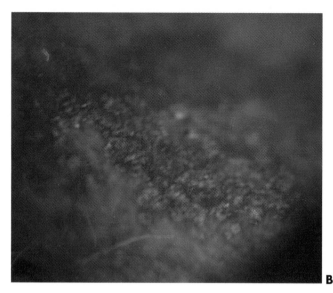

FIG. 14-10
A, A red-brown patch of erythrasma located on the inner thigh. **B**, Coral red fluorescence of erythrasma.

Differential diagnoses include tinea cruris, seborrheic dermatitis, and psoriasis.

Treatment

Recommend that the patient keep the area cool and dry and avoid tight synthetic clothing. The following drugs are also recommended:

Triclosan (Tersaseptic) wash bid plus
Erythromycin 250 mg qid po × 2 weeks plus
Erythromycin 2% to 4% in an alcoholic solution topically bid × 2 weeks

Syphilis

Syphilis (Lues) is an infectious disease caused by *Treponema pallidum*, a small spiral spirochete, that is sexually transmitted (except in the congenital form). Approximately 30% of those exposed become infected. It has gradually increased in incidence with AIDS and IV drug use.

Primary Syphilis

About 14 to 28 days after exposure to an infected individual, a little asymptomatic chancre develops at the point of inoculation. If the chancre is secondarily infected it can be painful. With no treatment, the lesion heals in 6 to 8 weeks.

Physical Examination

The chancre, usually solitary, starts as a small papule that breaks down into a painless round or oval 1 to 2 cm ulcer with a raised sharply demarcated border and little exudate (Fig. 14-11, A). The labium major is the most frequent site involved, although cervical lesions, anal ulcers, etc. may occur depending on the portal of entry. Regional lymph nodes are enlarged.

Diagnosis

The clinical picture plus dark-field examination and serologic testing confirm the diagnosis. The Rapid Plasma Reagin (RPR) is positive by the 14th day of the chancre. The Venereal Disease Research Laboratory (VDRL) test does not become reactive that early. The Fluorescent Treponema antibody-absorption test (FTA-ABS) becomes positive at the time of appearance of the chancre and is more specific than the VDRL. Biopsy of the genital ulcer, stained with Warthin-Starry silver, demonstrates the spirochetes.

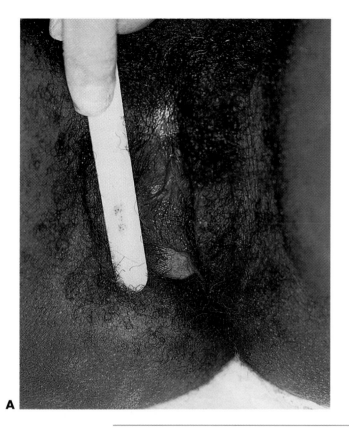

A

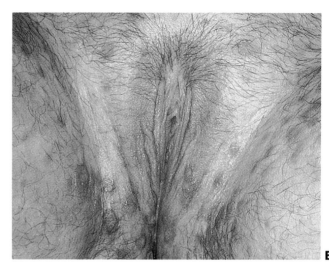

B

FIG. 14-11

A, Syphilitic chancre on labium major. **B**, Secondary syphilis with papulosquamous eruption plus small condylomata lata.

(**B**, Courtesy Dr. N.J. Fuimara.)

Syphilis must be considered and ruled out in the diagnosis of any ulcerative anogenital lesion, for example, chancroid, genital herpes, fixed drug eruption, lymphogranuloma venereum, traumatic ulcer, aphthous ulcer, and granuloma inguinale.

Treatment

Benzathine penicillin G 2.4 million units IM (1.2 million units per buttock) is prescribed.

Repeat 2.4 million units (as above) 1 week later for a total of 4.8 million units.[1]

For penicillin allergic patients use the following:

Doxycycline 100 mg orally bid × 14 days or

Erythromycin 40 mg/kg up to 500 mg qid × 14 days

Repeat serology at 1, 3, 6, 12, and 24 months and a CSF examination if there are any neurologic signs or the patient is HIV positive.

Secondary Syphilis

Most women are unaware of the primary chancre. Secondary syphilis develops about 10 weeks (2 to 6 months) after the primary chancre. A flulike illness onsets with headache, sore throat, arthralgias, low-grade fever, and lymphadenopathy. Skin complaints at this stage are rash and hair loss.

Physical Examination

The lesions develop slowly and can persist for weeks or months with few symptoms. In order of frequency the following signs may be observed:

Maculopapular/papulosquamous (Fig. 14-11, *B*) and a somewhat psoriasiform rash over the torso, arms, and legs, typically with involvement of the palms and soles.

An irregular, "moth-eaten" alopecia of the beard, scalp, and eyelashes.

Moist wartlike papules develop in the vulvar and perianal areas—condylomata lata (see Fig. 14-11, *B*).

Mucous patches in the form of grayish white round papules and thin plaques in the mouth and on the vulvar and perianal area.

Generalized lymphadenopathy usually occurs, sometimes with pharyngitis, iritis, periostitis, hepatosplenomegaly, nephritis, and gastritis.

Diagnosis

A positive dark-field examination of the mucous membrane lesions is diagnostic. The RPR and VDRL serology shows high or rising titers. In early secondary syphilis the tests may be falsely negative (the prozone phenomenon) resulting from a high antigen level. Special dilutional prozone testing needs to be done. If these tests are negative and there remains clinical suspicion, then an FTA-ABS test is required.

Differential diagnoses include pityriasis rosea, viral exanthem, infectious mononucleosis, psoriasis, tinea corporis and versicolor, scabies, lichen planus, drug reactions, and condyloma acuminata.

Treatment

In early secondary syphilis of less than 1 year's duration, the treatment is the same as for primary syphilis.

For latent syphilis of more than 1 year's duration prescribe the following:

Benzathine penicillin G 2.4 million units IM weekly × 3 weeks or

Doxycycline 100 mg bid × 4 weeks

The titre of the RPR or VDRL and the clinical symptoms must be followed after treatment to detect treatment failure.

A CSF examination should be carried out if VDRL is equal to or greater than 1:16 in the latent stage and if there are any neurologic signs. Generally HIV patients are treated with the same treatment regimen as for primary and secondary syphilis.[2]

HIV patients need careful follow-up for relapse.

All patients with syphilis should be tested for HIV.

Gonorrhea

Gonorrhea is a sexually transmitted bacterial disease of the vulvovaginal area in women. It may go unnoticed. The synonyms for gonorrhea are the clap and GC. The causative organism, *Neisseria gonorrhea,* is a gram-negative intracellular diplococcus that is spread sexually in young adults.

Seveny-five percent to 80% of infected women are asymptomatic. They may complain of some vaginal discharge, dysuria, or post-coital bleeding. Most frequently they may have painful infected Bartholin's vestibular glands. Rectal involvement produces itching, discharge, bleeding, and sometimes pain and tenesmus. Disseminated gonorrhea (gonococcemia, gonococcal arthritis—dermatitis syndrome) is beyond the scope of this text.

Physical Examination

Classically there is an endocervical discharge and a scant to copious mucopurulent vaginal discharge (Fig. 14-12). The cervix is almost always involved, but may show no typical changes. The

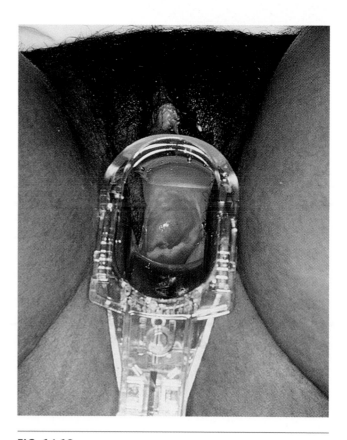

FIG. 14-12
Purulent cervical discharge in gonorrhea.
(Courtesy Dr. N.J. Fuimara.)

vulva may be red, swollen, and inflamed, but this may clear as the infection becomes more chronic. If there is a urethritis, there may be erythema and a purulent discharge from Skene's ducts. The inflammation of the Bartholin's glands may cause very marked swelling and abscess formation. About 35% to 50% of involved women may have a proctitis.

Diagnosis

The clinical picture and Gram stain showing the typical gram-negative intracellular diplococci in the exudate diagnostic. The organism grows on chocolate blood agar. Differential diagnoses include genital herpes, chlamydia, trichomonas, and bacterial vaginosis.

Treatment

Gonorrhea is usually treated with the following:
Ciprofloxacin 500 mg orally as a single dose or
Cefixime 400 mg orally as a single dose or
Ceftriaxone 125 mg IM as a single dose
For penicillin-allergic patients prescribe the following:
Ciprofloxacin 500 mg orally as a single dose or
Ofloxacin 400 mg orally as a single dose
▲ All regimens are followed by doxycycline 100 mg po bid × 7 days or azithromycin 1 g po as a single dose. ▼

Chancroid

Chancroid is an acute sexually transmitted disease caused by *Hemophilus ducreyi* that causes a very painful ulcer and suppurative regional lymphadenopathy. Synonyms for chancroid include soft chancre, chancre mou, and ulcus molle. Chancroid usually affects young adults.

Haemophilus ducreyi is a gram-negative rod. This is a sexually transmitted organism that is most common in tropical and subtropical climates. It is responsible for up to 60% of genital ulcers in Africa and Asia. After contact with an infected individual, a painful ulcer develops 4 to 7 days later, and a painful unilateral inguinal lymphadenitis occurs 1 to 2 weeks later in up to 50% of patients. Sometimes the ulcers can be present for months with little to no symptomatology.

Physical Examination

The first sign is a papule on the vulva in the area of the labia, posterior commissure, or vestibule. This becomes pustular and ulcerates. The ulcer has a grayish surface, an irregular border, and surrounding erythema. One third of patients may have multiple lesions (Fig. 14-13). The associated lymphadenopathy may progress in 50% of patients to bubo formation and may rupture, yielding a chronic sinus.

Diagnosis

Diagnosis is by clinical presentation. A smear of the ulcer reveals the typical short, plump gram-negative rods, often in streptobacillary chains. These are found in clusters outside the white cells, looking like a "school of fish." The organism can be cultured on selective media. Differential diagnoses include

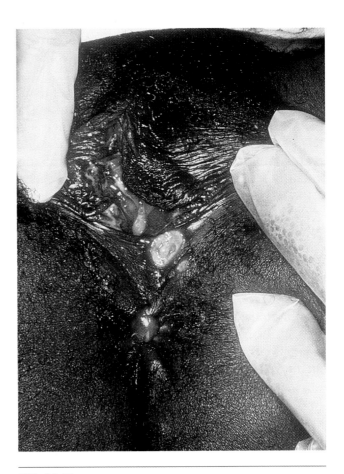

FIG. 14-13
Multiple discrete ulcers located on the vulva and perianal area in chancroid.
(Courtesy Dr. N.J. Fuimara.)

herpes simplex, syphilis, granuloma inguinale, lymphogranuloma venereum, and trauma.

Drugs prescribed include the following:

Erythromycin 500 mg qid × 7 days
Ceftriaxone 250 mg IM once
Azithromycin 1 g oral once
Ciprofloxacin 500 mg bid × 3 days

Patients with vulvar ulcerations should have HIV testing.

Lymphogranuloma Venereum

A rare sexually transmitted disease, lymphogranuloma venereum (LGV) is caused by L-serovars of *Chlamydia trachomatis,* immunotypes L1, L2, L3. It results in regional lymphadenitis, fistulas, and strictures. The synonym for LGV is lymphogranuloma inguinale. It usually occurs between the ages of 20 and 50 years. It is most commonly found in Africa, India, some parts of Asia, and the Caribbean. A history of sexual exposure to an infectious partner from an endemic area may be elicited. Incubation period is three days to three weeks.

In the primary stage there is a small relatively painless ulcer or abrasion in the genital area. The secondary stage occurs about one to four weeks later as these patients go on to develop a cervicitis and salpingitis with tender inguinal lymphadenopathy accompanied by fever, malaise, headache, arthralgia, and nausea. There may be severe lower abdominal and pelvic pain. In the third stage the resulting chronic edema and scarring can cause discomfort, dyspareunia, etc.

Physical Examination

First Stage. There is a small erosion or ulcer or even a group of ulcers like herpes simplex around the clitoris, vulvar introitus, or sometimes on the vaginal wall. There may be a mucopurulent cervical discharge.

Second Stage. Lymphadenopathy is the main feature of this disease, and the enlarged nodes are often perirectal in women, as opposed to inguinal in men. They can break down, creating rectovaginal and anal fistulas, giving gastrointestinal symptoms rather than genital ones. This is referred to as the anogenitorectal syndrome. In the inguinal area the enlarged buboes can cause an inflammatory mass of lymph nodes separated by a depression or groove made by Poupart's ligament, giving the typical "groove" sign (Fig. 14-14, *A*).

Third Stage. Chronic genital edema results from long-standing lymphatic inflammation and scarring, yielding vulvar elephantiasis (Fig. 14-14, *B*). Fistulae and abscesses may be difficult to manage.

Diagnosis

Serologic tests can confirm the diagnosis. A complement-fixation test demonstrates a titer of greater than 1:64 in active disease. A microimmuno-fluorescence test demonstrates a rising titer, which generally supports the diagnosis.

Differential diagnoses include the following:

First stage: Primary syphilis, chancroid, genital herpes

Second stage: Genital herpes, syphilis, bacterial infections, chancroid, Hodgkin's disease. In the anogenitorectal syndrome, differentiate from ulcerative colitis, Crohn's disease, etc.

Third stage: See Vulvar edema

It is important that this disease may be diagnosed early to avoid the scarring and chronic lymphedema.

Treatment

The following drugs may be prescibed for LGV:

Doxycycline 100 mg bid × 21 days or
Erythromycin 500 mg qid × 21 days or
Sulfisoxazole 500 mg qid × 21 days

During the third stage surgical management may be necessary.

Granuloma Inguinale

Granuloma inguinale is a mildly contagious, chronic, destructive sexually transmitted disease that results in ulcerative lesions that gradually enlarge, causing secondary scarring and boggy swelling. Synonyms for granuloma inguinale are granuloma venereum and Donovanosis. The etiology is *Calymmatobacterium granulomatsis,* an encapsulated gram-negative rod. This infection is found endemically in subtropical environments: India, the Caribbean, Africa, and rarely in North America or Europe. The patient's history usually reveals a sexual exposure to a contact in or from an endemic area. The nonhealing ulcer may be tender or painless. Secondary infection increases the discomfort. Late in the disease the patient's complaints center on scarring and distortion.

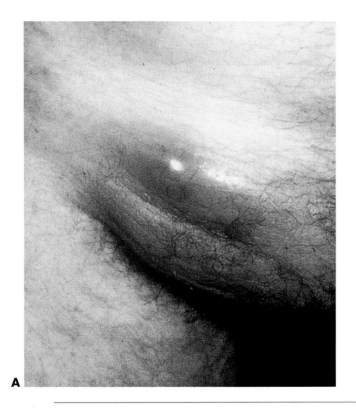

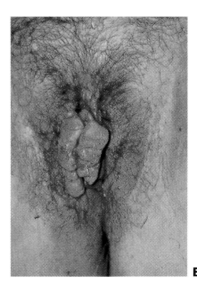

A

B

FIG. 14-14
A, "Groove sign" in the right inguinal area from lymphogranuloma venereum (LGV).
B, Chronic edema of the labia in LGV.
(**A**, Courtesy Dr. N.J. Fuimara. **B**, From Black MM, McKay M, Braude P: *Color atlas and text of obstetric and gynecologic dermatology*, London, 1995, Mosby.)

Physical Examination

The patient develops a papule after 1 to 12 weeks. It will eventually undergo central necrosis, forming a clean, sharply demarcated, granulomatous ulcer with a beefy red base that bleeds on contact. The lesions may be multiple and can develop in a variety of patterns: nodular with bright red granulating bases, hypertrophic with large vegetating masses, ulcerative (a combination of the two) (Fig. 14-15), or cicatricial with spreading scar tissue. The ulcers can be anywhere on the vulva, perianal area, vagina, or cervix. A degree of lymphedema causes vulvar distortion. If left untreated, the areas of involvement may develop squamous cell carcinoma.

Diagnosis

Diagnosis is clinical, confirmed by a tissue smear stained with Giemsa or Wright's stain. The Dono-van bodies are seen intracellularly and look like safety-pins. Biopsy and Warthin-Starry silver stains also can be used. Differential diagnoses include herpes simplex ulcers, syphilitic chancre, chancroid, lymphogranuloma venereum, cutaneous tuberculosis, and squamous cell carcinoma.

Treatment

The following are prescribed to treat granuloma inguinale:

Erythromycin 500 mg qid × 7 days or
Tetracycline 500 mg po qid × 3 to 4 weeks or
Chloramphenicol 500 mg q8h × 10 to 14 days or
Trimethoprim/sulfamethoxazole 2 tablets q12h × 10 days

In chronic disease do an appropriate biopsy to rule out squamous cell carcinoma.

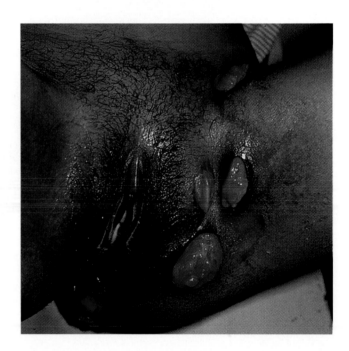

FIG. 14-15
Multiple, beefy-red, thick, granulating ulcers in granuloma inguinale.
(Courtesy Dr. J. Keystone.)

SUGGESTED READINGS

Human Papilloma Virus

Ling MR: Therapy of genital human papilloma virus infections. Part I: Indications for and justification of therapy, *Int J Dermatol* 31(10):682-686, 1992.

Ling MR: Therapy of genital human papilloma virus infections. Part II: Methods of treatment, *Int J Dermatol* 31(11):769-776, 1992.

Sawchuk WS: Vulvar manifestations of human papillomavirus infection, *Dermatol Clin* 10(2):405-414, 1992.

Herpes Simplex

Maccato ML, Kaufman RH: Herpes genitalis, *Dermatol Clin* 10(2):415-422, 1992.

Pereira FA: Herpes simplex: evolving concepts, *J Am Acad Dermatol* 35:503-520, 1996.

Herpes Zoster

Boon RJ, Griffin DR: Famciclovir: efficacy in zoster and issues in the assessment of pain, *Adv Exp Med Biol* 394:17-31, 1996.

Smiley ML, Murray A: Acyclovir and its l-valyl ester, valacyclovir, *Curr Probl Dermatol* 24:209-218, 1996.

Volmink J, Lancaster T, Gray S, Silagy C: Treatments for postherpetic neuralgia: a systematic review of randomized controlled trials, *Fam Pract* 13(1):84-91, 1996.

Candidiasis

McKay M: Vulvodynia, *Dermatol Clin* 10(2):423-433, 1992.

Sobel JD: Vulvovaginitis, *Dermatol Clin* 10(2):339-359, 1992.

Cellulitis/Erysipelas

Sachs MK: Cutaneous cellulitis, *Arch Dermatol* 127(4):493-496, 1991.

Syphilis

Fuimara NJ: Genital ulcer infections in the female patients and the vaginitides, *Dermatol Clin* 15(2):223-245, 1997.

Kraus SJ: Diagnosis and management of acute genital ulcers in sexually active patients, *Semin Dermatol* 9(2):160-166, 1990.

Krieger JN: New sexually transmitted diseases treatment guidelines, *J Urol* 154(1):209-213, 1995.

Moreland AA: Vulvar manifestations of sexually transmitted diseases, *Semin Dermatol* 13(4):262-268, 1994.

Nandwani R: Modern diagnosis and management of aquired syphilis, *Br J Hosp Med* 55(7):399-403, 1996.

Rolfs RT: Treatment of syphilis: 1993, *Clin Infect Dis* 20(suppl 1):523-538, 1995.

Gonorrhea

Elgart ML: Sexually transmitted diseases of the vulva, *Dermatol Clin* 10(2):387-403, 1992.

Chancroid

Margolis RJ, Hood AF: Chancroid: diagnosis and treatment, *J Am Acad Dermatol* 6(4 PT 1):493-499, 1982.

Lymphogranuloma Venereum

Buntin DM, Rosen T, Lesher JL Jr, et al: Sexually transmitted diseases: bacterial infections, *J Am Acad Dermatol* 25(2 Pt 1):287-299, 1991.

Elgart ML: Sexually transmitted diseases of the vulva, *Dermatol Clin* 10(2):387-403, 1992.

Granuloma Inguinale

Sehgal VN, Prasad AL: Donovanosis: current concepts, *Int J Dermatol* 25(1):8-16, 1986.

Wysoki RS, Majmudar B, Willis D: Granuloma inguinale (donovanosis) in women, *J Reprod Med* 33(8):709-713, 1988.

SCABIES

Scabies is a highly contagious, itchy, skin infestation caused by the mite *Sarcoptes scabiei* (Fig. 15-1, *A*). A synonym for scabies is "seven-year itch." It occurs in children, young adults, and the institutionalized elderly. The mites spread by skin-to-skin contact but also by fomites such as clothing, toilet seats, etc. The onset is insidious with minor irritation and slightly itchy skin that gradually worsens. It takes 6 weeks from direct contact to develop a full-blown infection. Nocturnal itching is typical.

Physical Examination

An examination shows typical tiny erythematous papules, vesicles, and small jagged linear burrows in body creases, particularly finger webs, wrists, and axillary folds. In women, the breasts, buttocks, and inframammary folds are commonly involved, but the vulva often escapes. As the condition becomes more chronic, the lesions can become papular and then nodular. Some of these nodules may persist even after treatment (Fig. 15-1, *B*). In infants there may be involvement of the scalp and face. In the elderly there may be more excoriations than true papules or nodules.

Diagnosis

The diagnosis rests on the clinical pattern, isolation of a mite and/or a confirmatory skin scraping. Use 10% KOH dropped on the skin scrapings on a glass slide under a cover slip. Examine the slide under the microscope for the typical mite and eggs. Differential diagnoses include folliculitis, neurodermatitis, atypical tinea, and contact dermatitis.

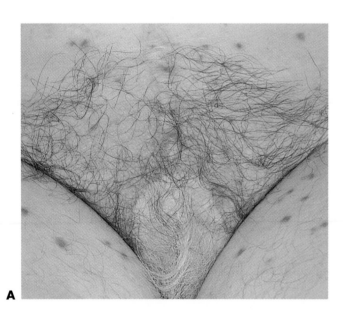
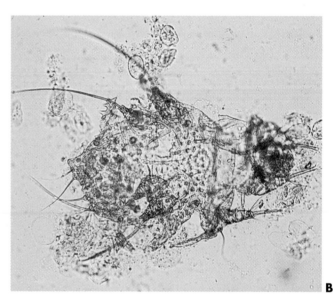

A   B

FIG. 15-1
A, Scabetic nodules in the groin of an elderly woman with vitiligo. **B,** *Sarcoptes scabiei* mite seen using potassium hydroxide preparation.
(**A,** Courtesy Dr. J. Walter.)

Treatment

All patient contacts need to be treated at the same time. All clothing, bedding, etc. is washed.

Options include:

Lindane 1% lotion is applied after a tub or shower and left on for 8 to 12 hours, then washed off. **This is not to be used in pregnant women** or in children under 2 years of age. It may be reapplied in 24 hours or in 7 days to minimize recurrences or failures.

Permethrin 5% (Nix or Elimite) cream is applied as for lindane.

Precipitated sulfur in petrolatum or a cold cream base (6% for children, 10% for adults) is applied from chin to toes twice a day for 2 days.

For the rash of scabies after the treatment, a mid-potency corticosteroid ointment can be used twice a day until the rash has subsided. An antihistamine such as hydroxyzine hydrochloride 10 to 25 mg qhs can be given for itching.

PEDICULOSIS

Pediculosis pubis is a louse infestation of the hairy regions of the body, most commonly the pubic area. Synonyms for pediculosis are pubic lice, crabs, and crab lice. *Phthirus pubis* is the crab or pubic louse (Fig. 15-2, *A*). It lives on humans and is spread by close physical contact either sexually or by fomites. It is an infestation of teenagers and young adults, occurring equally in men and women. The patient may be asymptomatic but usually there is mild to moderate itching for months, involving the hairy areas of the groin but also other areas—axilla, body, eyebrow, and eyelash hairs.

Physical Examination

Small, red, primary papules (bites) may be found, but secondary changes from scratching with some serous crusts are usually more obvious. Very careful inspection reveals the 1 to 2 mm louse, attached to the base of the pubic hair. It appears as a small tan or brown speck along with the nits (eggs) attached to the lower portion of the hair shafts (Fig. 15-2, *B*). Maculae ceruleae (taches bleues), slate gray macules 0.5 to 1 cm in diameter, seen on the abdominal wall, buttock, and thigh represent louse bites.

Diagnosis

Diagnosis is clinical. The louse can be identified under a microscope. Differential diagnoses include tinea, folliculitis, scabies, or eczema.

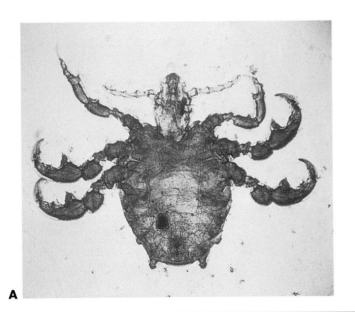
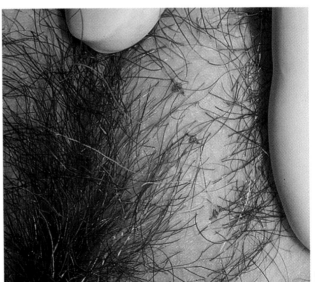

A   B

FIG. 15-2
A, *Phthirus pubis* (crab or pubic louse). **B,** Pubic lice seen attached to the hair on the mons pubis.
(**A,** Courtesy Dr. P. Lynch; **B,** courtesy Dr. L. Edwards.)

Treatment

All contacts need to be treated. All personal belongings must be washed. Treatments are listed in order of preference:

Permethrin (Nix) 1% cream rinse applied to hairy areas for 10 minutes and rinsed off. This should be repeated 1 week later, although some patients opt to shave the areas to make sure there are no nits left.

Pyrethrins (Rid) applied for 10 to 15 minutes and rinsed off.

Lindane 1% cream or lotion applied for 10 minutes and rinsed off or left on for 8 to 12 hours. It may be repeated once, 7 days later.

Petrolatum tid for 5 days or baby shampoo on a cotton swab tid for 5 days is applied to involved eyelashes.

TRICHOMONIASIS

This is a common sexually transmitted vaginal infection that causes a smelly discharge leading to secondary vulvar burning and itching. Of infected women, 80% have partners with the *Trichomonas* organism. A synonym for trichomoniasis is trich. It commonly occurs at 20 to 29 years of age, caused by *Trichomonas vaginalis,* a unicellular flagellate. The classic malodorous discharge that is worse after intercourse occurs in only 10% of affected patients. Pruritus and some degree of dyspareunia are seen in 25% to 50% of the patients. Urinary symptoms, dysuria, and frequency sometimes occur. Rarely there is lower abdominal pain.

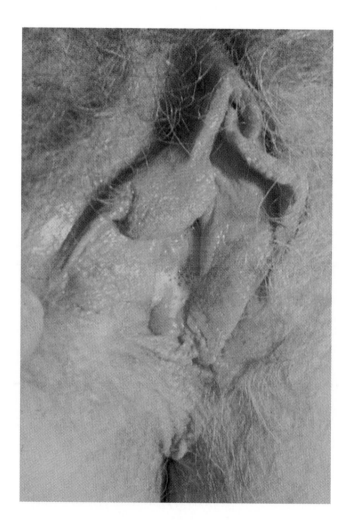

FIG. 15-3
Frothy discharge on labia minora in trichomoniasis.
(Courtesy Dr. P. Bryson)

Physical Examination

A diffusely red vestibule with an abundant, frothy, homogeneous, greenish discharge is observed (Fig. 15-3).

Diagnosis

Identification of the organism on a wet mount of the vaginal secretion with an associated high pH (above 5) leads to a diagnosis. On a smear of this secretion, multiple white cells, epithelial cells, and the typical tear-drop shaped, motile protozoan with its five small flagella are observed. The jerky movements of these protists are easy to recognize as they move across the slide. The addition of KOH to a wet smear gives a typical "fishy" odor, referred to as the positive "whiff" test. The organism can be cultured using Diamond's medium.

Differential diagnoses include moniliasis, bacterial vaginosis, gonorrhea, and foreign body.

Treatment

Treatments are in order of preference. Treat all sexual partners.

Metronidazole (Flagyl) 2g orally as a single dose or 1g bid in 1 day

Alternate regimens include the following:

Metronidazole (Flagyl) 500 mg orally bid × 7 days or

Metronidazole (Flagyl) 250 mg orally tid × 7 days or

Clotrimazole (Canesten) 1% cream or vaginal troche 100 mg qhs × 6 days (cure rate 48% to 66%)

CHAPTER 16

Inflammatory Diseases of the Vulva

ATOPIC DERMATITIS

This eruption, usually symmetric, consists of a dry, itchy, skin rash that occurs in patients with a personal or family history of one or more of the atopic conditions: asthma, hay fever, eczema. It is not common in the vulva. Synonyms for atopic dermatitis are eczema and neurodermatitis.

This condition is related to a cutaneous hypersensitivity associated with defective cell-mediated immunity and over production of B-cell IgE. Airborne allergens such as house dust, mites, molds, and grasses may play a role. Certain foods may also be a factor. Atopic individuals have very sensitive skin and are susceptible to irritation by soaps, cleansers, lotions, perfume products, and sanitary napkins. Most atopic patients have only intermittent eczematous rashes in the vulva. In some patients the itching and scratching sets up an "itch-scratch-itch cycle" that results in the development of lichen simplex chronicus.

There is often a background history of childhood eczema, hay fever, asthma, and dry skin. The vulvar complaints are those of itching, burning, or dryness.

Physical Examination

The vulvar eruption is usually subacute or chronic, with mild redness, dryness, and fine scaling (Fig. 16-1). With time, excoriation leads to lichenification and secondary infection with honey-colored crusting. The area of involvement may be ill-defined but usually involves the labia majora and variably the labia minora and inner thighs. This may evolve into the typical picture of lichen simplex chronicus (see the following discussion).

Diagnosis

The diagnosis is made on the personal and family history and the clinical pattern of atopy. Histology is seldom necessary. Differential diagnoses include psoriasis, seborrheic dermatitis, contact dermatitis, and eczematous candidiasis.

Treatment

Local. The avoidance of harsh irritating soaps, lotions, detergents, and feminine hygiene products is recommended. No perfumed products should be used in the vulva. Ventilated undergarments of natural fibers, preferably cotton, are best. If acute, a sitz bath or compresses with Burow's solution 1:40 once or twice daily will help relieve symptoms.

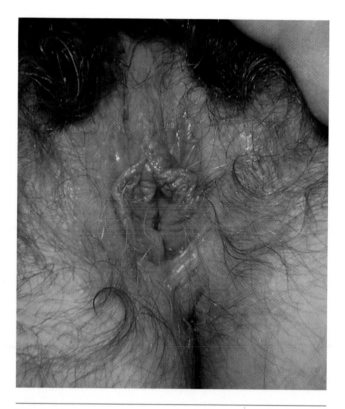

FIG. 16-1
Subacute dermatitis of the vulva in an atopic individual with early lichen simplex chronicus.

For mild gentle cleansing recommend that the patient use Cetaphil cleanser or Basis soap.

Specific. Rule out secondary infection—bacteria or yeast—with an appropriate culture.

Use topical steroids as follows:

Betamethasone-17-valerate 0.1% ointment bid × 7 to 14 days then hydrocortisone 1% ointment prn

Antibiotics for secondary infection include:

Cefadroxil 500 mg bid × 5 days or Azithromycin dihydrate 250 mg, 500 mg on day 1 then 250 mg/day × 4 days

If concurrent candidiasis exists, use terconazole vaginal cream qhs × 1 week.

For severe nocturnal itch, use hydroxyzine 25 to 75 mg po at 6:00 to 7:00 PM.

For severe cases, see treatment section on lichen simplex chronicus.

CONTACT DERMATITIS

Contact dermatitis is an inflammation of the skin resulting from an external agent that acts either as an irritant or an allergen, producing a rash that can be acute, subacute, or chronic. ▲ **It is important to work with the patient to determine if the agent is an irritant or an allergen. Find out precisely what products the patient uses and how often.** ▼

Primary irritant contact dermatitis is due to prolonged or repeated exposure to irritating products such as soaps or feminine hygiene products. Here, the problem is the caustic or physically irritating effect of the substance.

Allergic contact dermatitis is an eczematous dermatitis caused by a frank allergy to a low dose of a chemical substance such as perfume, benzocaine, or poison ivy. Allergic contact dermatitis is due to a type IV delayed hypersensitivity reaction. Primary irritant dermatitis is due to irritation without immune reactivity (Box 16-1).

The patient's main complaints are of itching, burning, and irritation that may be sudden in onset or gradual and cumulative depending on the etiology. The patient might be well aware of the product (e.g., clothing, sanitary napkins) that precipitated the problem. It may worsen with heat and moisture.

> **BOX 16-1**
>
> **List of Allergens and Irritants in Vulvar Contact Dermatitis**
>
> **Allergens**
> antibiotics—neomycin
> anesthetics—benzocaine
> preservatives—parabens, imidazolidinylurea
> perfumes—balsam of Peru
> moisturizers—lanolin
> plants—poison ivy
> rubber—gloves, condoms, and diaphragms
>
> **Irritants**
> soaps and detergents
> fabric softeners
> feminine hygiene products—pads, diapers, wipes, feminine deodorant sprays
> physically abrasive contactants—face cloths, sponges, etc.
> thermally damaging—hot water bottles

In irritant dermatitis there is a history of repeated use of the product. This is particularly true of the soap and feminine hygiene products. Some patients are obsessive cleansers of the vulvar area and seriously irritate their skin in the process. Elderly women may use normally harmless products that, when combined with napkins for incontinence or panty hose or girdles, can produce a reaction equivalent to a chronic irritant "diaper dermatitis" in infants.

In acute allergic contact dermatitis, the sudden development of itching, swelling, and irritation may pinpoint the precise cause such as exposure to latex in a condom or a particular cream or ointment used. If the condition is severe, there may be pain and burning on micturition.

Physical Examination

Acute involvement of the vulvar area can cause swelling, vesiculation, erythema, and weeping. Scratching may cause secondarily infected excoriations with crusting. The pattern may be subacute with some degree of erythema, swelling, erosion, and crustiness, or chronic with lichenification, induration, erythema, and either hypopigmentation or hyperpigmentation (Fig. 16-2).

Diagnosis

History and clinical pattern help determine the diagnosis. To investigate allergic contact dermatitis, patch testing is done by a dermatologist or allergist. Differential diagnoses include atopic dermatitis, psoriasis, intertrigo, and tinea.

Treatment

The most important treatment is to stop exposure to the allergen or irritant. For extensive allergic reactions, a dermatologist or allergist should be consulted.

Local care for weeping irritated skin and severe pruritus is covered in Appendices C and I. Sitz baths or cold compresses and ventilated cotton clothing are recommended to relieve the symptoms.

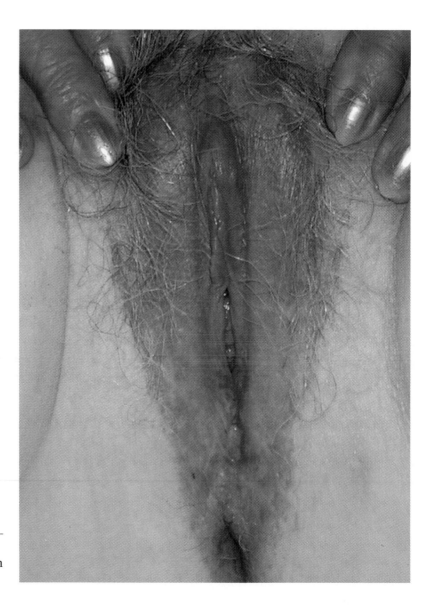

FIG. 16-2
Subacute contact dermatitis resulting from perfume in a feminine deoderant spray.

Topical corticosteroids that can be prescribed include the following:

Betamethasone-17-valerate 0.1% ointment bid

Triamcinolone acetonide 0.1% ointment bid

If the symptoms are severe, consider the following:

Prednisone 0.5 to 1 mg/kg/day decreased over 14 to 21 days

Triamcinolone acetonide 40 mg/mL (Kenalog 40) 1 mg/kg IM single dose

Antihistamine (as sedative)—hydroxyzine 25 to 75 mg qhs

Note: *Once the symptoms are controlled, the frequency of application and the potency of the cortisone can be gradually reduced, as indicated, moving from the midpotencies down to a mild steroid such as 1% to 2.5% hydrocortisone or desonide 0.05% ointment. Avoid creams.*

LICHEN SIMPLEX CHRONICUS

Lichen simplex chronicus (LSC) of the vulva is the end stage of the itch-scratch-itch cycle. Chronic intense pruritus results in repetitive scratching and rubbing so that the skin becomes thickened in the typical lichenified pattern. Synonyms for lichen simplex chronicus are hyperplastic dystrophy, neurodermatitis, and squamous cell hyperplasia. In LSC the skin is normal at the outset. The patient experiences itching, worse with stress, and persistent habitual scratching (the itch-scratch-itch cycle) results in lichenification. Secondary lichenification of the vulvar skin can occur associated with the following conditions:

Infections
  Candida
  Tinea cruris
Dermatoses
  Lichen sclerosus
  Atopic dermatitis
  Psoriasis
  Contact dermatitis
  Lichen planus
Neoplasia
  Vulvar intraepithelial neoplasia
Metabolic
  Diabetes
  Iron deficiency

The patient complains of years of constant itching that is often worse with stress. "Nothing helps," and the patient has often seen many physicians. Itching awakens patients at night and is worse with stress, menstrual periods, heat, and sanitary napkins.

Physical Examination

The vulvar skin, particularly over the labia majora, is diffusely thickened, with increased skin markings. This is called lichenification. The plaques may be bilaterally symmetric or unilateral, and the skin may be hyperpigmented or hypopigmented (Fig. 16-3, *A*). It may show a variety of shades of pink, red, ruddy brown, or purplish, with secondary excoriations, erosions, and crusting (Fig. 16-3, *B*). Active rubbing results in considerable swelling and, with time, causes the lichenification and broken off hairs.

Diagnosis

Diagnosis is clinical. Biopsy can rule out other conditions. Differential diagnoses include the causes of secondary lichenification listed earlier, and these should be ruled out since they can all present with this almost identical pattern. Extramammary Paget's disease may appear eczematous, like this condition.

Treatment

The treatment aim is to stop the chronic itch-scratch-itch cycle. Consult the section on severe pruritus and weeping irritated skin in Appendices C and H.

Control the itch by using
  Ice or cold gel packs
  Antihistamines—hydroxyzine or doxepin 25 to 75 mg qhs
Cleansing
  Be gentle; do not use a wash cloth
  If mild, use a product such as Cetaphil cleanser or Basis soap
  If severe, use sitz baths with Burow's solution (see Appendix I)
  Wear cool ventilated cotton clothing, and avoid pads if possible

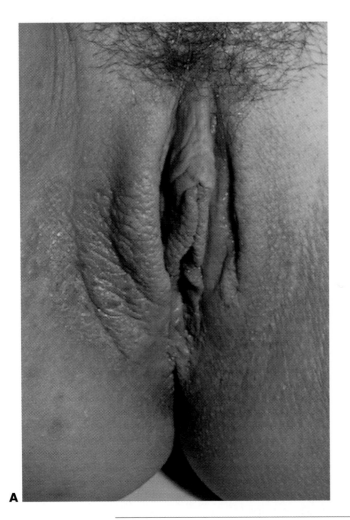
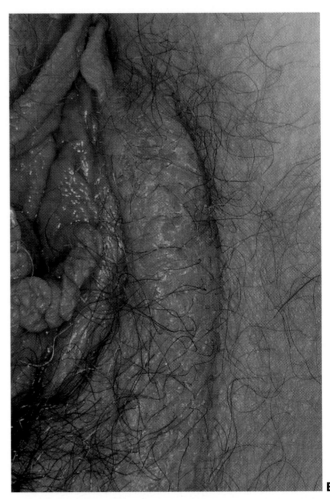

FIG. 16-3
Lichenification. **A**, Lichenification and swelling in a localized plaque of lichen simplex chronicus. **B**, Marked lichenification, erosions, and crusting in lichen simplex chronicus of left labium major.

Topical treatment
  Clobetasol or halobetasol 0.05% ointment bid for 2 weeks, once a day for 2 weeks, then Monday, Wednesday, Friday for 2 weeks, then on an intermittent basis, reducing potency for long-term care to desonide 0.05% ointment or 1% hydrocortisone in pramoxine cream.
  For marked thickness, inject one part triamcinolone acetonide (Kenalog 10) diluted with two parts of normal saline using a 30-gauge needle. The use of EMLA (a topical anesthesia cream applied in a thick film under plastic wrap for 15 to 20 minutes) makes this procedure almost painless. These injections can be repeated at 2 to 3 week intervals.
  It is necessary to treat any concurrent secondary infections—yeast or bacterial—to help stop the itching.
These patients need to be seen frequently and given general support.

Note: *Watch out for combinations of problems, for example, secondarily infected contact dermatitis with underlying psoriasis. Consider patch testing if the patient is not responding.*

APHTHOSIS

Aphthosis is a condition of single or multiple painful canker sores on the oral and genital mucosa. Synonyms include aphthous ulcers, canker sores on the vulva, Lipschütz ulcers, and ulcus vulvae acutum. The etiology is unknown. There may be an association with autoimmune disease. Patients complain of episodes of solitary or multiple painful vulvar ulcers. There seem to be two groups of patients with this condition. The first group is young, virginal girls with a history of fever and malaise who develop a sudden onset of very painful vulvar ulcers that are self-limited and clear in a few weeks. The other group is older women with a relapsing pattern like a partial Behçet's syndrome. In either group the pain may be incapacitating.

Physical Examination

A punched-out, shallow, well-defined ulcer with a fibrinous base and somewhat erythematous border is observed. The ulcers may be single or in groups and located around the vulvar vestibule. Occasionally a large deep punched-out destructive (giant) aphthous ulcer develops (Fig. 16-4).

Diagnosis

Diagnosis is by exclusion, following appropriate biopsies and cultures to rule out other conditions. Differential diagnosis is similar to Behçet's disease (see the following section). With time, the older patients with recurrent ulcers may develop Behçet's syndrome or inflammatory bowel disease.

Treatment

Management is the same as for limited ulcers in Behçet's disease (see the following section).

General comfort measures should be recommended, including gentle cleansing, sitz baths, and the avoidance of irritants.

Topical superpotent steroids, such as clobetasol or halobetasol 0.05% ointment twice a day, reducing as possible, can be prescribed. Intralesional steroid using triamcinolone acetonide (Kenalog 10), 10 mg/mL diluted 1:1 with saline and using a 30-gauge needle for injection, is used to control symptoms. Oral colchicine and dapsone have also been used for recurrent disease.

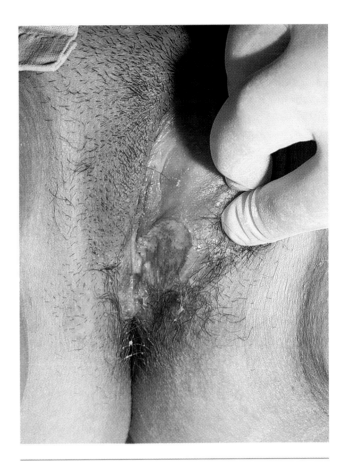

FIG. 16-4
Acute punched-out aphthous ulcer.

BEHÇET'S DISEASE

Behçet's disease is a rare, multi-system disorder that classically consists of the triad of oral ulcers, genital ulcers, and uveitis but is known to involve almost any organ system. Its etiology is unknown but probably involves altered immunity in genetically predisposed individuals. It is most commonly found in the Orient and Middle East, particularly Japan and Turkey, with the age of occurrence usually between 30 and 40 years.

The most common presentation is multiple, recurrent, painful, oral aphthous ulcers (100% of cases). In the vulva, the presenting complaint may be dyspareunia with recurrent crops of multiple, very tender, genital ulcers that take 2 to 4 weeks to heal. The onset of the oral and genital ulcers can be associated with fever, malaise, and arthritis. Elsewhere on the skin, folliculitis, furuncles, and a pustular dermatitis occur wherever there is skin trauma. Erythema nodosum and erythema multiforme have also been associated with this condition. More serious associations are thrombophlebitis and central nervous system changes such as stroke, paralysis, nerve palsies, and psychosis.

Physical Examination

Aphthous ulcers in the mouth present typically as small punched-out canker sores on the buccal mucosa and tongue and can be extensive (even on the pharynx) with a pseudomembranous coating. On the vulvar area, the 2 mm to 30 mm lesions can be individual and punched-out, but often form multiple contiguous (Fig. 16-5), sharply demarcated ulcers with fibrinous bases and considerable under-

mining that can eventually lead to sinus formation, fenestration, and partial or complete destruction of the labia.

Diagnosis

Diagnosis is made on the fulfillment of clinical criteria—recurrent oral ulceration plus two of the following:

recurrent genital ulceration

eye lesions (uveitis or retinovasculitis)

skin lesions (erythema nodosum, folliculitis, acneiform nodules)

positive pathergy tests (intradermal injection of sterile water that results in the formation of a papule or pustule in 48 hours).

Differential diagnoses include Crohn's disease, herpes simplex in the immunosuppressed, chancroid, granuloma inguinale, tuberculosis, syphilis, and lymphogranuloma venereum.

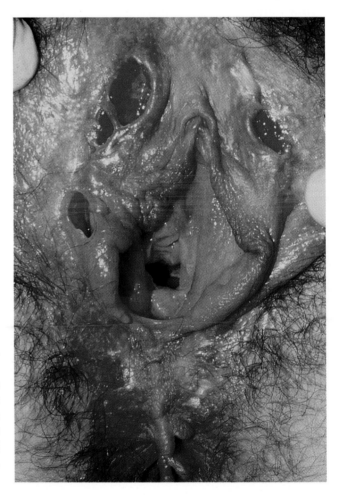

FIG. 16-5

Deep punched-out vulvar ulcers (all connected with sinuses on the right labium major) in Behçet's. This 16 year old had had painful ulcers for 3 years with what she thought was a sexually transmitted disease. She finally presented when she could not walk. She had had oral aphthae for years. She had small gastrointestinal ulcers on sigmoidoscopy, synovitis, and a positive pathergy test.

Treatment

Management depends on the extent of involvement. Treatment should be guided by an experienced dermatologist or gynecologist.

Local care for erosive and blistering diseases of the vulva is covered in Appendices D and I.

For mild vulvar ulceration, recommend gentle cleansing with Cetaphil cleanser or Basis soap to be followed by a superpotent steroid (halobetasol or clobetasol 0.05% ointment bid for 1 to 2 weeks or more). For local discomfort, the patient can use a topical EMLA cream applied for 15 to 20 minutes under plastic wrap occlusion. Sitz baths with Buro-Sol or Domeboro can be used for open ulcers.

Specific Treatment. The following treatments have been used separately and in combination.

For localized involvement, use intralesional cortisone, triamcinolone acetonide (Kenalog-10) mixed 1:2 with saline and injected after the EMLA topical anesthesia.

Prednisone 20 to 60 mg/day.

Colchicine 0.6 mg tid or less is good for limited disease and as a steroid sparer.

Dapsone 100 mg/day. It can be used along with colchicine or by itself as a steroid sparer. Before use check the patient's glucose-6-phosphate dehydrogenase (G-6-PD) level to rule out G-6-PD deficiency.

Azathioprine 1 to 2 mg/kg/day for patients unresponsive to prednisone.

Thalidomide (available on a restricted basis) 50 to 200 mg/day.

Methotrexate 7.5 to 20 mg/week for resistant disease.

Cyclosporine 3 to 5 mg/kg/day.

Note: *All cytotoxic drugs require careful adherence to monitoring guidelines.*

CROHN'S DISEASE

Crohn's disease is a chronic, granulomatous, inflammatory bowel disease that rarely can involve the vulva and groin, either primarily or secondarily. The etiology is unknown. Proposed causes include an unrecognized infectious agent or a disturbed immunologic reaction to an intestinal organism in a genetically predisposed individual.

Crohn's disease commonly occurs between the ages of 20 to 30 years. Of women with Crohn's disease, 2% have associated vulvar involvement.

Anogenital patterns of Crohn's disease include the following:

Contiguous: in this form there is a direct extension from the involved intestine with the formation of sinuses/fistulae to the skin or other organs

Metastatic (noncontiguous): very rare, with ulcers and swelling in the vulvar area

Nonspecific mucocutaneous lesions: aphthous ulcers, pyoderma gangrenosum

The patient presents with painful, thickened swelling of the vulvar or perianal area with or without draining sinuses/fistulous tracts. If present, these tracts may or may not connect directly to the gastrointestinal tract. Simple painful swelling may be the sole complaint, but ulcerated lesions cause pain and dyspareunia.

Physical Examination

The physical examination varies depending on the type of vulvar involvement. Labial edema may be localized or generalized and may or may not be inflammatory (Fig. 16-6, *A*). The severity of erosions and ulceration varies. The classic ulcerations associated with this condition are called "knife cut" linear fissures and are located along the labiocrural fold (Fig. 16-6, *B*). The ulcers may be solitary, deep, and necrotic and may lead to fistulae (Fig. 16-6, *C*). The area of involvement may extend to the perineal and perianal area.

Note: *The cutaneous changes can occur before the onset of bowel symptoms, and inguinal lymphadenopathy is absent in this situation.*

Diagnosis

The diagnosis is clinical. Biopsy shows the typical granulomatous change. Differential diagnoses include hidradenitis suppurativa, Behcet's disease, lymphogranuloma venereum, granuloma inguinale, and genitourinary tuberculosis. In a patient with biopsy-proven granulomatous vulvitis, consider Crohn's disease.

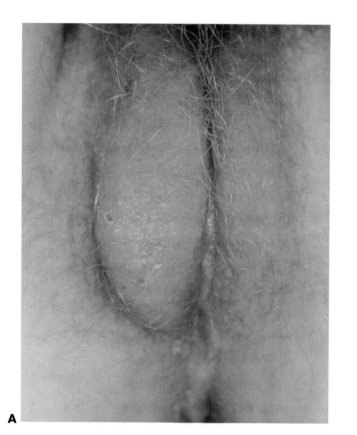

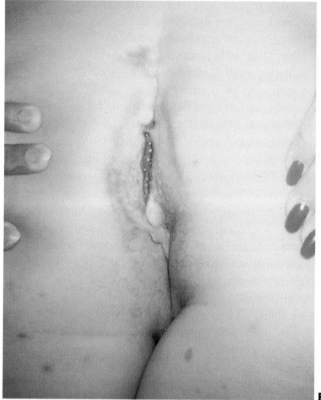

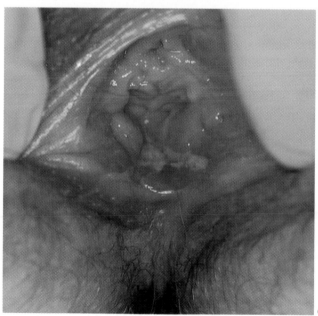

FIG. 16-6

Crohn's Disease. **A**, Labial edema and induration in Crohn's disease. **B**, "Knife cut" ulcer of perianal area/perineum in Crohn's disease. **C**, Ulcer with necrotic base on the perihymenal area at the 6 o'clock position in Crohn's disease.

(**A**, Courtesy Dr. M. Moyal-Barracco.)

Treatment

Treatment depends on the extent of involvement of the perineal area and the associated bowel disease. A team consisting of a dermatologist, gynecologist, and gastroenterologist is needed to successfully manage the condition.

Local care for erosive and blistering diseases of the vulva is covered in Appendices D and I.

Topical steroids must be superpotent, for example, clobetasol or halobetasol 0.05% ointment twice a day. A bland barrier ointment or paste can be used for protection. Intralesional triamcinolone (Kenalog-10) diluted 1:1 with saline injected using a 30-gauge needle is useful for small ulcers, erosions, and swollen granulomatous areas.

Specific therapy is best directed at control of the gastrointestinal disease and, ultimately, bowel resection for the control of severe cases must be considered. The following drugs can be prescribed:

Metronidazole 250 to 500 mg tid (with alcohol avoidance)

Prednisone 50 to 60 mg/day and slowly decreasing

Sulfasalazine 500 mg, 2 tablets tid to qid and up to 4 tablets tid to qid in severe cases

Azathioprine 1 to 2 mg/kg/day

Cyclosporine

FIXED DRUG ERUPTION

Fixed drug eruption is a cell-mediated allergic drug reaction causing formation initially of a single lesion and occasionally multiple lesions. It recurs in the same site on reexposure. This is an uncommon condition on the vulva. Barbiturates, acetaminophen, phenolphthalein, sulfonamide, tetracycline, and nonsteroidal antiinflammatories are the most common offending drugs.

The main complaint is burning in the area of involvement, but some cases are asymptomatic or just mildly itchy. The symptoms recur every time the offending chemical is ingested.

Physical Examination

Initially there is a well-circumscribed erythematous circular or oval plaque. It may swell, blister, or become eroded (Fig. 16-7). It fades over 7 to 10 days

after discontinuation of the precipitant, leaving hyperpigmentation.

Diagnosis

Made on the basis of the clinical appearance and history, diagnosis may be confirmed by challenge with the offending chemical. Differential diagnoses include recurrent herpes simplex, lichen planus, and bullous pemphigoid.

Treatment

Identifying the offending chemical and stopping its use is the basis of treatment. Bland symptomatic topical care is usually all that is needed.

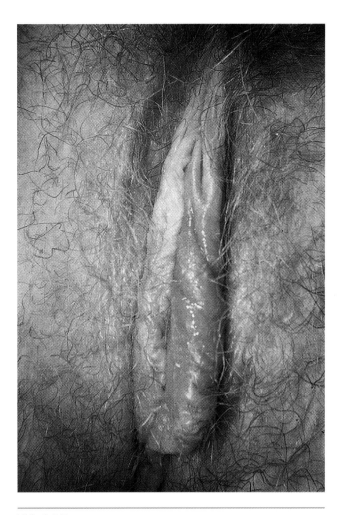

FIG. 16-7

Recurrent red, swollen, burning lesion localized always to the same area of the labium minor caused by pyridium in a fixed drug reaction.

INTERTRIGO

Intertrigo is a mechanical inflammatory dermatosis in the skin folds caused by friction, sweating, heat, and occlusion. Two skin surfaces rubbing together, with the addition of sweat, results in maceration, then dermatitis, fissuring, and secondary infection. It is worsened by obesity, tight synthetic clothing, incontinence, and any factors that increase heat, sweating, or wetness in the area.

Patients present with itching, burning, and malodor in the labiocrural fold, inguinal fold, and in the fold under the abdominal pannus.

Physical Examination

Erythema, maceration, fissuring, and sometimes frank weeping may be accompanied by considerable odor (Fig. 16-8). The surrounding skin may show reactive post-inflammatory hyperpigmentation.

Diagnosis

The clinical pattern makes the diagnosis. Differential diagnoses include the following conditions that may be associated with an intertriginous component: psoriasis, seborrheic dermatitis, lichen sclerosus, and familial benign pemphigus (Hailey-Hailey disease).

Treatment

The aim is to stop the friction. Patients should avoid tight, hot, synthetic clothing and keep the area cool and dry. Diabetes and obesity should always be aggressively managed.

For mild involvement, gentle cleansing may be all that is necessary. Washing with triclosan 0.5% cleanser or chlorhexidine 0.05% solution, rinsing thoroughly, patting the area dry, and using an absorbent powder such as Zeasorb helps to relieve the symptoms. Hydrocortisone 1% powder in miconazole 2% cream can be applied in a thin film as necessary.

For severe irritation, use Buro-Sol compresses bid (see Appendix C). For the breakdown under a heavy abdominal pannus, use a thin 100% cotton tea towel or cotton flannelette square. Place against the skin in the fold to absorb the moisture. Change twice a day to stop the friction and prevent recurrences of the problem.

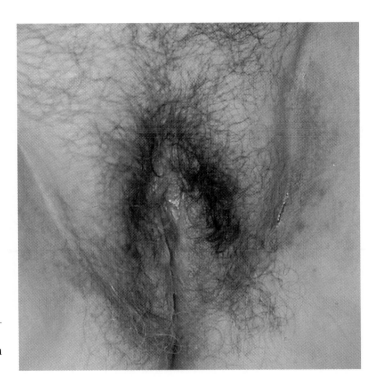

FIG. 16-8
Acute intertrigo with erythema and fissuring in labiocrural fold.

FOX-FORDYCE DISEASE

Fox-Fordyce disease is an uncommon, very itchy papular eruption of the axillary and anogenital regions, related to apocrine sweat duct occlusion.[1] The etiology is unknown. The apocrine sweat gland ducts become plugged, resulting in papular inflammation. It is more common in women than men and more common in black individuals.

Itching and irritation in the vulvar area and axillae can be acute, intense, and sometimes cyclic. The itching may improve with pregnancy and oral contraceptives. This annoying condition starts in puberty and ends with menopause.

Physical Examination

Monomorphous, skin-colored to slightly hyperpigmented, dome-shaped folliculopapules are observed in the axillae and in the anogenital region, mainly involving the mons pubis and labia majora areas (Fig. 16-9).

Diagnosis

Clinical presentation and biopsy define the diagnosis. Differential diagnoses include syringomata and folliculopapular lichen simplex chronicus.

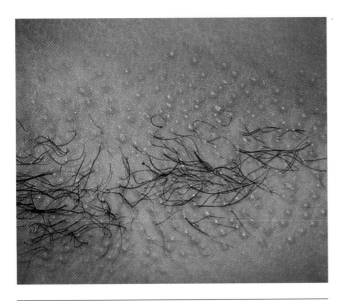

FIG. 16-9
Dome-shaped, follicular papules in Fox-Fordyce disease. (Courtesy Dr. P. Lynch.)

Treatment

Local. Cold gel packs are useful when the patient's itching is intense. Pramoxine HCl 1%, menthol ¼%, camphor ¼% in a cream base 3 to 4 times a day can be used as a nonspecific antipruritic.

Specific Treatment. Oral contraceptives[2] can be very effective. Hydrocortisone 1% cream or ointment with ¼% camphor used bid to tid prn is prescribed for mild cases. Superpotent corticosteroids, for example clobetasol or halobetasol 0.05% cream, twice a day for 10 to 14 days intermittently may be needed for resistant cases. Caution the patient that overuse can cause thinning of the skin. Topical tretinoin (Retin-A) 0.025% or 0.05% cream is another alternative provided there is no excessive irritation.

For severe cases, surgical excision is an option of last resort.

HIDRADENITIS SUPPURATIVA

Hidradenitis suppurativa is a chronic, acneiform eruption involving the axillary, inframammary, and anogenital areas manifested by deep painful cystic nodules, sinuses, and scarring.[3] This is an acute and chronic follicular occlusive process, just like acne vulgaris, and is analogous to acne mechanica. It is related to androgen excess, onsets at puberty, and typically flares with menstruation. It can be improved with antiandrogen treatment. Familial cases indicate that genetic factors also play a role. It is worse with sweating and heat, particularly in those individuals who are obese. It is far more common in women than in men (3:1).

Lesions onset after puberty as painful "boils" in the groin, axillae, or both. These typically flare with menstruation. A single lesion may be recurrent for months or years, or the patient may have crops of lesions coming and going. Some patients have only occasional lesions; others are severely and chronically involved.

Physical Examination

Erythematous acneiform papules, nodules, and cysts are scattered among multiheaded comedones (Fig. 16-10). The cysts may rupture spontaneously, leaving sinuses draining purulent yellow material that is usually sterile. Groups of nodules may form

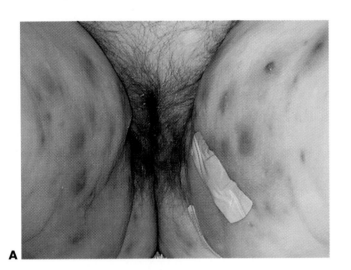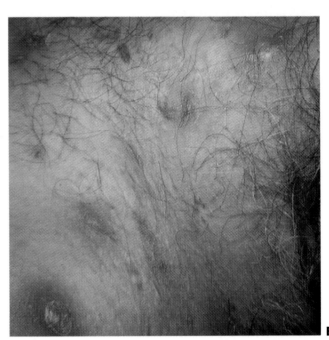

A   B

FIG. 16-10
A, Multiple acneiform papules and nodules of hidradenitis suppurativa. **B**, Scars, nodules, and cysts in right inguinal area in hidradenitis suppurativa.

conglobate lesions with resulting interconnecting sinus tracts. These sinuses can start anywhere in the anogenital region and may track beyond the mons pubis, past the crural folds, and onto the thighs, perineum, and buttocks. The resulting scarring can be extensive and destructive.

Diagnosis
Diagnosis is clinical. Differential diagnoses include bacterial infections (boils and carbuncles), Crohn's disease, and lymphogranuloma venereum.

Treatment
Treatment can be very difficult and requires a dermatologist. A surgeon will be needed for extensive disease.

Avoid any pressure and friction from panty hose, girdles, or other garments rubbing in the area. The use of ventilated cotton clothing (e.g., cotton boxer shorts) is essential.

The patient is instructed in gentle cleansing with triclosan solution once or twice a day. Topical 2% clindamycin in a mixture of isopropyl alcohol and propylene glycol bid is prescribed to avoid minor folliculitis.

An intralesional injection of triamcinolone 40 mg/mL (Kenalog-40) diluted 1:1:1 with lincomycin (Lincocin) sterile solution 300 mg/mL and sterile saline is injected with a 30-gauge needle into early individual nonfluctuant cysts every 2 to 3 weeks.

Antiandrogen treatment may be necessary.[4] Newer oral contraceptives with desogestrel or norgestimate provide less androgenic effects. Spironolactone 100 to 150 mg a day can be added to these or to regular birth control pills for additional or long-term control. In Europe a truly androgen-

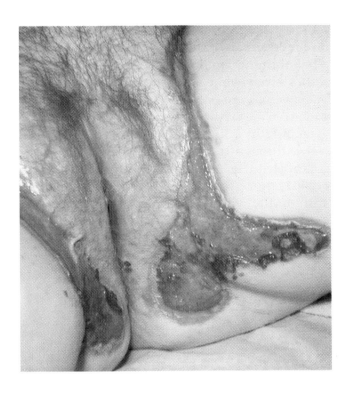

FIG. 16-11

The type of extensive surgery needed for multiple connecting sinuses in long-standing draining hidradenitis suppurativa. This patient had this surgery at age 18, after 6 years of problems and five other limited (and ultimately unsuccessful) surgical procedures to remove areas of sinus formation under general anesthetic. Her disease is quiet 10 years later on antiandrogens.

blocking combination of ethinyl estradiol 35 µg and cyproterone acetate 2 mg (Diane 35) is available and is very effective.

Tetracycline 500 mg bid to qid or minocycline 100 to 200 mg/day is used as for acne vulgaris.

For severe disease, isotretinoin (Accutane) 1 mg/kg/day for 16 to 20 weeks or longer (pregnancy must be avoided) can be prescribed.

Surgery for this condition must be directed at thorough detection and unroofing of all interconnecting sinuses.[5] This technique results in quite acceptable scars from healing by secondary intent. Minor incision and drainage of these lesions simply results in recurrences. En bloc excision results in unnecessary tissue destruction and may miss or transect some sinus tracts. An experienced dermatologic or general surgeon is invaluable. For persistent lesions, surgery is the only option (Fig. 16-11).

PSORIASIS

Psoriasis is a common, hereditary, papulosquamous disease of the skin characterized on most of the skin surface by typical well-defined, reddish papules and plaques with a silvery white scale.[1,6] In the inguinal and crural areas the characteristic scale may be missing, a variant called psoriasis inversus or flexural psoriasis.

The exact etiology is still speculative. It is a condition of epidermal hyperproliferation and dermal inflammation, probably the result of dysregulation of keratinocyte formation complicated by disordered immunity in genetically predisposed individuals. Trauma, whether physical (scratching), chemical (soaps and perfumes), or biologic (bacterial or yeast superinfection) triggers more psoriatic activity, a process known as Koebnerization. The end result is rapidly turning over keratinocytes and inflammation.

Irritation or itching is the presenting complaint in the vulvar area. The patient may or may not have a history or obvious lesions in the other typical areas of psoriasis—scalp, elbows, knees, ears, and nails. When the perineum and gluteal cleft are involved, fissuring, pain, and burning may occur. Symptoms are made worse with stress, heat, humidity, the use of sanitary napkins, tight synthetic clothing, and irritating soaps.

Physical Examination

The picture is variable. Papulosquamous lesions can be scattered throughout the mons pubis and labia majora areas. In some cases, there are thin salmon pink lesions of varying size and shape with minor scaling. In other cases, thick confluent plaques cover all of the labia majora and the mons pubis forming almost a solid horseshoe pattern with a silvery-white adherent scale (Fig. 16-12, *A*). The inverse form occurs in a bilaterally symmetric pattern, with erythema, maceration, and fissuring extending in a linear fashion from the inguinal crease through the labiocrural fold and into the gluteal cleft (Fig. 16-12, *B*). The gluteal cleft fissuring may be very difficult to manage. The mucosal area of the vulva is not involved. Secondary changes such as excoriations, lichenification, crusting, and bacterial and yeast infections confuse the classic picture in many patients.

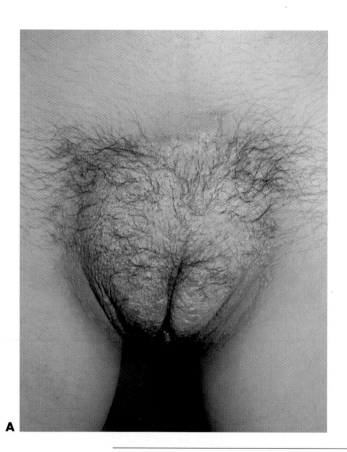

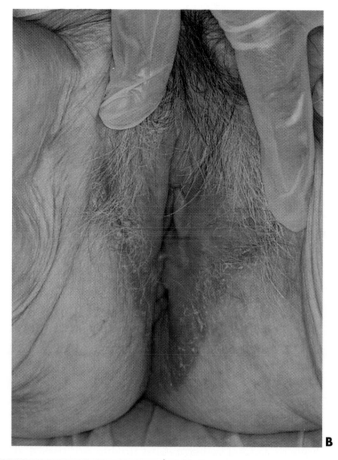

A

B

FIG. 16-12

Psoriasis. **A,** Thick plaque of psoriasis with silver adherent scale. **B,** Red, macerated psoriasis extending from the vulva to the perianal area.

Diagnosis

Diagnosis is clinical and should include a family history. Biopsy is seldom needed. Check other parts of the patient's body (scalp, ears, elbows, knees, nails for pitting, etc.) for typical psoriasis to confirm the diagnosis. Differential diagnoses include seborrheic dermatitis, monilial or dermatophyte infection, lichen simplex chronicus, and contact dermatitis.

Treatment

Nonspecific. Patients need to be instructed to avoid trauma, including all irritating soaps, lotions, detergents, and synthetic clothing. To control the itch, patients can use ice or cold gel packs.

Cleansing should be gentle, without the use of a wash cloth and with a product such as Cetaphil cleanser or Basis soap. If eczematous, recommend the patient use sitz baths or compresses with Buro-Sol 1:40 using cool water once or twice a day. The area should be patted (not rubbed) dry (see Appendices C and H).

An antihistamine—hydroxyzine or doxepin 25 to 75 mg qhs—may be prescribed for the itch.

Specific. For mild to moderate psoriasis:
Gently cleanse daily.

Desonide 0.05% ointment twice a day or 1% hydrocortisone in pramoxine cream bid × 2 to 3 weeks, then a milder topical prn.

For severe psoriasis:

Clobetasol or halobetasol 0.05% ointment bid × 2 weeks, once daily × 2 weeks, then Monday, Wednesday, Friday × 2 weeks.

Alternate with low-potency topicals and switch to intermittent low-potency preparations for long-term care.

Calcipotriene (Dovonex) 50 µg/g ointment[7] can be used as an alternate to topical steroids, bid × 3 to 6 weeks, or consider the calcipotriol in the morning and topical steroid at nighttime.

For marked thickness:

Triamcinolone acetonide (Kenalog-10) diluted one part with two parts of normal saline for injection using a 30-gauge needle. The use of EMLA, a topical anesthestic cream applied in a thick film under plastic wrap for 15 to 20 minutes, makes this procedure almost painless. It can be repeated at 2 to 3 week intervals.

For concurrent secondary infection:

To cover yeast and/or bacterial superinfection, it may be best to combine antiyeast cream (e.g., ketoconazole 2%) with an antibacterial (e.g., mupirocin ointment). Use these with the topical steroids in stubborn cases.

For severe generalized psoriasis:

Consult with a dermatologist to consider systemic therapy with retinoids, methotrexate, or even cyclosporine, subjects beyond this text.

LICHEN PLANUS

Lichen planus is a relatively common condition that presents as a papulosquamous skin eruption with or without mucous membrane involvement. It probably involves the vulva much more commonly than previously suggested,[8-10] involving patients 30 to 60 years old. The cause is unknown. It is probably a disorder of altered immunity. Some drugs induce lichen planus–like (lichenoid) eruptions. Synonyms for vulvovaginal lichen planus are erosive vaginal lichen planus, desquamative inflammatory vaginitis, vulvovaginal-gingival syndrome, ulcerative lichen planus, and LP.

The disease occurs in three patterns: (1) The papulosquamous form presents with the five P's—pruritic, purple, polyhedral, papules, and plaques—and classically involves the wrists and ankles. Here the vulvar involvement is part of a generalized disease with the papules and plaques on the labia and mons pubis. There is no atrophy or scarring. (2) The vulvovaginal gingival syndrome is an erosive and destructive form of lichen planus involving the mucous membranes of the mouth and vulvovaginal area with atrophy and scarring. (3) The hypertrophic is the least common form. It presents with extensive white scarring of the periclitoral area extending along the interlabial sulcus to the introitus with variable degrees of hyperkeratosis. It looks like lichen sclerosus but is treatment resistant.

There is a history of severe itching in the papulosquamous form but limited involvement in the vulvar area. The patient may be unaware of involvement in either the mouth or vulvar area (both areas should always be checked). Likewise the hypertrophic form may be very itchy. Dyspareunia is a problem when there is scarring.

In the erosive or ulcerative form, itching is rare but pain, burning, and irritation occur and may be responsible for severe dyspareunia and dysuria. Extensive vaginal involvement results in a purulent, malodorous discharge. The dyspareunia leads to depression, anger, frustration, and marital distress. This can severely compromise the therapeutic relationship.

Physical Examination

In the papulosquamous form the pruritic, polyhedral, purple papules and plaques are rarely found on the mons pubis, thighs, and labia majora. The trauma of scratching spreads the papules, a phenomenon termed *Koebnerization.*

In the erosive form there may initially be no erosions, just simply tiny white 1 mm papules, often in a linear or fernlike or lacy reticular pattern on the buccal mucosa or along the edges of the vulvar trigone (Figs. 16-13, *A* and *B*). The degree of erosion is variable in either site. In extensive disease the whole vulvar trigone and vaginal area

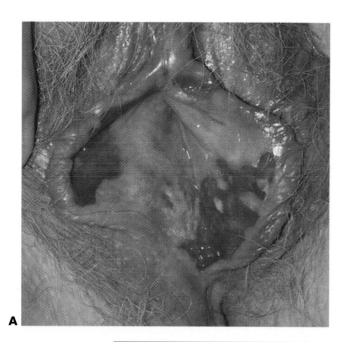

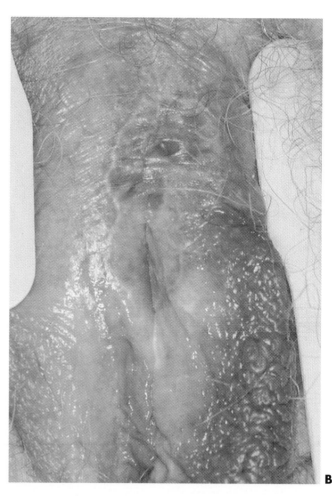

A　　　　　　　　　　　　　　　　　　　　　　　**B**

FIG. 16-13
Lichen Planus. **A**, Eroded ulcers of the vulva in lichen planus. **B**, Lacy reticulated pattern of lichen planus with periclitoral scarring in a 71-year-old woman who has had oral lichen planus for 10 to 15 years, cutaneous lichen planus of arms and legs for 18 months, and bouts of erosive vaginal lichen planus with scarring and partial vaginal stenosis.

may be denuded and open with a weeping discharge (Fig. 16-13, *C*). Over time there is scarring with loss of the clitoris and labia minora with vaginal adhesions. Ultimately there is gradual but progressive destruction of the vagina. This form is very chronic, destructive, debilitating, and difficult to treat. The hypertrophic form looks very much like lichen sclerosus. When chronic, there is burying of the clitoris, loss of labia minora, and introital stenosis.

Diagnosis

For the papular form and nonerosive disease, the clinical diagnosis can be confirmed by biopsy.

In extensive erosive disease biopsy may help but is not always confirmatory. Demonstration of typical oral changes carries more diagnostic weight than biopsy.

Differential diagnoses of the papulosquamous form include psoriasis, dermatophyte infection, lichen simplex chronicus and lichen sclerosus. For erosive disease, the differential diagnoses include lichen sclerosus, cicatricial pemphigoid, pemphigus, lupus erythematosus and bullous pemphigoid.

Treatment

Treatment requires the expertise of a dermatologist or gynecologist. No single agent has proven universally effective. Treatments are listed in order of preference.

1. Papulosquamous disease: Aim to manage the itching and the scratching as in lichen simplex chronicus (see appropriate section).
2. Erosive lichen planus of the vulva (Appendices D and I):

   Avoidance of irritants

   Cool, ventilated clothing

   Pain control

       Acetaminophen plus codeine

       Topical EMLA may be utilized

   Sitz baths or compresses with Burow's solution 1:40

Specific Treatment

Topical steroid

    Clobetasol, halobetasol 0.05% ointment bid

    Secondary candidiasis or bacterial infection must be managed appropriately.

Intravaginal steroid

    Clobetasol or halobetasol 0.05% ointment 2 g intravaginally qhs

    Clobetasol or halobetasol 0.05% ointment mixed 50:50 with bioadhesive compound (Replens Vaginal Moisturizer) 2 to 4 g, q2-4h

    Hydrocortisone acetate in a foam (Cortifoam) using 40 to 80 mg qhs or in suppository form (Cortiment) 20 to 40 mg qhs

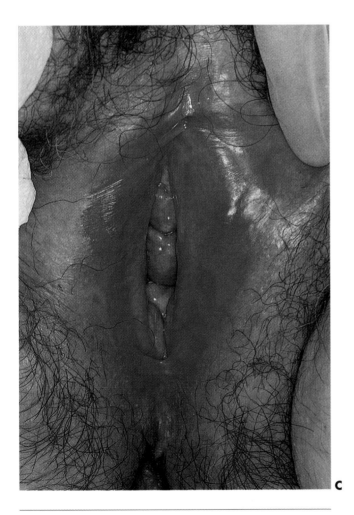

C

FIG. 16-13, cont'd
C, Extensice erosion of the vulva with loss of the clitoris and labia minora.

Other

Oral prednisone 50 to 60 mg/day, gradually decreasing

Intralesional triamcinolone 10 mg/mL (Kenalog-10) diluted 1:2 with saline and repeated every 2 to 3 weeks using a 30-gauge needle

Chloroquine phosphate 250-500 mg/day or hydroxychloroquine sulfate (Plaquenil) 200 to 400 mg/day

Azathioprine has been used

Oral retinoids—acitretin 10 to 30 mg/day or etretinate 25 mg 3 to 5 day/week given with fatty foods—a major teratogen

Topical cyclosporine is investigational[11]

3. Hypertrophic disease: Use the same local care as above plus topical superpotent and intralesional steroids (20 mg/mL triamcinolone may be needed). Oral retinoids may be very helpful.

Special Situations. For vaginal vault adhesions and scarring, Lucite vaginal dilators[12] coated with corticosteroid ointment or foam are used two or three times a day depending on the patient's tolerance. The area can be pretreated with EMLA. If suppression of menses is required, use medroxyprogesterone (Depo-Provera) 150 mg q3mon.

Emotional Support. These patients need help and understanding. They must be involved, along with their partner, in psychosexual counseling for this difficult and chronic condition. Realistic expectations must be defined to avoid disappointment with therapy and dissatisfaction with the therapists.

LUPUS ERYTHEMATOSUS

Lupus erythematosus (LE) is a multisystem disorder. Numerous associated autoimmune phenomena affect the connective tissue of many organ systems. Mucosal surfaces, usually the mouth, may be affected.[13] Genital involvement is uncommon. The etiology is unknown. Autoimmunity plays an important role in pathogenesis. This is modified by a variety of hereditary and environmental factors. It is most common in females and in the black population.

Lupus is classified according to the degree of systemic involvement. Vulvar manifestations may be different in each type.

Discoid Lupus Erythematosus— Chronic Cutaneous Lupus Erythematosus

In this form, only the skin (and rarely mucous membrane) is involved. Vulvar involvement is rare. On exposed skin, there is photosensitivity, resulting in scarring skin lesions. There may be no symptoms. Of these patients, 1% to 5% may develop systemic lupus erythematosus.

Physical Examination

Typically the lesion is a scarred plaque of variable size with marked peripheral hyperpigmentation, with or without central ulceration, anywhere on the vulva or perineum (Fig. 16-14).

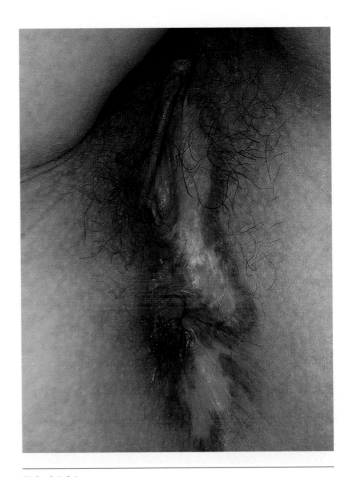

FIG. 16-14
Well-circumscribed scarred plaque of discoid lupus erythematosus on left perineum extending from interlabial sulcus to anus. Note central hypopigmentation and scarring with hyperpigmented border.

Subacute or Acute Lupus Erythematosus

In this variant there is systemic involvement. In the subacute form of lupus erythematosus the involvement is less serious, compared to the acute form in which the condition can be life-threatening. These patients may have vulvar involvement with an asymptomatic lacy pattern like lichen planus, or painful punched-out ulcers on the vestibule or in the vagina with variable scarring. Very rarely there is an erosive, destructive vulvovaginitis as in lichen planus.

Diagnosis

Clinical pattern, histopathology and immunohistopathology define the diagnosis. Differential diagnoses include genital ulcers or erosive vulvovaginitis (see Appendix F).

Treatment

Teamwork is needed with dermatology, rheumatology, and internal medicine expertise, depending on the systems involved. Patient education and support are very important.

Ulcerative disease is covered in Appendices D and I. For limited disease recommend the following:

Gentle cleansing

Avoid irritants—pads, clothing, topical products, etc.

Superpotent steroids—halobetasol or clobetasol 0.05% ointment bid × 3 to 4 weeks and reassess

Intralesional triamcinolone (Kenalog-10) 10 mg/mL diluted 1:2 with saline, injected with a 30-gauge needle, repeated in 3 to 4 weeks

Antimalarials—chloroquine 250 to 500 mg or hydroxychloroquine (Plaquenil) 200 to 400 mg daily with appropriate eye examinations

The treatment of systemic/extensive subacute or acute lupus erythematosus with gold, azathioprine, and cortisone is beyond the scope of this text.

VULVAR VESTIBULITIS SYNDROME

This syndrome consists of severe pain on vestibular contact or attempt at vaginal entry plus point tenderness and erythema in the vulvar vestibule around the openings of the minor vestibular glands.[14-18] The common age of occurrence is 35 to 40 years. The etiology is unknown. Possible etiologic factors suggested as resulting in vestibulitis include:

Contactants—Irritants like calcium oxalate in the urine, and chemicals like 5-fluorouracil

Trauma—Laser, previous surgery, lack of lubrication

Infections—In some series up to 80% of patients have had candida preceding the onset. Candidiasis organisms have been proposed as a direct cause or as an indirect cause resulting from local vulvar hypersensitivity. Human papilloma virus was considered to play a role, but this has not been confirmed.

Other—Genetic, hormonal

Classically, there is vulvar burning and pain when the area is touched, as with wiping, intercourse, or insertion of a tampon. The pain is enough to make intercourse uncomfortable or completely impossible. There may be associated deep pain from secondary vaginismus. Varying degrees of sexual dysfunction may be understandably followed by depression and anxiety (Table 16-1).

Physical Examination

Erythema surrounds the vulvovestibular gland openings and may extend around the vulvar trigone (Fig. 16-15). When a cotton-tipped applicator gently touches these areas, there is an exquisitely, painful response. There may be marked secondary vaginismus, but examination of the vagina shows no vaginitis.

Diagnosis

Diagnosis is clinical, other causes of chronic vulvar pain having been ruled out. (See section on vulvodynia.) The diagnosis rests on the pain, not the erythema. Normal women may have erythema in

Table 16-1   Staging of Vestibulitis

Stage of Vestibulitis	Degree of pain	Sexual Dysfunction
Stage I	Mild	Sex possible
Stage II	Moderate	Sex uncommon
Stage III	Severe	No sex

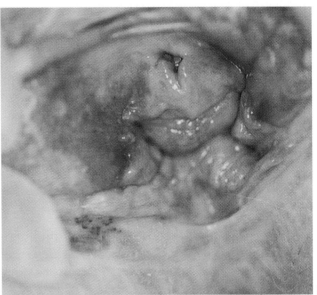

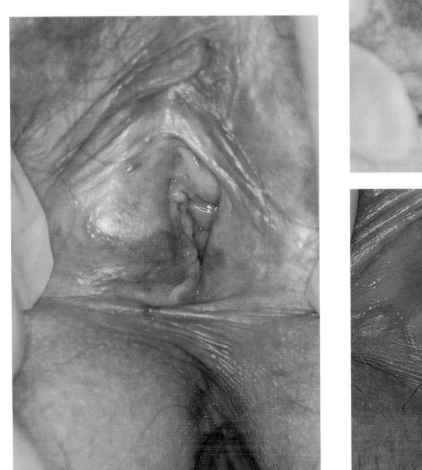

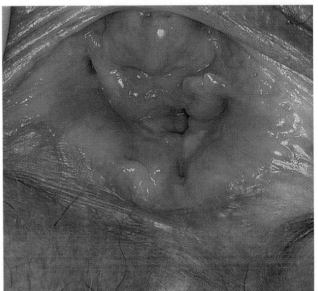

FIG. 16-15

Vulvar Vestibulitis. **A,** Redness localized to right Bartholin duct opening and, below it, vulvar vestibulitis. **B,** Discrete localized red periglandular erythema in vulvar vestibulitis in a 60-year-old woman. **C,** Diffuse erythema in perihymenal area in vulvar vestibulitis.

the vulvovestibular area without tenderness or discomfort. Differential diagnoses include cyclic monilial vulvovaginitis and dysesthetic vulvodynia (painful erosive causes of vulvar disease are ruled out on physical examination).

Treatment

Management is best coordinated with a knowledgeable dermatologist or gynecologist. The treatment of this condition is evolving as specialists in this field develop new concepts of pathogenesis and new medical and surgical therapeutic approaches.

Nonsurgical. Emotional support is very important and should be combined with patient education. Instruct the patient to avoid irritating soaps, detergents, and sanitary napkins and to wear ventilated cotton clothing. Also recommend gentle cleansing with Cetaphil cleanser and a mild lubricant—light mineral oil or olive oil—to be applied daily. The following medications are prescribed in various combinations:

Conjugated estrogen cream 0.625 mg/g or estradiol 0.01% cream can be used bid for atrophy or dryness

Ketoconazole 2% cream tid for 6 to 8 months— use if history of candidiasis.

Calcium oxalate–restricted diet for at least 6 to 9 months along with calcium citrate (200 mg Ca^{++}/950 mg citrate) 2 tablets po tid[19] to decrease calcium oxalate crystals in urine.

EMLA applied under Saran wrap for 20 minutes will relieve pain for 1½ to 2 hours at a time and may allow intermittent sexual intercourse

Amitriptyline 10 to 150 mg qhs or trazodone 25 to 150 mg qhs or sertraline 50 to 150 mg/day. Start low and go slow.

Biofeedback[20] techniques and physiotherapy for the pelvic floor muscles must be utilized if vaginismus is present. Active patient cooperation is essential. Psychosexual counseling is also very important for these patients. Treat *Candida* infections aggressively.

Note: *Up to 60% of patients improve with amitriptyline 10 to 75 mg/day for 6 months.*

Surgical. For selected patients who do not have significant vaginismus and who are unresponsive to conservative measures after 1 year, surgery[21] should be considered. Vestibulectomy with vaginal advancement has a success rate of 83% to 88%. The outcome is better in those who have had a shorter duration of pain.

REFERENCES

Fox-Fordyce Disease
1. Lynch PJ, Edwards L: *Genital dermatology,* Baltimore, 1995, Churchill Livingstone.
2. Kronthal HL, Pomeranz JR, Sitomer G: Fox-Fordyce disease: treatment with an oral contraceptive, *Arch Dermatol* 91(3):243-245, 1965.

Hidradenitis Suppurativa
3. Wilkinson EJ, Stone IK: *Atlas of vulvar disease,* Baltimore, 1995, Williams & Wilkins.
4. Camisa C, Sexton C, Freidman C: Treatment of hidradenitis suppurativa with combination hypothalamic-pituitary-ovarian and adrenal suppression, *J Reprod Med* 34(8):543-546, 1989.
5. Banerjee AK: Surgical treatment of hidradenitis suppurativa, *Br J Surg* 79(9):863-866, 1992.

Psoriasis
6. Pincus SH: Vulvar dermatoses and pruritus vulvae, *Dermatol Clin* 10(2):297-308, 1992.
7. Kienbaum S, Lehmann P, Ruzicka T: Topical calcipotriol in the treatment of intertriginous psoriasis, *Br J Dermatol* 135(4):647-650, 1996.

Lichen Planus
8. Edwards L: Vulvar lichen planus, *Arch Dermatol* 125(12):1677-1680, 1989.
9. Eisen D: The vulvovaginal-gingival syndrome of lichen planus: the clinical characteristics of 22 patients, *Arch Dermatol* 130(11):1379-1382, 1994.
10. Lewis FM, Shah M, Harrington CI: Vulval involvement in lichen planus: a study of 37 women, *Br J Dermatol* 135(1):89-91, 1996.

11. Borrego L, Ruiz-Rodriguez R, Ortiz de Frutos J, et al: Vulvar lichen planus treated with topical cyclosporine, *Arch Dermatol* 129(6):794, 1993.

12. Walsh DS, Dunn CL, Konzelman J Jr, et al: A vaginal prosthetic device as an aid in treating ulcerative lichen planus of the mucous membrane, *Arch Dermatol* 131(3):265-267, 1995.

Lupus Erythematosus

13. Burge SM, Frith PA, Juniper RP, Wojnarowska F: Mucosal involvement in systemic and chronic cutaneous lupus erythematosus, *Br J Dermatol* 121(6):727-741, 1989 and 131(3):265-267, 1989.

Vulvar Vestibulitis Syndrome

14. Bergeron S, Binik YM, Khalife S, Pagidas K: Vulvar vestibulitis syndrome: a critical review, *Clinical J Pain* 13(1):27-42, 1997.

15. Mann MS, Kaufman RH, Brown D Jr, Adam E: Vulvar vestibulitis: significant clinical variables and treatment outcome, *Obstet Gynecol* 79(1):122-125, 1992.

16. Marinoff SC, Turner ML: Vulvar vestibulitis syndrome, *Dermatol Clin* 10(2):435-444, 1992.

17. Morrison GD, Adams SJ, Curnow JS, et al: A preliminary study of topical ketoconazole in vulvar vestibulitis syndrome, *J Dermatol Treat* 7:219-221, 1996.

18. Paavonen J: Diagnosis and treatment of vulvodynia, *Ann Med* 27(2):175-181, 1995.

19. Solomons CC, Melmed MH, Heitler SM: Calcium citrate for vulvar vestibulitis: a case report, *J Reprod Med* 36(12):879-882, 1991.

20. Glazer HI: Treatment of vulvar vestibulitis syndrome with electromyographic biofeedback of pelvic floor musculature, *J Reprod Med* 40(4):283-290, 1995.

21. Goetsch MF: Simplified surgical revision of the vulvar vestibule for vulvar vestibulitis, *Am J Obstet Gynecol* 174(6):1701-1707, 1996.

SUGGESTED READINGS

Lichen Simplex Chronicus

Lynch PJ, Edwards L: *Genital dermatology,* New York, 1995, Churchill Livingstone, 34-41.

Pincus SH: Vulvar dermatoses and pruritus vulvae, *Dermatol Clin* 10(2):297-308, 1992.

Atopic Dermatitis

Cooper KD: Atopic dermatitis: recent trends in pathogenesis and therapy, *J Invest Dermatol* 102(1):128-137, 1994.

Lynch PJ, Edwards L: *Genital dermatology,* New York, 1994, Churchill Livingstone, 27-55.

Pincus SH: Vulvar dermatoses and pruritus vulvae, *Dermatol Clin* 10(2):297-308, 1992.

Ridley CM: *The vulva,* Edinburgh, 1988, Churchill Livingstone, 138-211.

Wilkinson EJ, Stone IK: *Atlas of vulvar disease,* Baltimore, 1995, Williams & Wilkins, 80-81.

Contact Dermatitis

Lynch PJ, Edwards L: *Genital dermatology,* New York, 1994, Churchill Livingstone, 27-34.

Marren P, Wojnarowska F, Powell S: Allergic contact dermatitis and vulvar dermatoses, *Br J Dermatol* 126(1):52-56, 1992.

Pincus SH: Vulvar dermatoses and pruritus vulvae, *Dermatol Clin* 10(2):297-308, 1992.

Aphthosis

Jorizzo JL, Taylor RS, Schmalstieg FC, et al: Complex aphthosis: a forme fruste of Behcet's syndrome? *J Am Acad Dermatol* 13(1):80-84, 1985.

Behçet's Disease

Mangelsdorf HC, White WL, Jorizzo JL: Behçet's disease: report of twenty-five patients from the United States with prominent mucocutaneous involvement, *J Am Acad Dermatol* 34(5 Pt 1):745-750, 1996.

Miyachi Y, Taniguchi S, Ozaki M, Horio T: Colchicine in the treatment of the cutaneous manifestations of Behçet's disease, *Br J Dermatol* 104(1):67-69, 1981.

Mizushima Y: Behçet's disease, *Curr Opin Rheumatol* 3(1):32-35, 1991.

Turner ML: Vulvar manifestations of systemic diseases, *Dermatol Clin* 10(2):445-58, 1992.

Crohn's Disease

Burgdorf W: Cutaneous manifestations of Crohn's disease, *J Am Acad Dermatol* 5(6):689-695, 1981.

Donaldson LB: Crohn's disease: its gynecologic aspect, *Am J Obstet Gynecol* 15;131(2):196-202, 1978.

Werlin SL, Esterly MB, Oechler H: Crohn's disease presenting as a unilateral labial hypertrophy, *J Am Acad Dermatol* 27(5 Pt 2):893-895, 1992.

Wilkinson EJ, Stone IK: *Atlas of vulvar disease,* Baltimore, 1995, Williams & Wilkins, 178-181.

Fixed Drug Eruption

Sehgal VH, Gangwani OP: Genital fixed drug eruptions, *Genitourin Med* 62(1):56-58, 1986.

Sehgal VN, Gangwani OP: Fixed drug eruption: current concepts, *Int J Dermatol* 26(2):67-74, 1987.

BENIGN FAMILIAL PEMPHIGUS

Benign familial pemphigus is a rare, autosomal dominant, superficial blistering disease of the intertriginous areas—usually groin and axillae. Synonyms for benign familial pemphigus are Hailey-Hailey disease and benign familial chronic pemphigus. It usually onsets early in adult life.

The multifactorial etiology includes an autosomal dominant predisposition to which the addition of minor friction, heat, dampness, and superimposed infection results in loss of keratinocyte cohesiveness with formation of small blisters and erosions.

In an environment of heat, sweating, and friction, patients complain of burning, soreness, and irritation in the axillae and groin associated with recurrent *Staphylococcus* and *Candida* infections.

Physical Examination

In the axillae and groin, annular and serpiginous groups of vesicles rupture and leave a rim of scaling and yellowish crusting and erosions. As these annular plaques extend, the central skin appears fissured and cracked and there may be a fair amount of maceration. Typically this is in the folds of the axillae. In the genital area, the inguinal crease is involved, with the lesions extending down along the edge of the labia majora and out onto the thighs (Fig. 17-1). There can also be involvement around the neck, trunk, and under the breasts. Bacteria or yeast superinfection is common, producing an unpleasant odor.

Diagnosis

Diagnosis is based on the clinical picture and histopathology. Differential diagnoses include intertrigo, Candidiasis, herpes simplex virus infections, secondarily infected eczema or psoriasis, and pemphigus.

Treatment

This requires a dermatologist. Management is aimed at control because there is no true satisfactory treatment, and these patients have flare-ups whenever they are in an environment of excess heat, moisture, and friction.

Nonspecific. Treatment is aimed at controlling the local environment and minimizing secondary superinfection. Recommendations to the patient include weight loss, avoidance of over-heating, and the use of loose ventilated clothing with layers of thin cotton between the skin folds to decrease moisture and friction.

Burow's compresses with a solution ratio of 1:40 can be applied for 10 to 15 minutes at morning and night. A topical antibiotic cream (e.g., fusidic acid or mupirocin) and an anticandidal cream (e.g., 2% miconazole) (see *Candida*) can be used together in a thin film twice a day with a light dusting (not enough to cause caking) of absorbent powder (Zeasorb). For secondary bacterial infections, appropriate systemic antibiotics may be necessary after the culture and sensitivity are obtained.

Specific. A topical corticosteroid, betamethasone-17-valerate cream 0.1% twice a day, can be useful for inflammation. Topical cyclosporine using the oral solution once a day has been used.

Local destructive measures—excision, carbon dioxide laser, split-thickness skin graft, and dermabrasion—have been used for chronic unresponsive areas.

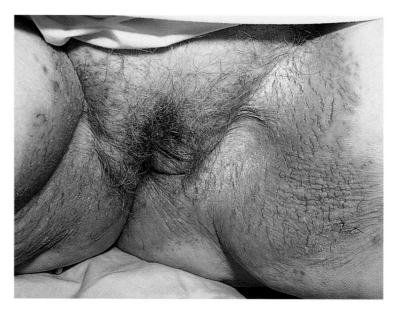

FIG. 17-1
Large plaque of erythema and fissuring on the inner thigh and in groin folds is observed in benign familial pemphigus.

BULLOUS PEMPHIGOID

Bullous pemphigoid is an uncommon autoimmune disorder of the elderly that results in tense bullae. Although it has been reported to occur in childhood, onset is usually after age 60.

An autoimmune disorder with autoantibodies directed against components of the basement membrane of the skin, this process causes tissue injury, inflammation, and dermoepidermal separation. The result is a tense subepidermal blister. There is often a prodromal phase of fixed urticarial plaques, with itching and irritation that can be present for several months. This eruption can be generalized. It is located most commonly in neck, axilla, groin, and the lower part of the abdomen. Mucosal sites in the mouth and the genitalia can occur in 50% of cases, causing labial erosions with or without discomfort.

Physical Examination

Firm vesicles and tense bullae of various sizes and full of straw-colored fluid develop on top of the erythematous, indurated, plaques formed during the prodrome. The size of the blisters ranges from 1 to 5 cm. When these blisters break, they leave raw denuded erosions (Fig. 17-2). Very uncommonly, bullous pemphigoid can be localized to the vulva.

When this occurs, it is most common on the hairy aspect of the labia majora and inner thighs. This is usually a nonscarring condition, but on occasion it can produce vulvar adhesions.

Diagnosis

Diagnosis is made on immunofluorescent histopathology, which shows the subepidermal blister with deposition of immunoglobulins along the basement membrane. Circulating anti–basement membrane antibodies can be found in 70% of patients' sera.

Differential diagnoses include pemphigus vulgaris, bullous drug eruptions, cicatricial pemphigoid, erythema multiforme, and lichen sclerosus.

Treatment

A patient who presents with this picture should be referred to a dermatologist who will, in turn, need to send specific biopsy specimens to a trained dermatopathologist for appropriate diagnosis to guide management.

Nonspecific care for the swollen and eroded vulva is discussed in Appendices D and I. Also recommend to the patient the following:

Gentle cleansing with Cetaphil cleanser
Avoid harsh, irritating soaps

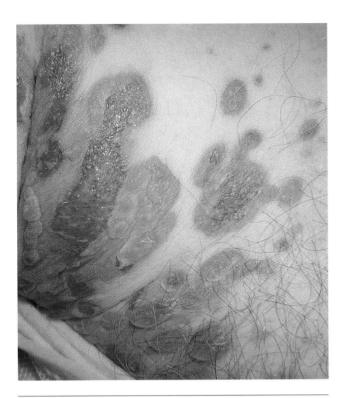

FIG. 17-2
Multiple flaccid bullae and erosions of bullous pemphigoid located on a buttock.

Wear loose ventilated clothing

For painful open areas, use Burow's 1:40 compresses or sitz baths

Specific treatment for the swollen and eroded vulva includes the following progressive therapeutic options:

Topical superpotent steroid (halobetasol or clobetasol) 0.05% ointment bid; can also be used with a Premarin applicator for intravaginal involvement (½ applicator full qhs)

Dapsone—after a negative G-6-PD screen, 50 to 200 mg a day

Tetracycline—1 to 2 g a day or minocycline 100 to 200 mg a day with niacinamide 1 to 2 g a day.

Systemic steroids—60 mg a day orally with gradually tapering doses depending on response

Azathioprine as a steroid sparer—1 to 2 mg/kg/day, carefully following the appropriate blood tests

Cyclophosphamide—1 to 2 mg/kg/day

CICATRICIAL PEMPHIGOID

Cicatricial pemphigoid is a rare, localized, scarring and blistering disease of mucosal surfaces of the elderly. Age at onset is between 50 and 70 years. It is an autoimmune condition with autoantibodies directed against the basement membrane zone with resulting inflammation and subepidermal splitting.

Patient history may not be impressive. Patients have involvement most commonly in the mouth (85%), in the eyes (65%), and on the skin (25%). About 50% of the patients have genital disease. There can be itching, vulvar pain, and dyspareunia. Purulent vaginal discharge may be present. Patients may have only mild oral or ocular complaints but may progress to very sore mouths and dry red eyes.

Physical Examination

The initial vulvar blister may never be seen. The patient usually presents with erosions involving the vulva or vagina, eventually showing scarring with loss of the labia and clitoris (Fig. 17-3). There may be considerable fragility of the vulvar skin, hypopigmentation, vaginal erosions, and desquamative vaginitis. This vaginitis produces a copious purulent discharge. Eventual vaginal scarring and obliteration can occur. At the same time, in the mouth, there may be a desquamative gingivitis and, in the eye, considerable destruction with severe ocular mucosal injury and even blindness. On the skin, rarely, scattered tense vesicles or bullae on a red base may occur, usually around the head and neck.

Diagnosis

Diagnosis is essentially clinical. A biopsy for routine and immunofluorescent histopathology is usually confirmatory. Differential diagnoses are similar to those for bullous pemphigoid and also include erosive lichen planus and lichen sclerosus.

Treatment

Management requires the care of a dermatologist working with a dermatohistopathologist.

Nonspecific care for erosive and blistering diseases of the vulva is discussed in Appendices D and I and includes the following:

Gentle cleansing with Cetaphil cleanser
Avoid harsh, irritating soaps
Wearing loose, ventilated clothing

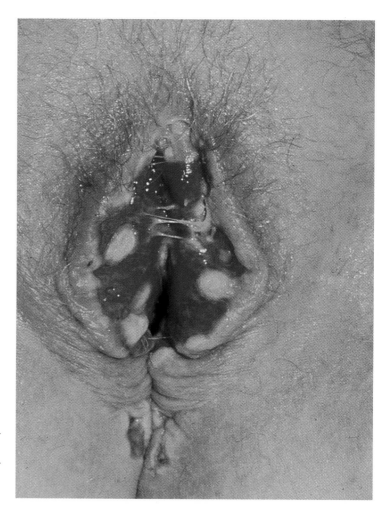

FIG. 17-3
Severe painful erosive vulvovaginitis with syne-
chiae in cicatricial pemphigoid.
(Courtesy Dr. A. Reicher.)

For painful open areas, compresses or sitz baths
using Burow's 1:40 solution are recommended to
the patient. Also suggested is the use of a bland barrier ointment—petrolatum, zinc-oxide ointment, or
Ihle's paste.

Specific treatment for erosive and blistering diseases of the vulva requires selecting appropriately
from the following:

High-potency corticosteroid, topical clobetasol
or halobetasol 0.05% ointment, bid; can also
be used with a Premarin applicator for intravaginal involvement (½ applicator full qhs)

Hydrocortisone acetate in a foam (Cortifoam)
using 40 to 80 mg qhs or in suppository form
(Cortiment) 20 to 40 mg qhs

Dapsone 100 to 200 mg daily after G-6-PD screen

Prednisone 80 to 100 mg od, depending on
severity

Steroid sparing doses of cyclophosphamide 1 to
2.5 mg/kg/day

Azathioprine 1 to 2 mg/kg/day

Intralesional triamcinolone 5 mg/mL via a 30-
gauge needle into small areas after topical
EMLA anesthestic cream and repeated every 2
to 4 weeks

If suppression of the menses is needed, use
medroxyprogesterone acetate 150 mg IM
q3mon

This can be a difficult, destructive, scarring
condition.

PEMPHIGUS VULGARIS

Pemphigus vulgaris is a rare, autoimmune, vesiculobullous disease of the skin and mucous membranes that, without treatment, is potentially fatal.[1]

The etiology involves an autoimmune process induced by a combination of endogenous and exogenous factors resulting in production of IgG autoantibodies directed against the intercellular substance and membrane antigens of epithelial cells. The resulting inflammation causes separation (acantholysis) of the epidermal cells as their intercellular bridges disintegrate in the suprabasal layers of both the epidermis and the mucous membrane areas. Age at onset is between 40 and 60 years.

The mouth is generally the first area involved, and patients complain of burning, soreness, irritation, and difficulty chewing. The vulva is affected in about 10% of cases, with complaints of soreness, burning, and irritation, as with any erosive vulvar condition.[2] The lesions in the vulva may be asymptomatic.

Physical Examination

Recurrent vulvar ulcers and erosions on the inner labia minora and vulvar vestibule are observed (Fig. 17-4). Long-term disease can result in scarring and loss of vulvar tissue, clitoris, and labia; and the vagina can also be involved, with subsequent scarring. Oral involvement is usually earliest and most difficult. Skin involvement elsewhere on the face and body causes open erosions and crusting.

Diagnosis

Clinical picture and biopsy with appropriate immunofluorescent testing defines the diagnosis. Differential diagnoses include cicatricial pemphigoid, lichen planus, erythema multiforme, bullous pemphigoid, drug reaction,[3] and paraneoplastic pemphigus.[4]

Treatment

This condition is managed by a dermatologist. With proper management, patients can really do quite well, but without treatment this is a life-threatening condition.[5]

Nonspecific care for the acute swollen vulva is discussed in Appendices D and I and includes the following:

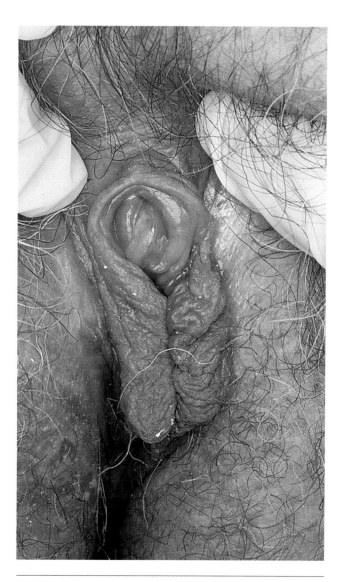

FIG. 17-4
Erosion of most of the clitoris plus an ulcer at the edge of the perineum in pemphigus vulgaris.

Gentle cleansing with Cetaphil cleanser
Avoidance of harsh, irritating soaps
Wearing loose, ventilated clothing

For painful open areas, compresses or sitz baths using Burow's 1:40 solution are recommended to the patient. Also suggested is the use of a bland barrier ointment as for pemphigus.

Specific treatment for the acute swollen vulva includes the following progressive therapeutic options:

Topical superpotent steroid (halobetasol or clobetasol) 0.05% ointment bid; can also be used with a Premarin applicator for intravaginal involvement (2 g qhs)

Corticosteroids—1 mg/kg/day prednisone, decreasing by 5 to 10 mg/day/month; at 20 mg/day of prednisone, add methotrexate 15 to 25 mg/week[6] or cyclophosphamide 1.5 to 2.5 mg/kg/day, gradually decreasing the prednisone by 5 to 2.5 mg/day/month.

Other choices as steroid sparing agents include azathioprine 1.5 to 2.5 mg/kg/day and dapsone 100 mg/day. Gold sodium thiomalate is sometimes prescribed for milder cases—after a test dose of 10 mg IM—at 25 to 50 mg IM weekly up to a cumulative dose of 1 g. Plasma exchange and extracorporeal photophoresis have also been used. Menses can be suppressed (as in cicatricial pemphigoid).

ERYTHEMA MULTIFORME MINOR

A cutaneous hypersensitivity reaction pattern that progresses to vesiculobullous lesions occurring in a symmetric pattern on the body in response to "bugs or drugs." Two forms of the condition exist, erythema multiforme minor and erythema multiforme major, the latter sometimes evolving into Stevens-Johnson syndrome (see the following discussion). A synonym for the condition is erythema multiforme simplex, and the age at occurrence is between 20 and 30 years.

The etiology includes infections, with the most common being herpes simplex, also streptococcus, mycoplasma, and histoplasma. Some of the drugs that cause this condition are sulfonamides, phenytoin, penicillin, and barbiturates. Approximately 50% of cases are idiopathic.

In the mild form there is a spectrum of involvement, from few to no symptoms to a prodrome of weakness, fever, and malaise with sore throat. If blistered, these lesions can be itchy, burning, or painful and may come and go in crops for over a month.

Physical Examination

In the minor form, hivelike macules, papules and occasional blisters develop in crops over distal arms and legs in a symmetric fashion. These lesions enlarge, forming secondary concentric rings giving the typical "target" or "iris" picture (Fig. 17-5). The lesions heal in 1 to 2 weeks, and the whole episode may last a month.

Diagnosis

Diagnosis is determined by clinical observation plus biopsy. Differential diagnoses include bullous diseases, urticaria, and drug rashes.

Treatment

The major goal of treatment is to define and remove precipitating factors. Mild cases are self-limited and require no treatment. **▼ There is a more vesiculobullous variant of the minor form that does not involve mucous membranes. Systemic steroids may be a consideration early in these cases. ▲**

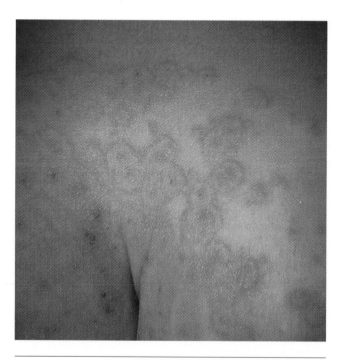

FIG. 17-5

Iris or target lesions of erythema multiforme located on a buttock.

ERYTHEMA MULTIFORME MAJOR

A cutaneous hypersensitivity reaction pattern with extensive blistering of the mucous membranes, widespread vesiculobullous eruption, and severe systemic symptoms caused by "bugs or drugs." Synonyms for erythema multiforme major include bullous erythema multiforme, severe erythema multiforme, and Stevens-Johnson syndrome.[7]

Age at onset is generally between 15 and 30 years. The etiology is the same as for erythema multiforme. Patients present with a history of fever, malaise, prostration, headache, cheilitis, photophobia, and sore throat that precede this blistering eruption by 2 to 3 days. In the vulva, pain, burning, and dysuria are prominent. These patients are acutely ill.

Physical Examination

Erosions in the mucous membranes of the throat, buccal mucosa, and lips produce cheilitis and stomatitis. Swelling, redness, and erosions can be seen in the vulvar area. Involvement of the vagina induces a purulent vaginal discharge caused by desquamative vaginitis. Associated with involvement of the mucous membranes in the genitalia, mouth, and eyes, there is a symmetric vesiculobullous eruption over the hands and feet, knees, and distal extremities (Fig. 17-6).

Diagnosis

Diagnosis is made on clinical pattern and is confirmed by biopsy. Differential diagnoses include bullous pemphigoid, pemphigus vulgaris, toxic epidermal necrolysis, and drug eruption.

Treatment

Identification and treatment of any underlying cause (i.e., stopping the medication or treating the underlying infection) is the primary course of action. A patient who presents with this picture should be referred to a dermatologist.

Nonspecific care for the erosive and blistering diseases of the vulva is discussed in Appendices D and I and includes the following:

Gentle cleansing with Cetaphil cleanser
Avoidance of harsh, irritating soaps
Wearing loose, ventilated clothing

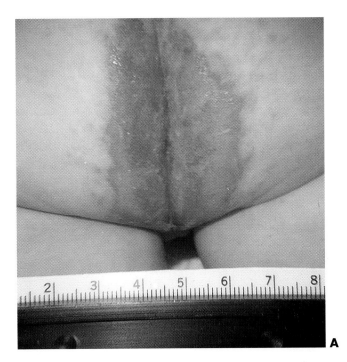

A

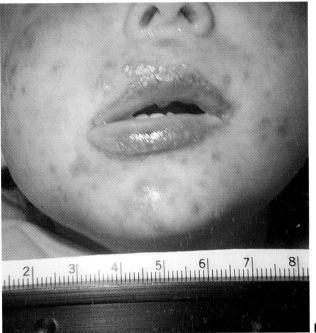

B

FIG. 17-6

A, Painful erythema and erosion of the perianal skin extending to the vulva in erythema multiforme. **B**, Same child showing blistering and erosions of lips and face

For painful open areas, use Burow's 1:40 compresses or sitz baths bid to tid plus a bland ointment—petrolatum, zinc oxide ointment or Ihle's paste.

Scarring, strictures, and adhesions need to be gently separated and, if vaginal involvement is extensive, the treatment recommended for erosive lichen planus could be utilized.

Systemic corticosteroid treatment is controversial.[8] Do not use after 72 hours from onset. Prednisone—0.5 to 1 mg/kg/day in divided doses and tapered over 7 to 10 days—can be prescribed. If suppression of menses is needed, prescribe medroxyprogesterone acetate as in cicatricial pemphigoid.

TOXIC EPIDERMAL NECROLYSIS

Toxic epidermal necrolysis is a serious, life-threatening cutaneous reaction pattern with full thickness loss of the epidermis, most often caused by drugs. The drug list is similar to that for erythema multiforme—antibiotics (40%), anticonvulsants (11%). In this condition there is sudden onset of generalized epithelial destruction, the mechanism of which is obscure.

As in erythema multiforme, there is usually a prodrome with fever, headache, and sore throat for a few days, and then sudden onset of a sore mouth and conjunctivitis that precedes the diffuse painful rash. Late symptoms resulting from scarring include dyspareunia and apareunia.

Physical Examination

A hot, confluent erythematous eruption starts in the body folds — neck, axillae, and groin. Within hours the skin becomes blistered and confluent sheets of skin peel off, leaving widespread denuded areas (Fig. 17-7). Mucous membranes (mouth, eye, vagina) are affected in 90% of cases and the genital area is affected in 70% of cases (11% vulvovaginal). The oral mucous membranes are involved most frequently. The vulvar area can develop blisters and very painful erosions causing difficulty in urination. Acutely, the vagina shows an erosive vaginitis. There is severe eye involvement, with a purulent conjunctivitis, photophobia, pain, crusting, and

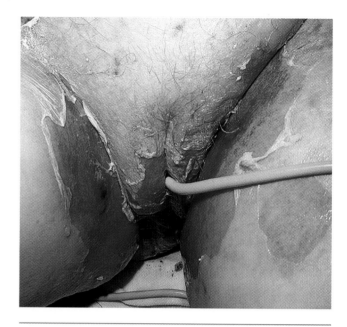

FIG. 17-7
Extensive denuded areas of skin in the inguinal and labiocrural folds in toxic epidermal necrolysis.

ulceration. These patients are seriously ill with a presentation much like a burn, with fluid loss and eventual sepsis and death in 35% to 40% of cases. After healing, the vulva may show atrophy, synechiae between the labia and in the posterior vestibule, vestibular stenosis, and vaginal synechiae and stenosis.

Diagnosis

Clinical picture and confirmatory skin biopsy define the diagnosis.

Treatment

This serious condition is managed in a hospital burn unit with a team that includes dermatology, plastic surgery, ophthalmology and internal medicine (infectious disease and an intensivist) specialists. Management of the eroded, painful vulvovaginal area is the same as for the other blistering conditions but is otherwise beyond the scope of this text.

REFERENCES

Pemphigus Vulgaris

1. Becker BA, Gaspari AA: Pemphigus vulgaris and vegetans, *Dermatol Clin* 11(3):429-452, 1993.
2. Edwards L: Desquamative vulvitis, *Dermatol Clin* 10(2):325-337, 1992.
3. Mutasim DF, Pelc NJ, Anhalt GJ: Drug-induced pemphigus, *Dermatol Clin* 11(3):463-481, 1993.
4. Mutasim DF, Pelc NJ, Anhalt GJ: Paraneoplastic pemphigus, *Dermatol Clin* 11(3):473-481, 1993.
5. Piamphongsant T, Ophaswongse S: Treatment of pemphigus, *Int J Dermatol* 30(2):139-146, 1991.
6. Lever WF, Schaumburg-Lever G: Treatment of pemphigus vulgaris: results obtained in 84 patients between 1961 and 1982, *Arch Dermatol* 120(1):44-47, 1984.

Erythema Multiforme Major

7. Assier H, Bastuji-Garin S, Revuz J, Roujeau JC: Erythema multiforme with mucous membrane involvement and Stevens-Johnson syndrome are clinically different disorders with distinct causes, *Arch Dermatol* 131(5):539-543, 1995.
8. Patterson R, Grammer LC, Greenberger PA, et al: Stevens-Johnson syndrome (SJS): effectiveness of corticosteroids in management and recurrent SJS, *Allergy Proc* 13(2):89-95, 1992.

SUGGESTED READINGS

Benign Familial Pemphigus

Burge SM: Hailey-Hailey disease: the clinical features, response to treatment and prognosis, *Br J Dermatol* 126(3):275-282, 1992.

Jitsukawa K, Ring J, Weyer U, et al: Topical cyclosporine in chronic benign familial pemphigus (Hailey-Hailey disease), *J Am Acad Dermatol* 27(4):625-626, 1992.

Kartamaa M, Reitamo S: Familial benign chronicus pemphigus (Hailey-Hailey disease): treatment with carbon dioxide laser vaporization, *Arch Dermatol* 128(5):646-648, 1992.

Wieselthier JS, Pincus SH: Hailey-Hailey disease of the vulva, *Arch Dermatol* 129(10):1344-1345, 1993.

Bullous Pemphigoid

Anhalt GJ, Morrison LH: Bullous and cicatricial pemphigoid, *J Autoimm* 4(1):17-35, 1991.

Crosby DL, Diaz LA: Bullous diseases: introduction, *Dermatol Clin* 11(3):373-378, 1993.

Paquet P, Richelle M, Lapiere CM: Bullous pemphigoid treated by topical corticosteroids, *Acta Derm Venereol* 71(6):534-535, 1991.

Saad RW, Domloge-Hultsch N, Yancey KB, et al: Childhood localized vulvar pemphigoid is a true variant of bullous pemphigoid, *Arch Dermatol* 128(6):807-810, 1992.

Thornfeldt CR, Menkes AW: Bullous pemphigoid controlled by tetracycline, *J Am Acad Dermatol* 16(2 Pt 1):305-310, 1987.

Cicatricial Pemphigoid

Ahmed AR, Kurgis CS, Rogers RS III: Cicatricial pemphigoid, *J Am Acad Dermatol* 24(6 Pt 1):987-1001, 1991.

Marren P, Walkden V, Mallon E, Wojnarowska F: Vulval cicatricial pemphigoid may mimic lichen sclerosus, *Br J Dermatol* 134(3):522-524, 1996.

Marren P, Wojnarowska F, Venning VA, et al: Vulvar involvement in autoimmune bullous diseases, *J Reprod Med* 38(2):101-107, 1993.

Toxic Epidermal Necrolysis

Avakian R, Flowers FP, Araujo OE, Ramos-Caro FA: Toxic epidermal necrolysis: a review, *J Am Acad Dermatol* 25(1 Pt 1):69-79, 1991.

Meneux E, Paniel BJ, Pouget F, et al: Vulvovaginal sequelae in toxic epidermal necrolysis, *J Repro Med* 42(3):153-156, 1997.

CHAPTER 18

Pigmentary Changes in the Vulva

HYPERPIGMENTATION

Pigmentation in the vulvar area is quite variable, depending on racial origin and hormonal status. Any inflammation in the vulvar area can result in hyperpigmentation or hypopigmentation. Benign and malignant tumors (e.g., seborrheic keratosis and basal cell carcinoma) can be hyperpigmented and are discussed elsewhere.

Acanthosis Nigricans

Acanthosis nigricans is a rare, nonspecific, cutaneous reaction pattern that results in a diffuse, dirty brown, velvety, or warty-surfaced skin change in the axillae and body folds. Etiology is considered in Box 18-1. Usually there is a gradual onset with no symptoms. The malignant form can be itchy or irritating.

Physical Examination

Hyperpigmentation gradually increases around the neck, in the axillae, in the labiocrural folds, and in the inguinal creases. The skin in the areas becomes thicker and velvety, even warty (Fig. 18-1). In the malignant form, very pronounced pigmentation changes occur and involve the mouth, lips, palms, and soles.

Diagnosis

Diagnosis is based on the clinical pattern.

Treatment

There is no specific treatment. If malignancy is suspected, a thorough investigation is indicated. Some cases may improve with weight loss and a subsequent change in androgen status. Alpha-hydroxy acid lotions with 12% lactic acid can be helpful when applied twice a day (Lac-Hydrin lotion). Topical adapalene (Differin) 0.1% gel has also been used with success. These products are best for thinning the thicker lesions and thus decreasing the hyperpigmentation.

BOX 18-1

Etiology of Acathosis Nigricans

Hereditary benign acanthosis nigricans—onsets in childhood.

Benign acanthosis nigricans is associated with endocrine disorders—diabetes, acromegaly, Cushing's disease, insulin resistance, and hirsutism.

Pseudoacanthosis nigricans is a complication of obesity.

Drug-induced acanthosis nigricans can be caused by nicotinic acid and stilbestrol.

Malignant acanthosis nigricans may be part of a paraneoplastic syndrome induced by adenocarcinoma or lymphoma.

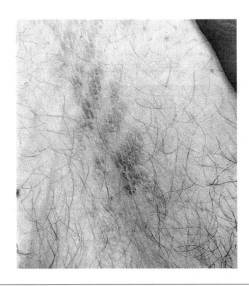

FIG. 18-1
Velvety patches of hyperpigmented hyperkeratosis in the left inguinal crease in early acanthosis nigricans. This 16-year-old woman has extensive hirsutism and acanthosis nigricans in the HAIR-AN syndrome.

Benign Vulvar Melanosis and Lentiginosis

Hyperpigmented macular freckling can occur as a single lesion (lentigo simplex) or as multiple lesions (benign vulvar melanosis). These are completely harmless macules or patches, but they can mimic melanoma.

These hyperpigmented lesions represent an unexplained accumulation of melanin within keratinocytes—simple, epidermal hyperpigmentation occurring usually between age 30 to 40 years. Patients present because of discovery during self-examination or a gynecologic examination.

Physical Examination

Irregular brown or black macules or patches with irregular margins scattered anywhere on the vulva—labia majora, minora, or the vestibule (Fig. 18-2, *A*). If the hyperpigmentation is less than 4 mm, it is termed *lentigo simplex.* Larger lesions, termed *vulvar melanosis,* can extend to 10 cm or more.

Diagnosis

Diagnosis is made on histopathology. Because the differential diagnoses include malignant melanoma and pigmented basal cell carcinoma as well as post-inflammatory hyperpigmentation, biopsy is strongly recommended.

Treatment

No treatment needed. Biopsy permits informed reassurance to the patient and is the only thing recommended.

Note: *Lentigines in the vulvar area may be found in some cutaneous syndromes (Fig. 18-2, B and Box 18-2).*

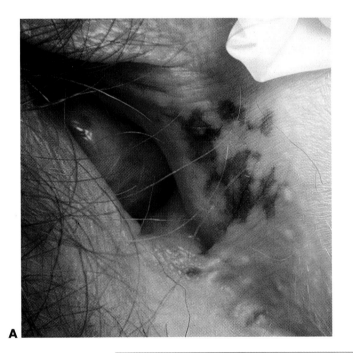
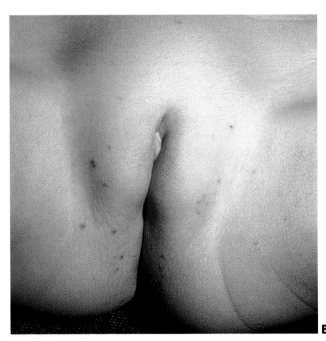

FIG. 18-2

A, Irregular pigmented macules in benign vulvar melanosis. **B,** Scattered lentigines on the vulva of a normal child.

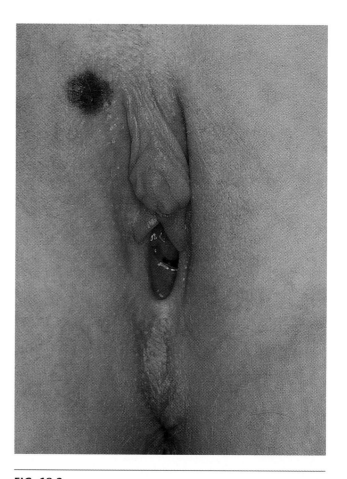

FIG. 18-3
Pigmented compound nevus on the edge of the vulva in a 4 year old.

BOX 18-2

Cutaneous Syndromes with Vulvar Lentigines

LAMB—Lentigines, atrial myxoma, and blue nevi
LEOPARD—Lentigines, electrocardiographic conduction defects, ocular hypertelorism, pulmonary stenosis, abnormalities of the genitalia, retardation of growth, and deafness

---

Melanocytic Nevus

A melanocytic nevus is a small, circumscribed, variably pigmented macule or papule made up of nests of melanocytic cells derived from the neural crest (Fig. 18-3). (See Benign Tumors p. 196.)

Postinflammatory Hyperpigmentation

Pigmented macules or patches can be seen on the skin after any inflammatory injury. Postinflammatory pigmentation refers to the end stage of a prior inflammatory process that deposits melanin in the dermis but gives no clues as to the nature of the original problem. Exogenous causes include physical or chemical agents used either topically or internally. Topical examples include soaps, cleansers, and topical allergens; internal causes are usually drugs (fixed drug eruption). Endogenous causes of inflammation include lichen planus, discoid lupus erythematosus, and psoriasis.

The patient gives a history of a preexisting inflammatory process or injury, although sometimes the history may be missed (e.g., in a fixed drug eruption when the patient noted little or no prior inflammation).

Physical Examination

Varying degrees of macular or patchy hyperpigmentation occur. The color can be brown to black, is usually irregular, and can also show scattered patches of hypopigmentation (Fig. 18-4). The pigment intensity depends on the severity of the original inflammation and the natural background pigmentation.

Diagnosis

Clinical picture and histopathology determine the diagnosis. Differential diagnoses include benign vulvar melanosis and vulvar intraepithelial neoplasia.

Treatment

No treatment is needed for this condition. Any inflammatory process that is ongoing should be treated. With time the pigmentation should fade.

HYPOPIGMENTATION

Pigment may be reduced or lost for various reasons. The most common reason is the destruction of melanocytes by inflammatory reactions (post-

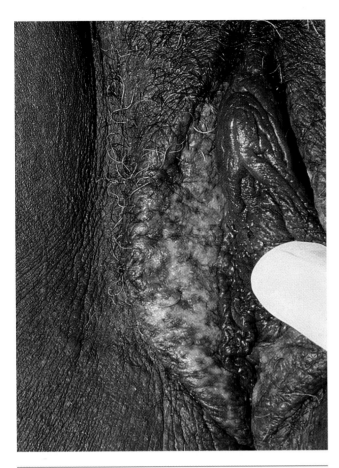

FIG. 18-4

Post-inflammatory hyperpigmentation of right interlabial sulcus and labium major with some hypopigmentation in lichen simplex chronicus.

(Courtesy Dr. L. Edwards.)

inflammatory hypopigmentation), either from autoimmune (vitiligo) or direct inflammatory mechanisms (lichen sclerosus and other dermatoses).

Lichen Sclerosus

Lichen sclerosus is a common mucocutaneous disorder of the genitalia and the skin, resulting in marked hypopigmentation, tissue thinning, and scarring.[1-5] Synonyms for lichen sclerosus are lichen sclerosus et atrophicus (LS & A), hyperplastic dystrophy, and kraurosis vulvae.

It is most common in middle-aged women, but lichen sclerosus can also occur in children from infancy on.[6,7] The etiology is unknown. It has been weakly linked with autoimmune disease.[8] Autoimmune diseases occur in 20% of patients and 22% of their families. Familial cases have been reported. Infectious organisms have been postulated but never confirmed.

The onset may be asymptomatic until the patient has sufficient scarring to produce dyspareunia or even urinary retention. Pruritus is the most common complaint, and it can be severe enough to wake the patient at night and to be socially incapacitating by day. Uncontrollable scratching may lead to open excoriations, pain, dysuria, and dyspareunia.

Physical Examination

Several patterns of lichen sclerosus exist. The classic lesions are circumscribed whitish papules and plaques covered with thin "cigarette paper" atrophic skin. This may start in the periclitoral area, spreading to involve the entire labia minora and interlabial sulcus and then extending down through the perineum and the perianal area, forming the typical figure-of-eight pattern (Fig. 18-5, *A*). With time, atrophy of all the subcutaneous tissue leads to gradual effacement and eventual complete disappearance of the clitoris and/or labia minora (Fig. 18-5, *B*). In end-stage disease the opening of the vagina may be stenosed or even closed (Fig. 18-5, *C*).

Patchy involvement of the vulva (Fig. 18-6, *A*) can occur, affecting the periclitoral area or the perineum and the perianal area. In mild cases there may be only simple hypopigmentation (Fig. 18-6, *B*). Sometimes only scattered white guttate papules are seen.

Secondary changes are common. Scratching produces varying degrees of purpura, erosions, and excoriation. Scarred areas may be torn by attempts at sexual intercourse. Some patients show Koebnerization (the induction of new lesions by physical trauma). Repeated scratching causes lichenification that can be frankly warty (Fig. 18-6, *C*). Five percent of cases of lichen sclerosus are associated with squamous cell carcinoma, and a mixed pattern of tumor and lichen sclerosus may be seen. Up to 20% of patients may have involvement of other body areas, especially the trunk and arms.

Note: *The mucous membrane of the vagina is not involved.*

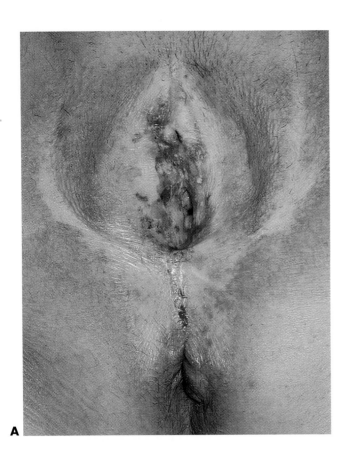

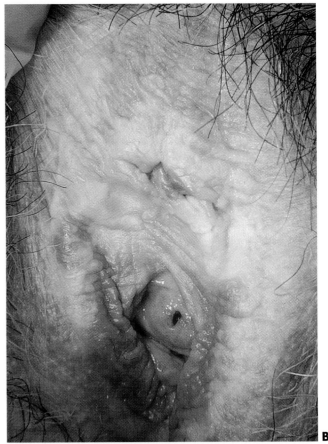

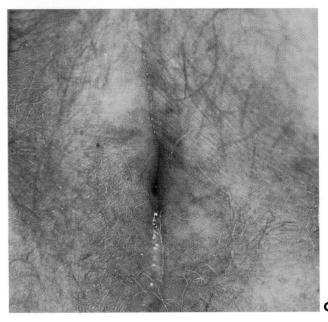

FIG. 18-5
Lichen Sclerosus. **A,** Figure-of-eight pattern of lichen sclerosus with labiocrural extensions. Notice the scarring, fissuring, and hematoma formation. **B,** Loss of most of the
clitoris and labia minora in lichenified lichen sclerosus.
C, End-stage scarred lichen sclerosus with urinary retention. This 76 year old had a problem for more than 40
years, undiagnosed.

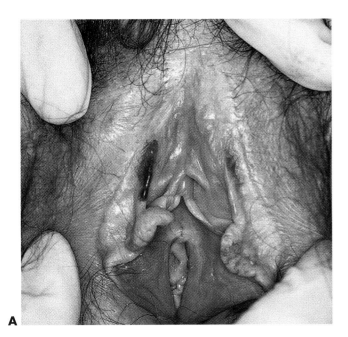

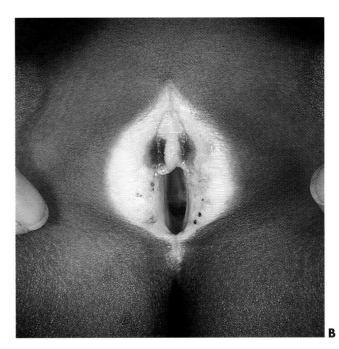

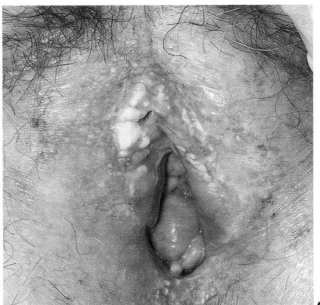

FIG. 18-6

A, Patchy involvement of frenulum, periclitoral and interlabial sulci with purpura.
B, Hypopigmentation in lichen sclerosus. **C,** Hyperkeratotic scarred lichen sclerosus.
This 72-year-old woman had severe itching. Three months after superpotent steroid
ointment, she was asymptomatic with resolution of hyperkeratotic areas but with
residual scarring.

(**B,** Courtesy Dr. B. Krafchik.)

Diagnosis
Clinical pattern and histopathology.

Note: *The clinical features are lost in the glare of over-bright lighting.*

Differential diagnoses include vitiligo, lichen planus, post-menopausal atrophy, cicatricial pemphigoid, pemphigus vulgaris, and sexual abuse (in children) (Fig. 18-7).

Treatment
Nonspecific treatment of lichen sclerosus.
Gentle cleansing with a very mild cleanser (Cetaphil cleanser)
Avoidance of strong soaps and detergents
Use of ventilated cotton clothing
Avoidance of panty liners
Use of a mild lubricant for sexual intercourse (e.g., a tiny dab of light olive oil)

If very itchy, use cool gel packs applied directly to the vulva for burning and itching (keep gel pack in refrigerator in a freezer bag with a zippered closure).
If the vulva is very itchy, irritated, or eroded, use Burow's' solution 1:40 (mix one packet or tablet of Domeboro or Bluboro in 500 mL cool water) in a sitz bath or as a cool compress 2 to 3 times a day.

Specific treatment for lichen sclerosus. Topical superpotent steroids are the most effective,[9] halobetasol or clobetasol 0.05% ointment bid for 6 to 8 weeks and then once a day for 6 to 8 weeks and then 1 to 3 times a week in a maintenance program. If the risk of secondary candidiasis exists, use topical nystatin ointment or ketoconazole cream over the steroid.

For major itching and lichenification, use intralesional triamcinolone (Kenalog-10) usually diluted 1:2 with saline. For very thick lesions use triamci-

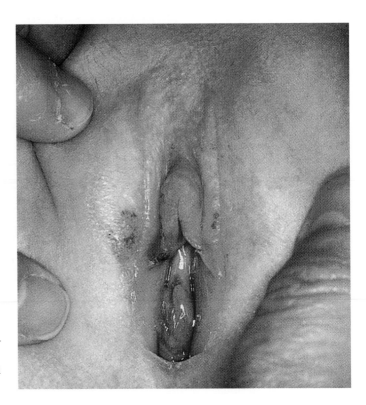

FIG. 18-7
Scarring and mild purpura in lichen sclerosus (mistaken for sexual abuse).

nolone up to 20 mg/mL by diluting triamcinolone (Kenalog-40) with saline. The injections are given using a 30-gauge needle over a 1 cm grid. Use EMLA anesthetic cream under plastic wrap for 20 minutes minimum to reduce the discomfort from the injections. Repeat the injections monthly depending on the response.

Some patients prefer ointments and others prefer creams. In children, mid-to-high-potency steroid can be chosen. With proper treatment, the response of lichen sclerosus is usually dramatic. Maintenance topical therapy is long-term. Over-use and thinning of the skin must be avoided.

Oral retinoids—etretinate 25 mg daily has been used for variable periods of time for thick hyperkeratotic lichen sclerosus.

Surgery may be necessary if there is serious introital stenosis.

Five percent of lichen sclerosus has been reported to progress to squamous cell carcinoma. Always biopsy any unusual change.

Postinflammatory Hypopigmentation

Any injury to the skin that causes disruption of the melanocytes and basement membrane can result in depigmentation or hypomelanosis, either temporary or permanent. The causes, as in postinflammatory hyperpigmentation, are exogenous (e.g., ionizing radiation) or endogenous (e.g., discoid lupus erythematosus). The inflammation results in loss of melanocytes resulting from damage or destruction. While precipitants should be sought, the patient may have forgotten any history of a preceding process.

Physical Examination

The skin color may be lightened (hypopigmented) or completely white (depigmented). The pattern on the vulva is variable, involving any portion, including the legs and thighs. It follows the shape of the original eruption and is much more noticeable in darker skin (Fig. 18-8).

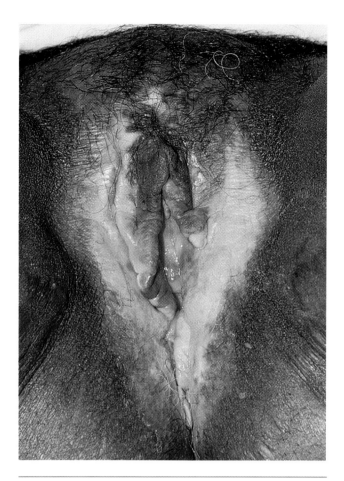

FIG. 18-8
Post-inflammatory hypopigmentation in lichen simplex chronicus.
(Courtesy Dr. L. Edwards.)

Diagnosis

Diagnosis is clinical, based on pattern and, if necessary, histopathology. Differential diagnoses include vitiligo and lichen sclerosus.

Treatment

No therapy is necessary. Treating the underlying cause, if it is still active, hastens resolution and the pigmentation often returns with time. Reassure the patient the condition is completely harmless.

Vitiligo

This is an acquired loss of pigmentation, probably on an autoimmune basis. It results in irregularly shaped patches of hypomelanosis and/or depigmentation of the skin. It is probably autoimmune, with a polygenic familial predisposition and positive family history of 30%. It is associated with other autoimmune conditions such as pernicious anemia and Addison's disease. There may be an intrinsic melanocyte dysfunction leading to death and/or dysfunction of melanocytes in the lesions. The patient develops gradually increasing asymptomatic white areas. The cosmetic defect is emotionally traumatic for darker skinned races.

Physical Examination

White macules appear most commonly over the extensor areas of the body, most usually at sites of trauma, including the backs of the hands, face, and body folds, including the genito-crural area in women. As the macules enlarge into spreading patches, the hair in the involved area also turns white (Fig 18-9). Patients seen in vulvar clinics may present solely with vitiligo limited to the genital area.

Note: *Vitiliginous lesions show no surface change, just color loss.*

Diagnosis

Diagnosis is clinical. Differential diagnoses include lichen sclerosus, postinflammatory hypopigmentation, piebaldism, and lupus erythematosus.

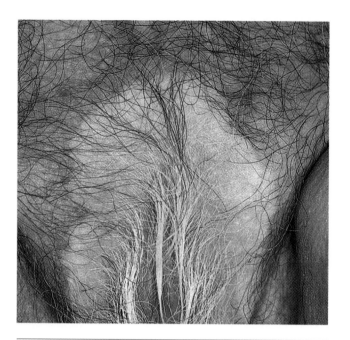

FIG. 18-9
Hypopigmented vulvar skin and hair in vitiligo.

Treatment

Treatment of vitiligo is difficult and often disappointing. For involvement of the vulvar area alone, no treatment may be recommended other than reassurance. A dermatologist is needed to supervise a trial of topical mild potency to midpotency corticosteroids. For extensive disease topical or systemic psoralens are being used, but this would not be recommended for localized vulvar vitiligo.

REFERENCES

Lichen Sclerosus

1. Meffert JJ, Davis BM, Grimwood RE: Lichen sclerosus, *J Am Acad Dermatol* 32(3):393-416, 1995.
2. Ridley CM: Lichen sclerosus, *Dermatol Clin* 10(2):309-323, 1992.
3. Ridley CM: Lichen sclerosus et atrophicus, *Semin Dermatol* 8(1):54-63, 1989.
4. Ridley CM: *The vulva,* Edinburgh, 1988, Churchill Livingstone, 173-193.
5. Lynch PJ, Edwards L: *Genital dermatology,* Baltimore, 1995, Churchill Livingstone.
6. Loening-Baucke V: Lichen sclerosus et atrophicus in children, *Am J Dis Child* 145(9):1058-1061, 1991.
7. Ridley CM: Genital lichen sclerosus (lichen sclerosus et atrophicus) in childhood and adolescence, *J R Soc Med* 86(2):69-75, 1993.
8. Meyrick Thomas RH, Ridley CM, McGibbon DH, Black MM: Lichen sclerosus et atrophicus and autoimmunity: a study of 350 women, *Br J Dermatol* 118(1):41-46, 1988.
9. Dalziel KL, Wojnarowska F: Long-term control of vulval lichen sclerosus after treatment with a potent topical steroid cream, *J Reprod Med* 38(1):25-27, 1993.

SUGGESTED READINGS

Acanthosis Nigricans

Grasinger CC, Wild RA, Parker IJ: Vulvar acanthosis nigricans: a marker for insulin resistance in hirsute women, *Fertil Steril* 59(3):583-586, 1993.

Hud JA Jr, Cohen JB, Wagner JM, Cruz PD Jr: Prevalence and significance of acanthosis nigricans in an adult obese population, *Arch Dermatol* 128(7):941-944, 1992.

Benign Vulvar Melanosis and Lentiginosis

Barnhill RL, Albert LS, Shama SK, et al: Genital lentiginosis: a clinical and histopathologic study, *J Am Acad Dermatol* 22(3):453-460, 1990.

Estrada R, Kaufman RH: Benign vulvar melanosis, *J Reprod Med* 38(1):5-8, 1993.

Kanj LF, Rubeiz NG, Mroueh AM, Kibbi AG: Vulvar melanosis and lentiginosis: a case report, *J Am Acad Dermatol* 27(5 Pt 1):777-778, 1992.

Rudolph RI: Vulvar melanosis, *J Am Acad Dermatol* 23(5 Pt 2):982-984, 1990.

Vitiligo

Grimes PE: Vitiligo: an overview of therapeutic approaches, *Dermatol Clin* 11(2):325-337, 1993.

Lynch PJ, Edwards L: *Genital dermatology,* Baltimore, 1995, Churchill Livingstone, 149-162.

Nordlund JJ, Ortonne JP: Vitiligo and depigmentation. In Weston WL, editor: *Current problems in dermatology,* St Louis, 1992, Mosby, 3-30.

BENIGN TUMORS

Acrochordon

An acrochordon is a very common benign, skin-colored, pedunculated, fibroepitheliomatous polyp found in intertriginous areas. Synonyms for acrochordon are skin tag, soft fibroma, papilloma, and fibroepithelial polyp.

The etiology is unknown. Hormonal or growth factors seem to play a role in obese and diabetic patients. Small acrochorda are referred to as skin tags. The large single lesion is a fibroepithelial polyp.

Asymptomatic unless they are traumatized, they can become inflamed, painful, and can even develop spontaneous necrosis if the pedicle is twisted (Fig. 19-1, *A*). The patient's usual complaint is that the lesions catch on their clothing.

Physical Examination

Multiple soft, brown, tan, or skin-colored lesions can be found in the groin and axilla, particularly in patients who are obese and/or diabetic (Fig. 19-1, *B*). Skin tags, the small ones, may be 2 to 4 mm in diameter and scattered around the sides of the mons pubis and inner thighs. The solitary fibroepithelial polyp is a fleshy, pedunculated mass and may be up to 1.5 cm long on a 2 to 3 mm stalk (Fig. 19-1, *C*).

Diagnosis

Diagnosis is clinical. Differential diagnoses include nevus, neurofibroma, molluscum, and neuroma.

Treatment

Electrodesiccate or snip off the polyps with scissors under local anesthesia. Asymptomatic lesions do not need treatment.

Angiokeratoma

This is a very common, small, harmless, papular blood vessel tumor with a keratotic surface. Patients with multiple angiokeratomas of the vulva may have underlying disorders of glycosphingolipid metabolism. A synonym for this condition is angiokeratoma of Fordyce. Patient history is asymptomatic vulvar papules. Occasionally a patient may pick at these, causing bleeding.

Physical Examination

These common vascular papules are 2 to 5 mm in diameter, range in color from dark red to purplish, and are scattered anywhere on the vulva (Fig. 19-2, *A*). There may be few or sheets of them, and the surface may range from slightly thickened to frankly verrucous.

Diagnosis

Diagnosis is a combination of clinical and histopathologic. Differential diagnoses include melanoma, vulvar warts, and nevi.

Fabry's disease (Anderson-Fabry disease or angiokeratoma corporis diffusum) can very rarely present with multiple angiokeratomas of the vulva. There is an X-linked deficiency of α-galactosidase-A, resulting in glycosphingolipid accumulation. The condition is mild in women, causing some renal, eye, and neurologic changes.

Fucosidosis is due to a deficiency of α-L-fucosidase resulting in abnormal glycosphingolipid metabolism. Multiple angiokeratomas appear in early childhood on the trunk, groin, upper legs, and in the vulva (Fig. 19-2, *B*). It is associated with severe mental retardation and is lethal.

Treatment

No treatment is needed for asymptomatic lesions. Destruction by electrodesiccation, laser ablation, or occasionally local excision can be considered.

Bartholin's Cyst

This is a common vulvar cyst (1% to 2% of women) that develops from blockage of one of the two major vulvar vestibular glands. This cyst forms

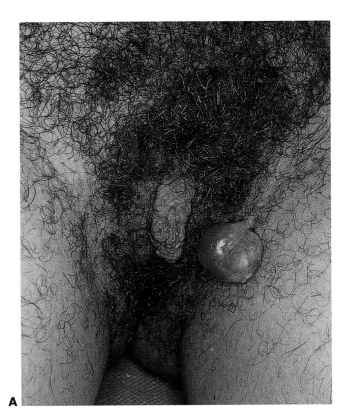

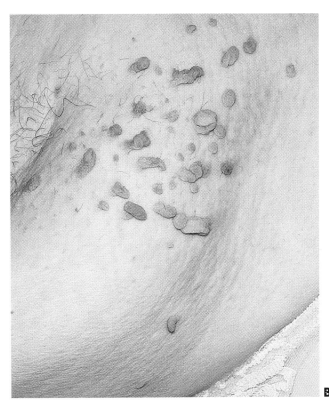

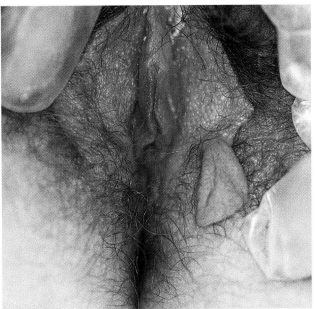

FIG. 19-1
Acrochordon. **A**, A skin tag with a twisted pedicle that resulted in considerable pain from swelling and ischemia. **B**, Multiple acrochordae on the inner thigh of a woman with diabetes. **C**, A skin-colored, fibroepithelial polyp on the edge of the labium minor.

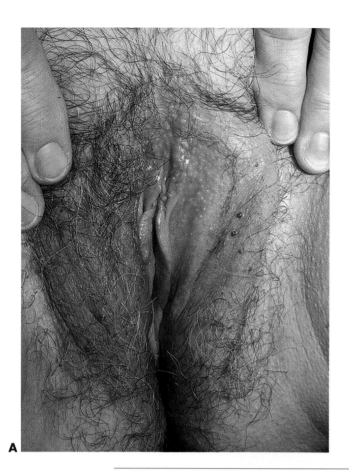
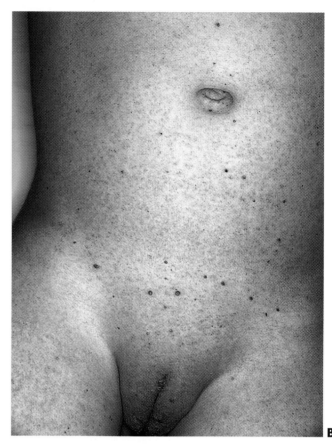

A

B

FIG. 19-2

Angiokeratoma. **A,** Purple, vascular papules on left labium major. **B,** Multiple angio-keratomata with a diffuse telangiectatic background on the body and vulva of a 5 year old with mental retardation resulting from fucosidosis.

when there is an obstruction to the Bartholin's gland duct. These common cysts, when small, may be asymptomatic. Symptoms develop as they enlarge or become infected. Sitting or walking may then be difficult because they are extremely painful. Signs of systemic infection may develop.

Physical Examination

These round or ovoid cysts, located at the 5 or 7 o'clock positions on the hymenal ring, are usually 1 to 4 cm but may become as large as 8 cm in diameter (Fig. 19-3, *A*). Infection with the usual skin organisms (and in some cases *Neisseria gonorrhoeae*) results in marked erythema and exquisite tenderness. The whole introital area can be blocked

with the edematous and erythematous swelling (Fig. 19-3, *B* and *C*).

Diagnosis

Diagnosis is clinical. Differential diagnoses include epidermal cyst, lipoma, and fibroma.

Treatment

Asymptomatic, small cysts require no treatment.

Symptomatic cysts or abscesses require surgery by a gynecologist. "Marsupialization" (actually unroofing) of the cyst or abscess cavity or complete removal of the cyst may be necessary. Bartholin's abscesses should be cultured for *Neisseria gonorrhoeae*. Antibiotics are needed for infected cysts.

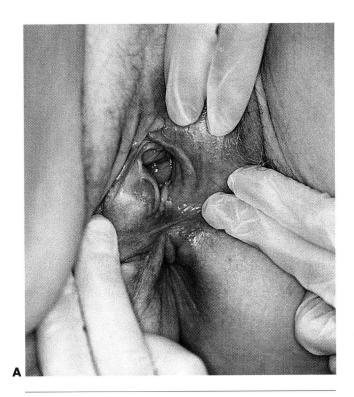

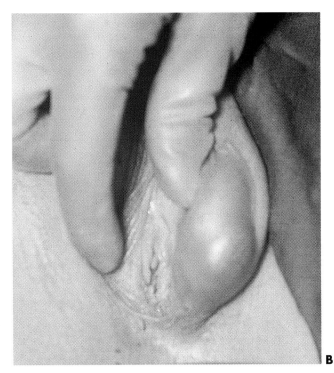

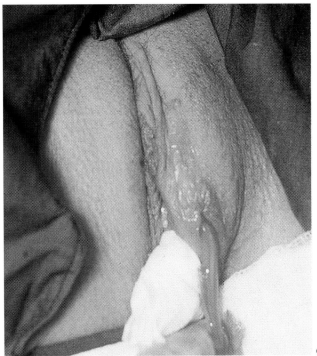

FIG. 19-3

Bartholin's Cyst. **A**, A swollen, tender Bartholin's cyst. **B**, A very painful, acute Bartholin's cyst before surgery. **C**, Same cyst as in *B* being draining before removal. (**B** and **C**, Courtesy Dr. P. Bryson.)

Capillary Hemangioma

Hemangiomas are benign tumors of the vascular endothelium characterized by a proliferative phase in infancy and involution at about 9 years of age. Synonyms for capillary hemangioma include strawberry nevus or mark and angiomatous nevus. Unknown factors initially cause very active capillary endothelial cell proliferation. With time, regression occurs with involution and fibrosis. Usually within days after birth, a small red patch appears and rapidly commences the first of three phases (Box 19-1).

The symptoms depend on the size of the lesion. Some of the lesions can reach enormous size (e.g., Klippel-Trenaunay-Weber syndrome). Magnetic resonance imaging (MRI) may be necessary to decide on the size of the lesion. The Kasabach-Merritt syndrome (thrombocytopenia and consumptive coagulopathy) can develop in large lesions (Fig. 19-5).

Physical Examination

Most genital hemangiomas involve the labia majora, but can involve the labia minora, perineum, and perianal area to a varying degree. Ulceration and bleeding may occur.

Diagnosis

Diagnosis is clinical.

Treatment

Treatment depends on the degree of involvement. For asymptomatic limited lesions, no treat-

---

BOX 19-1

Three Phases of Capillary Hemangioma

Proliferative phase
Lasts about 8 or 9 months, during which time the lesion grows at a faster rate than the body, with the development of a bright red nodular lesion. Genital hemangiomas may cause difficulty because of erosion of the rapidly growing tumor, secondary infection, and discomfort. Chronic ulceration can produce bleeding and pain (Fig. 19-4).

Stationary phase
Finds the lesion indolent for several months.

Involution phase
Starts at about 2 years of age and 90% of lesions involute by 9 years of age.

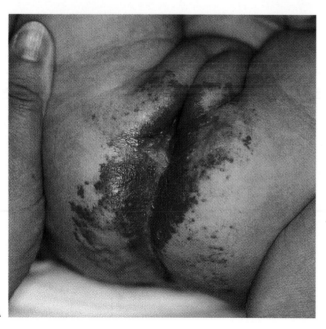

A

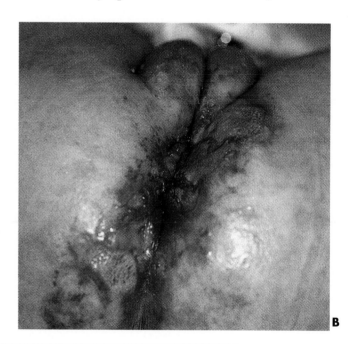

B

FIG. 19-4
For legend see opposite page.

ment, other than reassurance, may be necessary. For complicated hemangiomas, expert advice from a pediatric dermatologist should be sought. For rapidly growing hemangiomas with bleeding and ulceration, pulsed dye laser treatment should be initiated as soon as possible. Cryotherapy, using a cryoprobe with repeated treatments every 4 to 6 weeks for 2 to 4 applications, is also effective. Oral, high-dose prednisone—1 to 2 mg/kg/day— is utilized if there is obstructive hemangioma-

tous growth or consumptive coagulopathy with Kasabach-Merritt syndrome.

Capillary hemangioma may be associated with an underlying subcutaneous or deep dermal cavernous hemangioma. The history is similar but on physical examination the vulvar lesions are deeper, purple, multilobular, and can involve large areas of the vulva with a tumor mass extending up into the vagina. Investigation with an MRI is essential. These tumors can last into adult life.

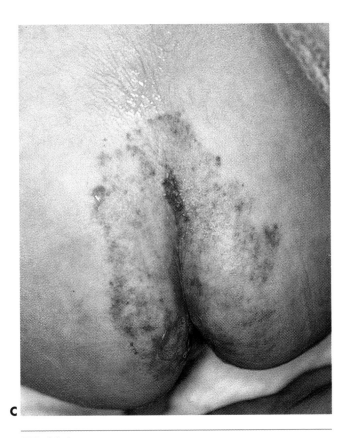

C

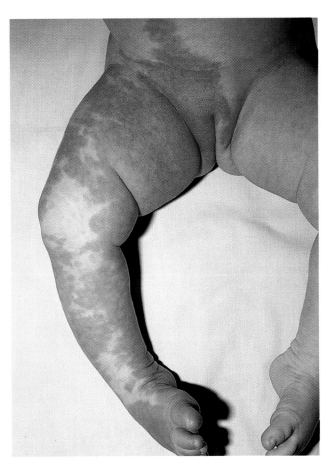

FIG. 19-4

A, Rapidly growing capillary hemangioma of the perineum in a 1-month-old baby. The lesion repeatedly ulcerated and bled. B, Eroded ulcerated perineum 10 days after the second pulsed dye laser treatment. The first pulsed dye laser treatment was at 1 month of age, the second at 2 months of age. After laser treatment, the ulcers resolved in 3 weeks. C, Result of the laser treatment at 6 months of age, 5 months after laser treatment. Note the marked resolution.

FIG. 19-5

A 2 month old with extensive capillary hemangioma of abdomen, vulva, and right leg with Klippel-Trenaunay-Weber syndrome.

Cherry Angioma

This is a common, red, domed, vascular lesion that can appear anywhere on the trunk or body. They appear at about age 40 and become more numerous with age. Synonyms for this condiditon are senile hemangioma, cherry hemangioma, and Campbell de Morgan spot. The etiology is unknown. These are simply a lobular proliferation of capillaries. Patient history is completely asymptomatic unless the lesions are traumatized and bleeding.

Physical Examination

Smooth, bright red to purplish, domed papules 1 to 8 mm in diameter (Fig. 19-6). They are soft, blanche with pressure, are often multiple, and can be found on the mons pubis or labia.

Diagnosis

Diagnosis is clinical. Differential diagnoses include angiokeratoma, pyogenic granuloma, and melanoma.

Treatment

If the papules are asymptomatic, no treatment is needed. The papules can be destroyed with electrodesiccation, shave excision, or laser therapy.

Epidermal Cysts

An epidermal cyst, the most common cutaneous cyst, is also the most common genital cyst in women. It consists of the subcutaneous enclosure by a stratified squamous epithelial of keratin and lipid-rich debris. The sac can rupture, causing pain. Synonyms for epidermal cysts are keratinous cyst, epidermal inclusion cyst, sebaceous cyst, wen, infundibular cyst, and epidermoid cyst. There is entrapment of epidermal cells in the dermis, probably secondary to trauma, or, more commonly, there is blockage of the pilosebaceous duct resulting in distention and cyst formation. These are single or multiple asymptomatic nodules within the vulvar skin. Their size is variable, and if the cyst is traumatized, the patient complains of pain and tenderness.

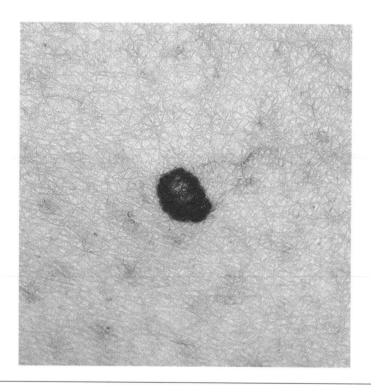

FIG. 19-6
Cherry Angioma. A bright red vascular papule is evident.

If the cyst ruptures, the complaint is that of an unpleasant, cheesy odor. There may be so many cysts that any pressure in the area can be quite uncomfortable. Some patients become very worried about these unexplained lumps.

Physical Examination

Single cysts are typically round, firm, and smooth, mobile, subcutaneous nodules and may have a barely visible, keratin-filled orifice. These dermal nodules range in size from 2 to 3 mm up to 1 to 2 cm and are located along the labia majora and, less commonly, the labia minora. They can be multiple, sometimes forming a cobblestone effect. The skin surface is smooth, and the skin is a yellowish color (Fig. 19-7, *A*). There may be an obvious comedo at the opening (Fig. 19-7, *B*). With pressure or with a minor incision, yellow, smelly, cheesy material can be expressed. If there has been trauma and rupture of the cyst, it may be erythematous and tender like a furuncle.

Diagnosis

Diagnosis is clinical and can be confirmed on biopsy. Differential diagnoses include neuroma, dermal nevus, xanthoma, furuncle, and hidradenitis suppurativa.

Treatment

Asymptomatic, indolent, vulvar cysts need no treatment. Reassure the patient that the cysts are harmless.

Symptomatic cysts are surgically removed under local anesthesia.

Inflamed cysts should not be excised. They may be infected or simply ruptured with foreign body reaction. They should be treated with a tetracycline antibiotic (partly as an antiinflammatory) and, if there is true infection with abscess formation, drainage should be carried out first.

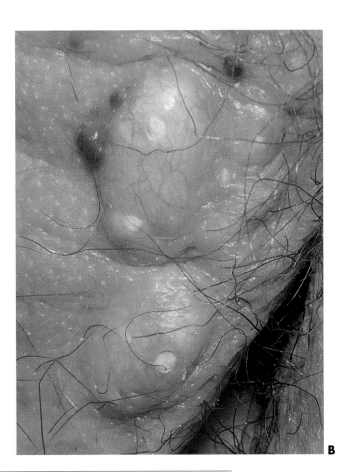

A **B**

FIG. 19-7
A, Yellow cysts of varying size along the edge of the labia minora. **B,** Two large cysts with a central yellow comedonal plug at each opening.

Hidradenoma Papilliferum

Hidradenoma papilliferum is an uncommon sweat gland tumor that develops on the inner aspect of the labium major in white women. The lesion is a tumor of sweat glands or ducts. Patient history is an asymptomatic vulvar papule.

Physical Examination

The tumor presents as a sharply circumscribed, skin-colored, 1 cm nodule on the interlabial sulcus or elsewhere on the labia majora (Fig. 19-8). The lesion is freely moveable.

Diagnosis

Diagnosis is made by biopsy. Differential diagnoses include nevus, cyst, and neuroma.

Treatment

No treatment is necessary if the tumor is asymptomatic. Excision is required if the tumor is symptomatic.

Lipoma

Lipoma is an uncommon hamartoma of fatty subcutaneous tissue. The patient notices a mass in the vulva that has grown in size but is usually asymptomatic.

Physical Examination

On the labium major there is a soft, sessile, or pedunculated mass varying in size from 1 cm to several centimeters in diameter (Fig. 19-9). Very large lesions may be ulcerated.

Diagnosis

Diagnosis is clinical and confirmed by biopsy. Differential diagnoses include hemangioma, fibroma, and Bartholin's cyst.

Treatment

Excision of the mass is necessary if it is symptomatic.

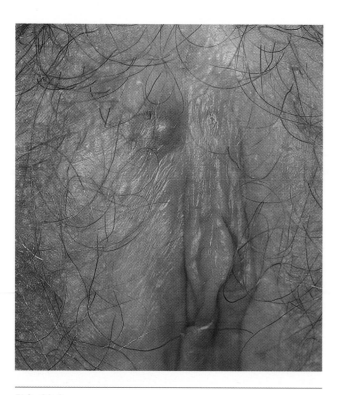

FIG. 19-8
Hidradenoma Papilliferum. An asymptomatic, skin-colored papule on the inner labium major.

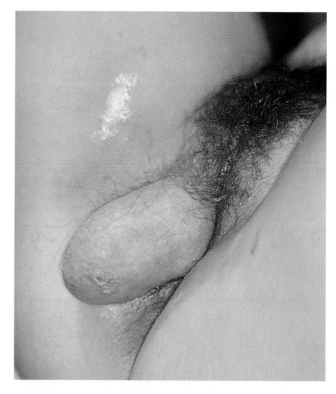

FIG. 19-9
Skin-colored pedunculated lipoma of labium major observed in a 15 year old.
(Courtesy Dr. G.D. Oliver.)

Lymphangioma

Lymphangioma (superficial lymphatic malformation) is a tumor of the lymphatic vessels, which can be either primary or secondary (lymphangiectasia). The disorder can present in either of the following two manners:

1. Lymphangioma circumscriptum, a hamartoma, is a developmental malformation of lymphatic tissue resulting in dilated superficial lymphatic and capillary channels of varying size.
2. Secondary lymphangiomas are due to obstruction of lymphatic drainage such as in a patient with a pelvic tumor after irradiation or surgery.

Lymphangioma circumscriptum lesions appear after birth. In the secondary type there is a history of surgery or irradiation in the pelvic or abdominal area with the subsequent formation of these lesions. Generally asymptomatic, these lesions can itch and burn. In the vulvar area they may rupture and discharge lymph, causing local irritation.

Physical Examination

In both types, the lesions appear like a mass of "frog's eggs" with groups of 1 to 5 mm translucent or hemorrhagic vesicles on skin-colored bases or a reddish-brown base (Fig. 19-10). There may be several groups of these vesicles. Leakage of lymph can be a problem but confirms the diagnosis (Fig. 19-11).

Diagnosis

Diagnosis is made on clinical observation and histopathology.

Treatment

Management is symptomatic. It usually is not possible to completely excise these. As it is impossible to delineate the edges and depth of the lesions, there is a high recurrence rate. Superficial laser destruction or electrodesiccation is useful in superficial lesions but rarely curative.

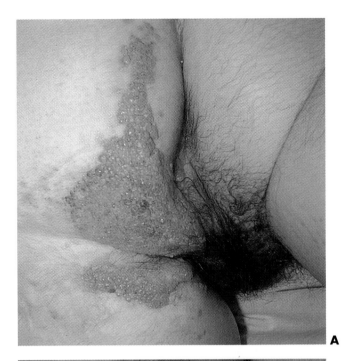

A

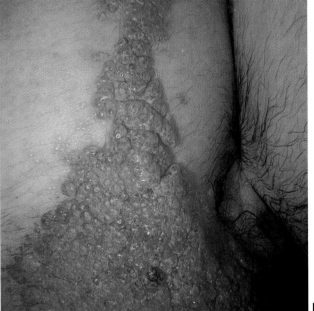

B

FIG. 19-10

Lymphangioma Circumscriptum. **A,** Reddish, cystic, perivulvar and perianal papulovesicles forming a large plaque in a 25 year old. **B,** Close up of *A* showing the dilated papulovesicles almost like red fish eggs.

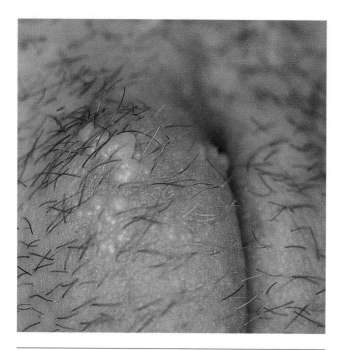

FIG. 19-11
Close up of milky lymphatic fluid-filled cystic vesicles on the edge of the labium major and on the mons pubis. This 17-year-old patient had radiation for a pelvic rhabdomyosarcoma at 3 years of age with resulting pelvic fibrosis. These lesions sporadically leaked lymph, causing pruritus and irritation.

BOX 19-2

Types of Melanocytic Nevi

Junctional Nevi—cells at the dermoepidermal junction above the basement membrane
Intradermal Nevi—cells in the dermis only
Compound Nevi—combination of junctional and intradermal nevi

BOX 19-3

Different Morphologic Types of Nevi

Flat Nevi—usually junctional
Slightly Elevated Nevi—compound
Papillomatous Nevi—mostly intradermal
Dome-Shaped Nevi—intradermal
Pedunculated Nevi—intradermal
Dysplastic Nevi—flat or elevated, speckled pigmentation, irregular shape, reddish hues, and indistinct margins (Fig. 19-12, *A*)
Giant Congenital Nevomelanocytic Nevi—a rare congenital nevomelanocytic nevus that presents at birth as a sharply demarcated hyperpigmented plaque studded with papules and nodules of varying sizes and degrees of pigmentation, usually over the lower back and hips, hence "bathing trunk" nevus (Fig. 19-12, *B*); melanoma risk is about 6.3%

Melanocytic Nevus

The melanocytic nevus is a very common hamartoma of melanocytic cells located within the dermis and epidermis. The types of melanocytic nevi are listed in Box 19-2.

Melanocytic nevi are very common on the skin surface but not in the vulvar area. Synonyms include nevocellular nevus, mole, nevus pigmentosus, and acquired melanocytic nevocellular nevus. Nevi are hamartomas of melanocytes derived from neural crest cells. Most are not present at birth but develop in childhood or adolescence.

Nevi are often noted not by the patient but by the caregiver, and the patient is referred to rule out neoplasia. The patients themselves may notice a lesion that is changing color or size. Occasionally the lesions may be traumatized and irritated by clothing, or accidentally scratched and ulcerated.

Physical Examination

There are several clinical types of nevi (Box 19-3). Nevi show varying patterns of pigmentation. The patterns can be found anywhere on the vulva. Benign nevi are uniformly pigmented, well circumscribed, and usually under 6 mm in diameter.

Junctional nevi are flat or slightly elevated and show uniform light-brown to brown-black pigmentation. Mucosal nevi are usually junctional. Compound nevi are papular, slightly elevated, dome-shaped (Fig. 19-13, *A*), flesh-colored to brown, and show a smooth or pebbly surface (Fig. 19-13, *B*). They are sharply margined with a variable degree of pigmentation and can be situated anywhere in the vulva but more commonly in the hair-bearing areas.

Intradermal nevi are brown to black and become lighter with age. They are often dome-shaped but they can be papillomatous or pedunculated.

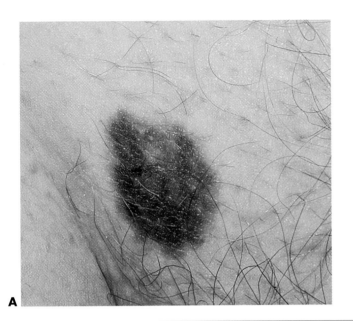
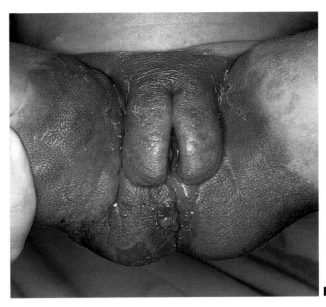

FIG. 19-12

A, Suprapubic dysplastic nevus with an irregular shape, reddish hue to the edges, and indistinct margins. **B,** Giant pigmented nevus of the vulva, thighs, and buttocks in a baby with an eroded diaper rash.

(**A,** Courtesy Dr. L. From.)

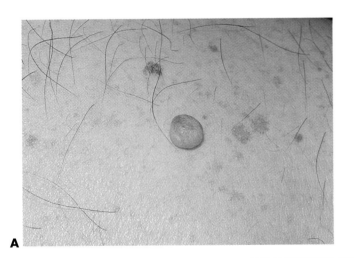
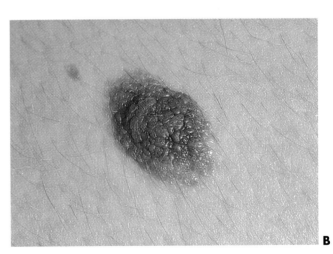

FIG. 19-13

A, Dome-shaped, skin-colored intradermal nevus. **B,** A papular compound nevus with a pebbly surface and very slight irregular pigmentation.

(Courtesy Dr. L. From.)

Diagnosis

Diagnosis is made on histopathology. Differential diagnoses include seborrheic keratoses, warts, VIN, melanoma, and basal cell carcinoma.

Treatment

No treatment is needed for obvious benign nevi unless there is repeated trauma resulting from their size and site. Then surgical removal is necessary. All suspicious lesions should be excised by either a shave excision or a simple excision with suture closure. Up to 20% of malignant melanomas arise in preexisting nevi, usually junctional or compound. If there is any question, always do an excisional removal for histopathology.

Seborrheic Keratosis

This is a very common, benign, warty-surfaced pigmented growth that can appear anywhere on the body after age 30, but uncommonly on the vulva. Synonyms for this condition are seborrheic wart and senile keratosis. The lesions are usually asymptomatic. Occasionally they are itchy and if scratched can become secondarily infected.

Physical Examination

The lesions are 0.25 to 1 cm in diameter and oval to round. They can be scattered anywhere on the lower abdomen and inner thighs or on the nonmucosal surface of the vulva. The lesions are tan colored to brownish black. Their surface may be somewhat smooth to frankly warty, with a somewhat "stuck on" appearance (Fig. 19-14).

Diagnosis

Diagnosis is clinical and histopathologic. Differential diagnoses include pigmented basal cell carcinoma, melanoma, and viral warts.

Treatment

Asymptomatic lesions need no treatment. Local destruction can be carried out using electrodesiccation, curettage, or cryosurgery with liquid nitrogen.

Skene's Duct Cyst

Skene's duct cysts are uncommon paraurethral duct cysts on the edge of or beside the urethral orifice.

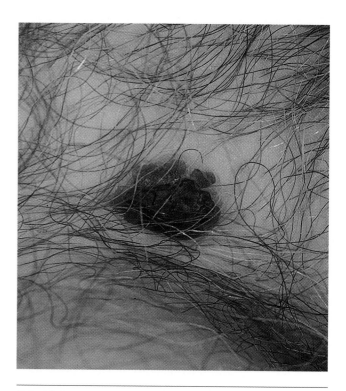

FIG. 19-14
Warty-surfaced, hyperpigmented papule on the right labium major showing the "stuck-on" appearance of a seborrheic keratosis.

Retention cysts form within the ducts resulting from ductal occlusion that may be caused by Skenitis (usually infection) or trauma. Small cysts are asymptomatic unless infected, when there is pain, urinary retention, and dyspareunia. Very large cysts can cause symptoms of obstruction including urinary retention. They are usually discovered during a routine pelvic examination or by self-examination.

Physical Examination

These cysts are usually less than 2 cm in diameter and are located at the edge of or beside the meatus. They are mobile and skin-colored or translucent (Fig. 19-15). Rarely they are large enough to partially block the urethral meatus.

Diagnosis

Diagnosis is clinical and histopathologic. Differential diagnoses include urethral diverticulum and mucous cyst.

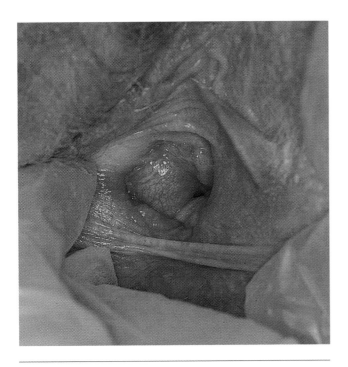

FIG. 19-15
Skin-colored, mobile Skene's duct cyst at the edge of the meatus.

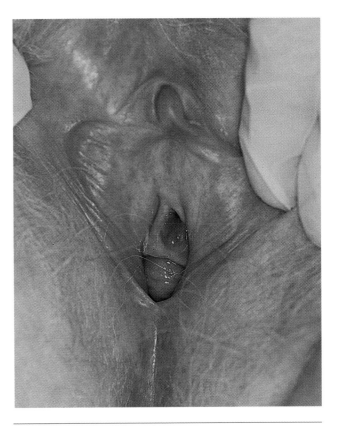

FIG. 19-16
Urethral Caruncle. Asymptomatic bright red papular lesion at the lower edge of the meatus in 65-year-old woman.

Treatment

For an asymptomatic cyst, no treatment but reassurance is necessary. Symptomatic cysts can be excised.

Urethral Caruncle

A urethral caruncle is a common, benign, polypoid growth derived from the posterior urethral mucosa. The etiology is unknown. It is believed to be an ectropion of the urethral mucosa. It may be related to trauma, altered environment, chronic irritation, or infection. Most lesions occur in menopausal women and are asymptomatic but they can cause pain, dysuria, and bleeding.

Physical Examination

It is a flesh-colored to red solitary polypoid tumor that is 0.5 to 1 cm in diameter and is usually seen as a bright red nodule at the urethral meatus (Fig. 19-16).

Diagnosis

Diagnosis is obtained with biopsy. Differential diagnoses include hemangioma, polyp, urethral prolapse, and urethral carcinoma.

Treatment

For small asymptomatic lesions no treatment is needed. Small symptomatic lesions can be destroyed with electrodesiccation, cryotherapy, or excision under local anesthesia. Larger lesions need the skills of a urologist and general anesthesia.

Vestibular Mucous Cyst

Vestibular mucous cysts are not uncommon. They are simple cysts within the vulvar vestibule and are composed of mucus-secreting epithelium. The exact origin of these cysts is disputed. They may be derived from urogenital sinus epithelium or from the obstruction of minor vestibular glands. These lesions are usually asymptomatic unless infected, when there is pain. Very large cysts can cause symptoms of obstruction. They are usually discovered on routine pelvic examination or by self-examination.

Physical Examination

These cysts vary in size from 0.5 to 1.5 cm in diameter and are located around the introitus. They are mobile, nontender, skin-colored, yellowish, or bluish/translucent with a smooth surface (Fig. 19-17). Rarely they are large enough to partially block the urethral meatus.

Diagnosis

Diagnosis is clinical and histopathologic. Differential diagnoses include Bartholin's duct cyst, Skene's duct cyst, and epidermal cyst.

Treatment

For an asymptomatic cyst, no treatment but reassurance is necessary. Symptomatic cysts can be excised.

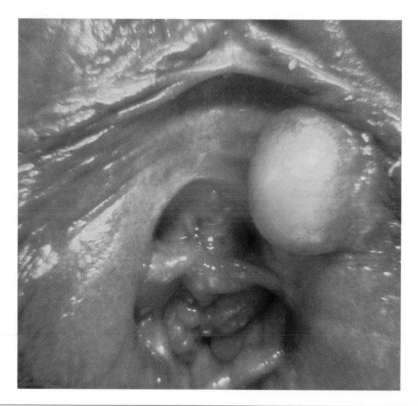

FIG. 19-17
A yellow, well-circumscribed, smooth-surfaced vestibular cyst on the left side of the vulvar vestibule.
(Courtesy Dr. G.D. Oliver.)

MALIGNANT TUMORS

Basal Cell Carcinoma

Basal cell carcinoma is a tumor of the epidermal basal cells. Although it is a very common skin cancer, it is an uncommon vulvar neoplasm[1-3] with a prevalence of 2.6% of vulvar neoplasms. There are no known predisposing factors. Ultraviolet light exposure plays a role in other areas of the skin. This is usually an asymptomatic tumor of postmenopausal women. There may be mild itching, irritation, or pain. The tumor may ulcerate and bleed with trauma.

Physical Examination

The early lesion is a small, firm, skin-colored, pearly, asymptomatic papule (Fig. 19-18, *A*). It is most frequently located on the hair-bearing area of the labium major. Pigmentation is variable. With time, the lesion ulcerates (Fig. 19-18, *B*).

Diagnosis

Diagnosis is made on histopathology. Differential diagnoses include molluscum contagiosum, intradermal nevus, neuroma, hidradenoma papilliferum, and squamous cell carcinoma.

Treatment

Complete destruction or removal of the lesions is necessary. For smaller lesions, curettage and electrodesiccation can be used. For larger lesions, surgical excision is used for removal. For lesions with questionable borders, Mohs' micrographic surgery is best.[4]

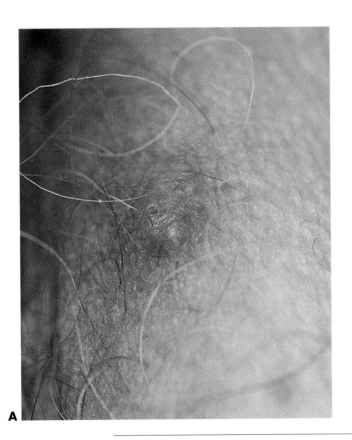
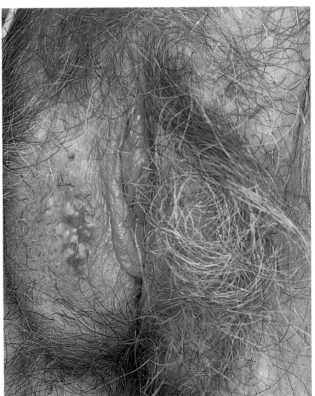

A   B

FIG. 19-18
Basal Cell Carcinoma. **A**, Asymptomatic, firm, cystic, slightly pigmented papule on labium major. This basal cell carcinoma in a 60 year old was found on routine pelvic exam. **B**, Ulcerated, irregularly outlined, itchy bleeding lesion in a 55-year-old woman. The diagnosis of basal cell carcinoma is made on biopsy.

Squamous Cell Carcinoma

Squamous cell carcinoma is a malignant tumor of the epidermal keratinocytes. It is the most common and important of the malignant tumors of the vulva, accounting for 85% to 90% of cases.

Squamous cell neoplasms are classified as intraepithelial or invasive.

Intraepithelial

Superficial squamous cell carcinoma is squamous cell carcinoma-in-situ (SCCIS). This is also referred to as intraepithelial neoplasia, and, on the vulva, vulvar intraepithelial neoplasia (VIN). This replaces the clinical terms Bowen's disease and Bowenoid papulosis.

The vulvar intraepithelial neoplasias have been formally grouped together and subclassified as VIN (agreed on by the International Society for the Study of Vulvovaginal Disease [ISSVD] and the International Society of Gynecologic Pathologists [ISGP]).[5,6]

According to their criteria, the histologic pattern of the disorganized epidermis shows variations in degree of dysplasia, cellular atypia, and mitotic activity (Box 19-4).

VIN III has been linked to human papillomavirus (HPV) types 16 and 18 (also 31, 33, 35, 51, and 52). Contributing factors in its development are age, immune status, and smoking.[7-9]

Note: *The terms Bowenoid papulosis, Bowenoid dysplasia, carcinoma simplex, and Bowen's disease are no longer recommended for clinical or pathologic use.*

There are two general patterns, the multifocal type that occurs in younger women ages 20 to 50 and the solitary lesions that occur in older women 60 to 70 years of age. The multifocal type can be itchy and irritating. The solitary lesions often have no symptomatology unless cracked and then they are painful, burning, or sore. Patients with these lesions are often asymptomatic. The lesions can grow insidiously over many years.

Physical Examination. Multlifocal lesions show sharply marginated, flat-topped papules or small plaques that are variably colored (Figs. 19-19, *A* and *B*). Often they can be reddish or pink, tan to gray-brown to darkly pigmented. The lesions can measure 2 to 3 cm and may be scattered in a few areas or extensively involve the vulva and perianal area. They look much like condylomata (Fig. 19-19, *C*).

The solitary lesions show a single, pink or reddish, sharply marginated patch or plaque. It can be skin-colored or red, shiny, and almost velvety looking on the surface. (Fig. 19-19, *D*).

Diagnosis. Diagnosis is clinical and histopathologic and can be improved with the use of a culposcope and/or acetowhitening. It is important to assess extent so multiple biopsies are needed in multifocal disease to rule out invasion. Differential diagnoses of the solitary lesion include condylomata, seborrheic keratosis, lentigo, and condylomata lata. For multifocal disease include condyloma acuminata and extramammary Paget's disease.

BOX 19-4

**Histologic Patterns of
Vulvar Intraepithelial Neoplasia (VIN)**

VIN I—mild dysplasia
VIN II—moderate dysplasia
VIN III—severe dysplasia, carcinoma in situ

FIG. 19-19
Vulvar Intraepithelial Neoplasia (VIN). **A,** Two small gray/white plaques with a velvety surface on either side of the clitoris in VIN III (best seen with acetowhitening). **B,** Extensive, pink, slightly eroded plaques of VIN III involving all of the right interlabial sulcus and the inner aspect of the labium minor, left side of the clitoris, and in the perianal area. This condition was very itchy. **C,** Hyperpigmented, multifocal, warty lesions of VIN III looking like condylomata acuminata. **D,** Isolated lesion of VIN III on the left lower edge of the labium minor in a patient who presented with dyspareunia.
(A, B, and C, Courtesy Dr. P. Bryson.)

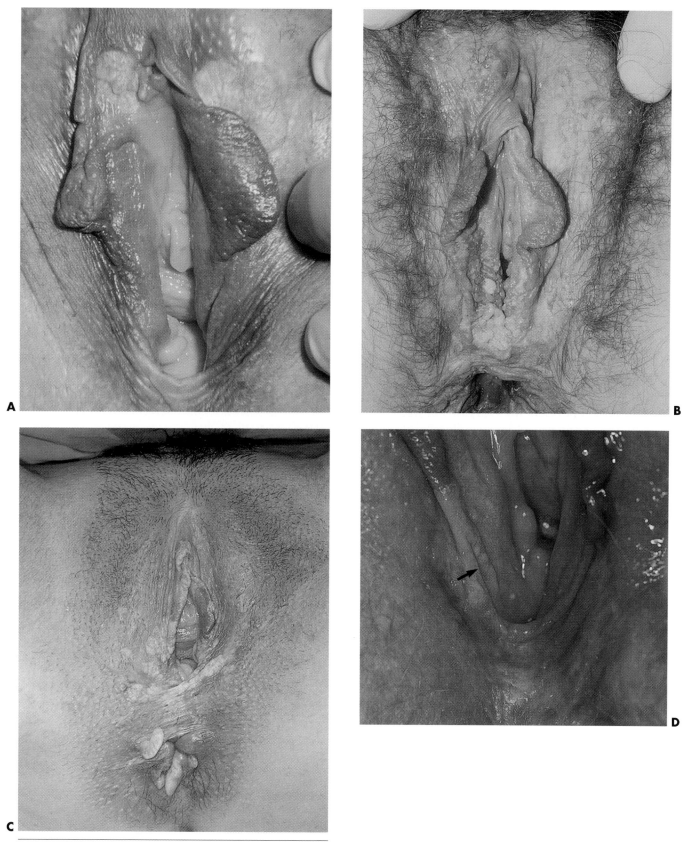

FIG. 19-19
For legend see opposite page.

Treatment. Depends on the location and extent of the lesion. Management should be overseen by an experienced dermatologist or gynecologic oncologist.

A solitary lesion can be removed by the following:

Local excision with 0.5 to 1 cm margin

Mohs' micrographic surgery if margins indistinct

Carbon dioxide laser destruction or electrosurgical destruction

Multifocal disease can be treated with the following:

Local excision with 0.5 to 1 cm margin

Mohs' micrographic surgery if margins are indistinct

Laser ablation

Cryosurgery

Topical 5-fluorouracil cream (Efudex) twice a day for 6 to 8 weeks (produces an inflammatory reaction that may not be tolerated)

Most procedures can be done with local anesthetic. For extensive disease general anesthesia is necessary.

Notes on Prognosis. The frequency of VIN progressing to invasive disease is not known precisely. Generally, women age 40 years or younger with VIN III have a 5% risk of developing invasive squamous cell carcinoma. Above age 40, a woman's risk increases to 15% to 20%.

In addition, there are two populations of VIN III patients: those age 45 years or younger whose lesions are usually associated with HPV (usually 16 to 18) and the more elderly patients with no associated HPV.

Relevant to VIN III with HPV, there is also an association with sexually transmitted diseases such as herpes simplex and syphilis, plus a higher incidence of cervical dysplasia and possibly invasive cancer of the cervix, all of which should be searched for in this group.

Invasive

This is an epidermal keratinocyte neoplasm that occurs as a solitary lesion on the vulva in patients older than 55 years. The lesion is usually asymptomatic but when exophytic, cracked, and ulcerated, it may bleed and can become itchy, sore, or painful. Complaints in advanced cases include discharge, dysuria, and foul odor.

This may occur on the background of other chronic vulvar diseases such as lichen sclerosus and lichen planus. These vulvar conditions have their own symptomatology—itching, burning, irritation, and years of dyspareunia. Of patients with lichen sclerosus, 5% develop squamous cell carcinoma of the vulva, but 30% to 40% of squamous cell carcinomas of the vulva are associated with surrounding lichen sclerosus.[10]

Physical Examination. Lesions of the vulva are usually unifocal and 1 to 2 cm in diameter. They may be nodular or ulcerated (Fig. 19-20, *A*). The color may vary from white to red. They are situated on the posterior fourchette, labia minora, or interlabial sulcus. As they become more exophytic and larger, the surface becomes eroded and ulcerated with a varying degree of bleeding. They may be associated with a background of lichen sclerosus (Fig. 19-20, *B*) in the vulva or, more rarely, lichen planus.

Note: *Early invasive squamous cell carcinoma can be associated with VIN III, as mentioned above. This is referred to as superficial invasive squamous cell carcinoma (SISCC) and is 2 cm or less in diameter and 1 mm or less in depth. The clinical presentation is an ulcerated or hyperkeratotic plaque.*

Diagnosis. Diagnosis is clinical with incisional or excisional biopsy. Culposcopic examination may be of additional value. Differential diagnoses include VIN, Paget's disease, amelanotic melanoma, chancroid, Crohn's disease, and metastatic carcinoma.

Treatment. Management involves the expertise of a gynecologic oncologist. The tumor has to be well assessed, staged, and then specific treatment planned for tumor removal. The details are beyond the scope of this text.

Malignant Melanoma

Melanoma is a malignant neoplasm of melanocytes. The majority of these develop de novo and 30% evolve from previous nevi. Melanoma accounts for 8% to 11% of vulvar malignancies and 2% to 3% of all malignant melanomas in females. Vulvar melanomas occur more commonly in white women after menopause and are thicker and larger at the time of diagnosis than melanomas diagnosed elsewhere (Box 19-5).

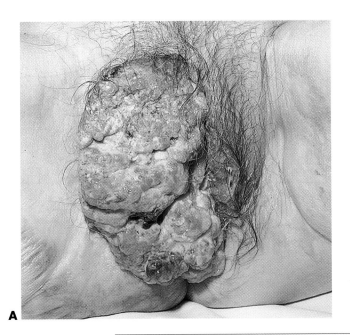

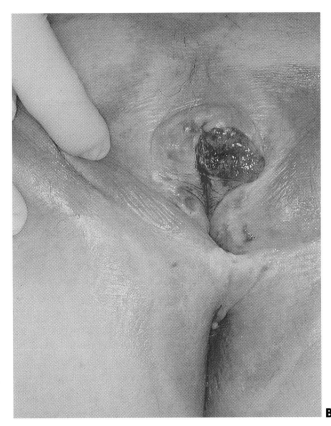

A

B

FIG. 19-20
A, Huge exophytic, exudative, squamous cell carcinoma destroying most of the vulva and extending anteriorly to the thigh and posteriorly to the perianal area in an elderly woman. **B**, Well-circumscribed ulcerated, bleeding, squamous cell carcinoma in a scarred lichen sclerosus.
(**B**, Courtesy Dr. P. Bryson.)

A patient with a vulvar melanoma is usually 45 to 65 years of age. Often patients do not notice the lesion until the melanoma reaches an advanced stage, presenting as a lump or mass, bleeding or itching. Less frequently, patients present with a "changing mole."[11,12]

Physical Examination

Melanomas can involve the vulva anywhere, but 80% are on the mucous membrane (vestibule, labia minora and clitoris). The lesions may be quite large when finally discovered and diagnosed.

Superficial Spreading Melanoma. This type appears as a flat, pigmented macule with a jagged border and a spectrum of colors—black, brown, red, gray. Nodular lesions may develop within the macule as time passes.

Nodular Melanoma. There is a simple dermal nodule, 0.5 to 1 cm, with a homogeneous to slightly variegated color, blue-black or reddish. These can ulcerate (Figs. 19-21 and 19-22).

Acral-lentiginous Melanoma. These look similar to lentigo maligna melanoma. They are initially flat with markedly variegated color (brown, black, blue, and depigmented areas) and ill-defined margins. Nodules eventually develop within the margins of the lesion. Margins are difficult to define for planning curative surgery.

BOX 19-5

Types of Melanoma

1. Superficial spreading melanoma—an elevated, variegated brown, blue-gray to black plaque with a very irregular border that typically has a slow horizontal growth phase then a vertical growth phase. It represents 50% of vulvar melanomas.
2. Nodular melanoma—a rapidly growing melanocytic tumor with no horizontal growth phase, an aggressive vertical growth phase, and a poor prognosis. The two variants (nodular and nodular polypoid) of nodular melanoma together make up 35% of vulvar melanomas.
3. Acral-lentiginous melanoma—a melanoma that occurs on palms, soles, nailbeds, and the mucocutaneous skin of the mouth, genitalia, and anus. It has a sometimes discontinuous horizontal growth phase and is aggressive but relatively rare in whites, occurring more commonly in Asians and in patients with brown or black skin. It comprises 15% of melanomas of the vulva.

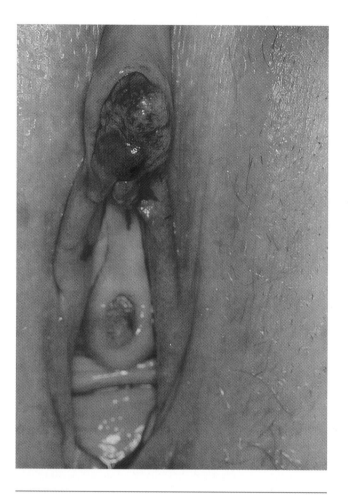

FIG. 19-21
Superficial spreading malignant melanoma of the periclitoral area with two nodules.
(Courtesy Dr. P. Bryson.)

Diagnosis

Clinical and histopathologic determine the diagnosis. Prognosis is decided on the basis of Clark's levels of invasion,[13] Breslow's direct thickness measurement,[14] and completeness of excision. Differential diagnoses include nevus, VIN, and mucosal melanotic macule.[15]

Treatment

Management and outcome depend on the histologic depth of the lesion and the completeness of removal. Treatment is surgical, requiring the expertise of the gynecologic oncologist. Frozen sections can be used to ascertain ulcer margins in recurrent acral-lentiginous lesions.

Early superficial spreading melanomas less than 1.5 mm in depth of invasion have a relatively good outcome with radical wide local resection. These patients have the best chance for "cure." Beyond that, surgery is combined with a variety of chemotherapeutic modalities. The best treatment is an early diagnosis and local removal. Surgery, radiation, and chemotherapy may provide some helpful palliative treatment for larger lesions. Palpably positive groin lymph nodes should be removed to prevent groin skin ulceration in the palliative phase of care of advanced disease.

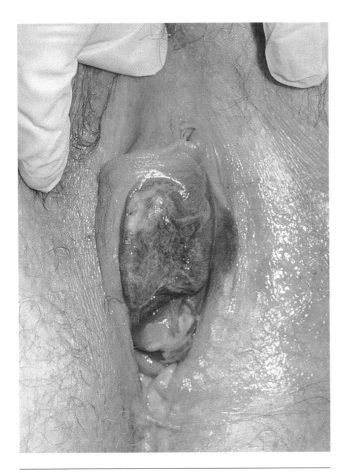

FIG. 19-22
Ulcerated malignant melanoma of the vulvar trigone and inner labium minor.
(Courtesy Dr. A. Covens.)

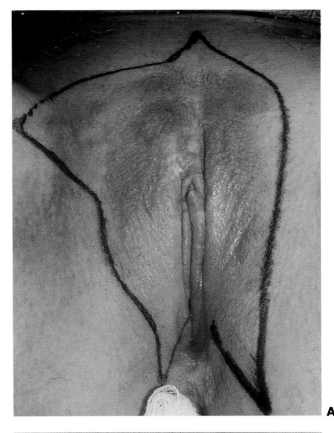

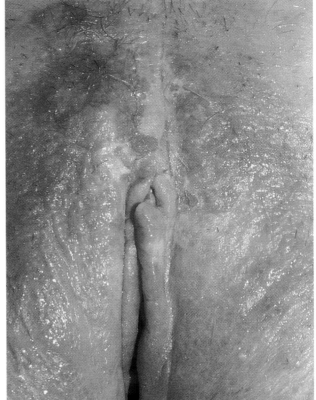

FIG. 19-23
A, Extensive, mildly eczematous erythematous plaque involving the labium major and extending up to the mons pubis. This case of Paget's disease was mildly itchy and had been called "eczema." **B,** Close up of *A* showing the erythema plus very superficial erosions around the clitoris.
(Courtesy Dr. P. Bryson.)

Extramammary Paget's Disease

Extramammary Paget's disease is a rare intraepithelial carcinoma of apocrine gland cells, found in the anogenital, umbilical, or axillary areas. The origin of the cancerous cells is variously thought to be from apocrine glands, anal or other mucosa, or epidermal cells with apocrine differentiation. A condition found on the vulva of elderly patients, it is usually asymptomatic but there may be some mild to moderate itching. On occasion, the patient presents because of an "itchy rash."

Physical Examination

The clinical picture is varied. Usually there is an eczematous, erythematous papule or plaque ranging in size from 1 to 10 cm with a variable degree of scaling and a sharply demarcated border (Fig. 19-23). The surface may show erosion or mild crusting. If the involvement is near the mucosa and the area is moist, the moist dysplastic keratin of the lesion is white. At times, the lesions may form gyrate multifocal plaques.

Diagnosis

Diagnosis is made on clinical suspicion supported by histopathology, including special stains. Differential diagnoses include malignant melanoma, VIN, psoriasis, Darier's disease, Hailey-Hailey disease, tinea cruris, and candidiasis.

Treatment

Efforts should be made to detect any underlying sweat gland carcinoma or adenocarcinoma. Distant neoplasia occurs in 10% of patients with vulvar Extramammary Paget's disease—breast, genitourinary, perianal, and anal carcinoma. Investigations should include breast examination with mammography, barium studies, and endoscopy of the entire gastrointestinal tract, IVP, and bladder cytology, plus thorough vaginal examination with colposcopy, cervical cytology, and endometrial biopsy.[16]

Local excision of all clinically involved skin is mandated. As this condition can be multifocal, Mohs' micrographic surgery is the treatment of choice. Recurrent extensive involvement needs the expertise of a gynecologic oncologist; details are beyond the scope of this book.

MALIGNANT TUMORS METASTATIC TO THE VULVA

Primary tumors elsewhere in the body can infrequently spread to the vulva with a resulting metastatic lesion. The most common tumors to metastasize to the vulva are squamous cell carcinomas of the cervix and adenocarcinomas of the endometrium. Tumors from the vagina, ovary, urethra, bladder, kidney, rectum, breast, and lung can spread to the vulva, as can choriocarcinoma, neuroblastoma, and melanoma. These tumors spread in their later stages when there is extensive lymphatic and blood vessel invasion.

The patient usually has obvious carcinoma in the primary organ. Less frequently the patient presents with sudden onset of a firm nodule or groups of firm nodules in the vulvar area years after the primary tumor has been dealt with.

Physical Examination

Vulvar metastases are usually around the labia minora and clitoris. Most commonly a single nodule exists, but there may be several nodules. The color is grayish to red and the tumors may be broken down and ulcerated (Fig. 19-24, *A*). Very rarely inflammatory carcinoma of the vulva mimics a cellulitis. Less frequently, multiple metastatic cutaneous nodules are seen on the vulva, mons, abdomen, or thighs (Fig. 19-24, *B*).

Diagnosis

The clinical picture and histopathologic examinations lead to diagnosis. Differential diagnoses include keloid, lymphoma, sarcoid, and leishmaniasis.

Treatment

Management depends on the original carcinoma. Vulvar metastases usually are associated with a poor prognosis.

Langerhans Cell Histiocytosis

Langerhans cell histiocytosis is a neoplastic proliferation of Langerhans cell histiocytes that can result in a spectrum of disease, one form of which can involve the genital area in children and young adults. Synonyms for Langerhans cell histiocytosis include histiocytosis X, eosinophilic granulomato-

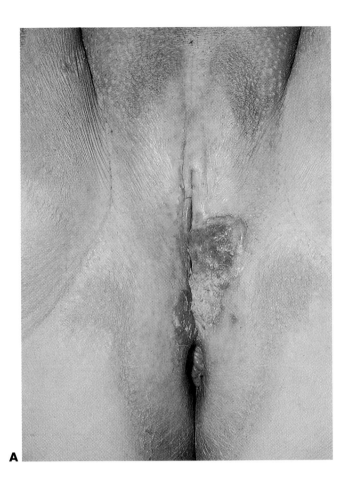

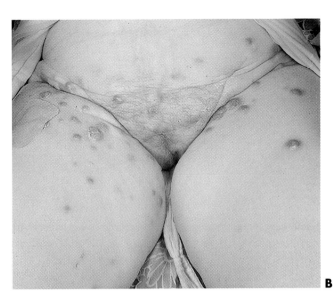

FIG. 19-24
A, Ulcerated, exophytic tumors on the vulva from endometrial carcinoma. **B,** Firm reddish subcutaneous nodules on the mons pubis, abdomen, and thighs from metastatic carcinoma of the cervix.
(Courtesy Dr. P. Bryson.)

sis, Type II histiocytosis, and nonlipid reticuloendotheliosis. The cause of the excess proliferation of these xanthohistiocytic cells is not known. These cells, along with other inflammatory cells, can produce indolent localized lesions or frankly disseminated fulminant disease. Whether this is a neoplastic or reactive condition remains in question.

This condition is rare in the vulvar area but can be seen at any age. In babies it presents as a diaper rash that is irritated, uncomfortable, itchy, sometimes painful, and won't heal. This may be part of the diffuse systemic form of this condition. In older children and adults the lesions may be itchy or painful papules, and older adults may be seen with somewhat itchy or frankly sore ulcers that are nonhealing.

Physical Examination

In babies and young children, the eruption is often confused with seborrheic dermatitis. Greasy, yellowish, scaly papules involve the diaper area and buttocks. Ulcers and some degree of purpura may appear in the inguinal area and elsewhere (Fig. 19-25). The same brown crusted papules also involve the scalp, behind the ears, and even the mouth.

In older children and adults, erosive hemorrhagic papules appear on the labia minora and majora, forming confluent sheets and eventually shallow, well-defined ulcers. A mixed pattern of lesions may occur, with vegetating plaques and occasional nodules. The vagina may be involved with erosion.

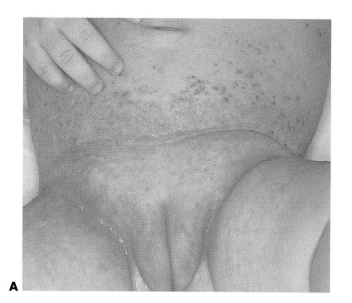

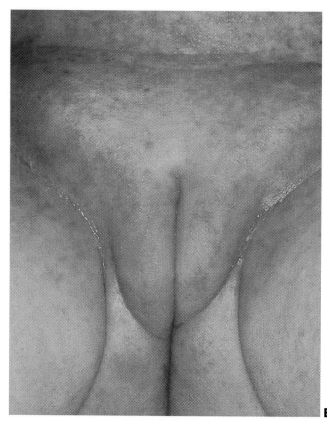

A **B**

FIG. 19-25
Langerhans Cell Histiocytosis. **A,** A baby with extensive erythematous papules on the lower abdomen, vulva, and inner thighs. Note petechiae on the left lower abdomen and marked erythema in the groin. **B,** Close up of *A* showing erosions in the inguinal creases.

Diagnosis

Diagnosis is by clinical pattern and histopathology. In adult diabetes insipidus, the vulvar eruption may be the sole clue to the underlying histocytic disease. Differential diagnoses include seborrheic dermatitis, napkin psoriasis, candidiasis, and atypical herpes simplex in the immunocompromised patient.

Treatment

Management is with chemotherapy with cytotoxic agents, under the guidance of an oncologist, and is beyond the scope of this text.

REFERENCES

Benign Tumors

1. Kaufman RH, Faro S: *Benign disease of the vulva and vagina,* ed 4, St Louis, 1994, Mosby.
2. Kharfi M, Mokhtar I, Fazaa B, et al: Vulvar basal cell carcinoma, *Eur J Dermatol* 2(2):81-84, 1992.
3. Stiller M, Klein W, Dorman R, Albom M: Bilateral vulvar basal cell carcinomata, *J Am Acad Dermatol* 28(5 Pt 2):836-838, 1993.

Malignant Tumors

4. Brown MD, Zachary CB, Grekin RC, Swanson NA: Genital tumors: their management by micrographic surgery, *J Am Acad Dermatol* 18 (1 Pt 1):115-122, 1988.

5. Wilkinson EJ: Normal histology and nomenclature of the vulva, and malignant neoplasms, including VIN, *Dermatol Clin* 10(2):283-286, 1992.

6. Wilkinson EJ: The 1989 presidential address: International Society for the Study of Vulvar Disease, *J Repro Med* 35(11):981-991, 1990.

7. Ansink AC, Heintz APM: Epidemiology and etiology of squamous cell carcinoma of the vulva, *Eur J Obstet Gyn Repro Biol* 48(2):111-115, 1993.

8. Kaufman RH: Intraepithelial neoplasia of the vulva, *Gynecol Oncol* 56(1):8-21, 1995.

9. Quan MB, Moy RL: The role of human papillomavirus in carcinoma, *J Am Acad Dermatol* 25(4):698-705, 1991.

10. Ridley CM: Lichen sclerosus, *Dermatol Clin* 10(2):309-323, 1992.

11. Look KY, Roth LM, Sutton GP: Vulvar melanoma reconsidered, *Cancer* 72(1):143-146, 1993.

12. Ronan SG, Eng AM, Briele HA, et al: Malignant melanoma of the female genitalia, *J Am Acad Dermatol* 22(3):428-435, 1990.

13. Clark WH, From L, Bernardino EA, Mihm M: The histogenesis and biologic behavior of primary human malignant melanoma of the skin, *Cancer Res* 29(3):705-726,1969.

14. Breslow A: Thickness, cross-sectional areas and depth of invasion in the prognosis of cutaneous melanoma, *Ann Surg* 172(5):902-908, 1970.

15. Rock B: Pigmented lesions of the vulva, *Dermatol Clin* 10(2): 361-370, 1992.

16. Chanda JJ: Extramammary Paget's disease: prognosis and relationship to internal malignancy, *J Am Acad Dermatol* 13(6):1009-1014, 1985.

ADDITIONAL READINGS

Benign Tumors

Kaufman RH, Faro S: *Benign disease of the vulva and vagina,* ed 4, St Louis, 1994, Mosby.

Lynch PJ, Edwards L: *Genital dermatology,* Baltimore, 1995, Churchill Livingstone.

Rock B: Pigmented lesions of the vulva, *Dermatol Clin* 10(2):361-370, 1992.

Wilkinson EJ, Stone IK: *Atlas of vulvar disease,* Baltimore, 1995, Williams & Wilkins.

Malignant Tumors Metastatic to the Vulva

Hewitt J, Pelisse M, Paniel BJ: *Diseases of the vulva,* London, 1991, McGraw-Hill.

Thomas R, Barnhill D, Bibro M, et al: Histocytosis-X in gynecology: a case presentation and review of the literature, *Obstet Gynecol* 67(Suppl):46S-49S, 1986.

VULVAR EDEMA

Edema of the vulva can be caused by inflammation, lymphatic obstruction, or many other conditions (Fig. 20-1, *A* through *D*).

The most common cause is an allergic reaction with systemic urticaria or an allergic contact dermatitis (e.g., reaction to latex in a condom). The causes of granulomatous inflammation are rare and can be identified with a biopsy. The infections are differentiated on clinical pattern and appropriate testing. Physical lymphatic obstruction is diagnosed with a thorough history and pelvic examination plus x-ray examinations, ultrasound, and magnetic resonance imaging (MRI).

Physical Examination

A thorough history and physical examination plus appropriate laboratory testing will usually define the cause of the edema (Box 20-1). Specific treatment can then be started.

Treatment

Recurrent streptococcal cellulitis can cause a progressive edema and vulvar distortion. A recurrent low-grade cellulitis with edema, redness, and irritation (itching or burning), usually with no systemic signs, leads to repeated lymphatic damage, resulting in stasis and susceptibility to more infection (Fig. 20-1, *E*). Management of this condition is usually handled with penicillin V potassium 300 to 500 mg qid for 3 to 4 weeks with a gradually decreasing dose over 6 months combined with prednisone 20 to 30 mg/day decreasing by 2.5 to 5 mg every 2 to 3 weeks over 3 to 6 months.

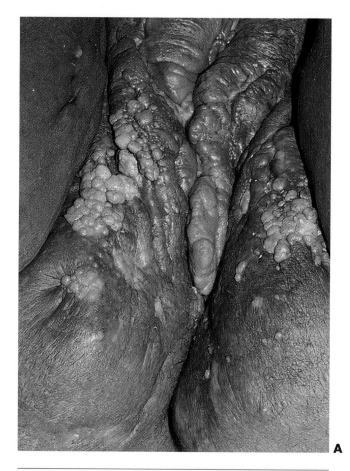

A

FIG. 20-1

A, Extensive scarring resulting in elephantiasis with papillomatous change as a result of chronic edema and fibrosis—all caused by Crohn's disease. **B,** Localized edema of left labia major and minor in Crohn's disease. **C,** Lymphedema of the labium minor resulting from chronic infection and lymphatic damage. **D,** Edema and distortion of the vulva caused by chronic excoriation with secondary infection. Note extensive erosive changes and hypopigmentation. **E,** Edema of labium as a result of recurrent streptococcal cellulitis.

(Courtesy Dr. L. Edwards.)

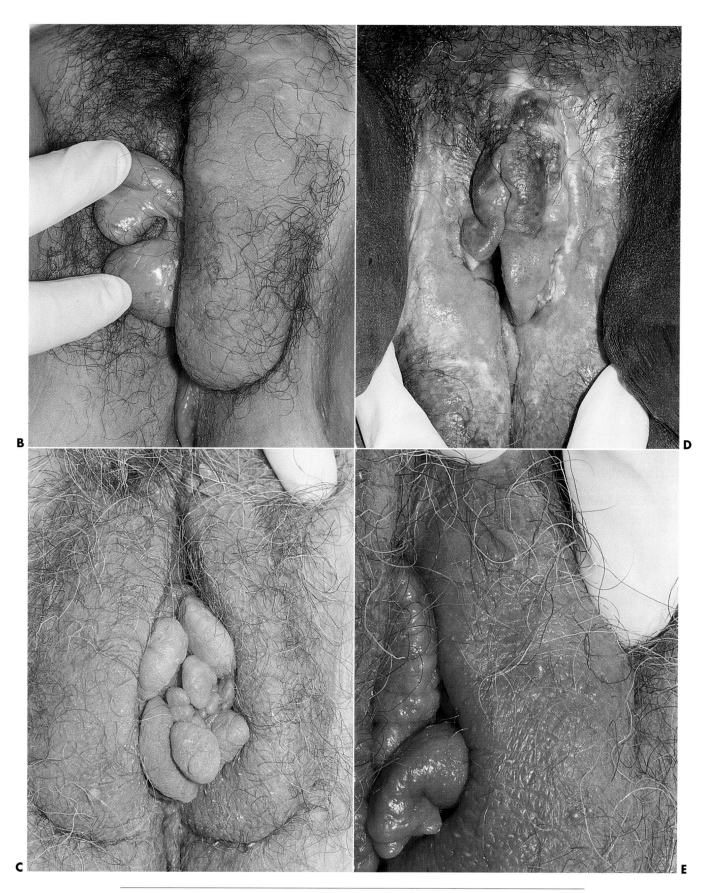

FIG. 20-1, cont'd
For legend see opposite page.

BOX 20-1

Causes of Edema of the Vulva

I Inflammatory edema
  A. Allergic/Immune
    1. Allergic reaction
      a. Angioedema with or without urticaria
      b. Allergic contact reaction (e.g., latex)
    2. Granulomatous inflammation
      a. Crohn's disease
      b. Melkersson-Rosenthal type syndrome
  B. Infectious—edema secondary to local infection
    1. Cellulitis—streptococcal
    2. Abscess—Bartholin's duct
    3. Candidiasis
    4. Rare
      a. Tuberculosis
      b. Actinomycosis
      c. Granuloma inguinale
      d. Amebiasis
      e. Blastomycosis
      f. Schistosomiasis

  C. Other
    1. Direct trauma
    2. Hidradenitis suppurativa

II Obstructive lymphedema
  A. Congenital—Milroy's disease (congenital lymphedema)
  B. Infection with secondary lymphatic damage
    1. Recurrent cellulitis—streptococcal
    2. Lymphogranuloma venereum
    3. Filariasis
  C. Physical lymphatic obstruction with mass or tumor or destructive process
    1. Pregnancy
    2. Pelvic or local trauma
    3. Pelvic tumor
    4. Irradiation

VULVODYNIA

Vulvodynia is defined by the International Society for the Study of Vulvovaginal Disease (ISSVD) as "chronic vulvar discomfort, with the patient's complaint of burning, stinging, irritation or rawness." *Vulvodynia is a symptom, not a disease.* It may lead to a complex, multifactorial clinical picture comprising vulvar pain, sexual dysfunction, and psychologic disability requiring a multidisciplinary approach.

Many vulvar conditions can be painful. The most problematic condition is dysesthetic vulvodynia. It is diagnosed by ruling out all the other conditions (Box 20-2).

Patients with vulvodynia complain of pain and burning. Burning alone may be the most important problem and may be further described as stinging, irritation, or rawness.

The pain may be sexually induced or physically provoked as in vestibulitis. It may be episodic as in herpes simplex; constant as in dysesthetic vulvodynia; or cyclic as in herpes simplex and cyclic *Candida* vulvovaginitis.

For all patients a thorough history and physical examination must be carried out, paying particular attention to precise details of the pain, which may include the following:
  duration and character
  previous treatments
  episodic nature
  other medical conditions
  precipitating factors
  menstrual association
  alleviating factors
  degree of incapacity

Physical Examination

This should include assessment of the whole patient including oral examination (e.g., lichen planus on the buccal mucosa may facilitate the diagnosis of vulvar lichen planus). The vulva must be thoroughly examined noting redness, fissures, blisters, erosions, or ulcers. The hymenal ring may show areas of erythema.

BOX 20-2

Differential Diagnosis of Vulvodynia

I Painful vulvar conditions—these show lesions on the cutaneous and/or mucosal surfaces

A Infections
Herpes simplex
Herpes zoster
Candidiasis
Impetigo
Streptococcal cellulitis
Chancroid
Lymphogranuloma venereum

B Trauma
Hymenal fissures
Trauma—abrasion/laceration
Split thick posterior commissure

C Miscellaneous
Atrophic vulvovaginitis
Fixed drug eruption
Steroid rebound dermatitis
Cystitis, bladder calculi, etc.

D Dermatoses
Lichen sclerosus
Lichen planus
Aphthosis/Behçet's
Bullous pemphigoid
Pemphigus vulgaris
Lupus erythematosus
Erythema multiforme
Toxic epidermal necrolysis

E Tumors
VIN/Squamous cell carcinoma
Basal cell carcinoma
Paget's disease

II Painful vulvar dermatoses—pain resulting from scratching and irritation
Psoriasis
Contact dermatitis (chronic)
Lichen simplex chronicus

III Causes of desquamative vulvovaginitis
Lichen planus (most common)
Bullous pemphigoid
Pemphigus vulgaris
Cicatricial pemphigoid
Langerhans cell histiocytosis (rare)
Erythema multiforme
Toxic epidermal necrolysis

IV Vulvar vestibulitis

V Neurologic problems resulting in vulvar pain/burning
Post-herpetic neuralgia
Pudendal neuralgia
Referred pelvic pain

VI Dysesthetic (essential) vulvodynia

Note: *Because of the exquisite pain of vulvar vestibulitis, this entity should be tested for before the vaginal examination. A cotton-tipped applicator should be used gently to pinpoint tender areas, especially at the site of the hymenal ring gland ducts.*

A vaginal examination should be gently carried out to rule out the causes of desquamative vulvovaginitis. Vaginismus must be noted. In patients with pelvic floor problems the transverse perineal and levator ani muscle must be palpated to localize the discomfort.

It may be possible to visualize the cause, as in the ulcerative conditions, or there may be no physical findings, as in some herpetic infections or in dysesthetic vulvodynia.

Diagnosis

It is essential to rule out the recognizable conditions in Box 20-2 before proceeding further. Vulvodynia may be triggered by more than one concurrent pathologic condition (e.g., vulvar lichen planus may be secondarily infected with yeast), so watch must be kept for more than one cause.

Infections with *Candida* and herpes simplex can be the most confusing. They both cause cyclic vulvar pain with pain-free days.

When caused by *Candida* (as discussed in Chapter 19) the flare is usually just before the menstrual period but this timing may vary. The pain is worse after intercourse. Cultures may not be helpful for the diagnosis. Clinically the vulva is usually just red and swollen with little to no discharge. It is believed this condition may represent an allergic hypersensitivity to small amounts of the organism.

Herpes simplex also causes cyclic pain, but there is usually a prodrome of itching, tingling, or burning. This condition also may flare with menstruation, and the patient may show no visible lesions (e.g., herpes simplex *sine eruptione* [without blisters]). In some patients persistent neuralgia may follow a severe primary herpes infection and last for months. In these cases amitriptyline or desipramine is useful, combined with long-term antiviral medication (Fig 20-2).

The most difficult of the vulvar pain conditions are the lesion-free types of pudendal neuralgia and dysesthetic vulvodynia.

PUDENDAL NEURALGIA

This very uncommon neuropathy of the nerve(s) serving the pudendal area causes continuous burning and deep aching. Pelvic nerves are subject to compression, stretching, entrapment, or transection, either directly (e.g., with tumor, degenerative disc disease, or pelvic or obstetric surgery) or indirectly (e.g., fall off a swing or down stairs onto the coccyx). Neuropathy also occurs in diabetes or postherpetic neuralgia. The pain is usually spontaneous and may be constant, deep, aching, burning, or lancinating. The genital area involved is dictated by the distribution of the affected nerve or nerve root and may include extension to the inner thighs. Anything touching the area of involvement (e.g., clothing) can make it worse. There may be associated dysuria and frequency.

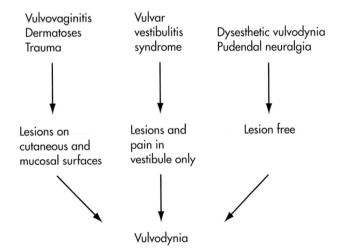

FIG. 20-2
Pathways to Vulvodynia.

Physical Examination

There are no visible physical changes. Neurologic examination may demonstrate hyperesthesia or hypoesthesia to touch; a touch may evoke either hyperalgesia or hypalgesia; and the sensation perceived (e.g., burning) may bear little relation to the stimulus applied (e.g., light touch)—a sensory misinterpretation termed *allodynia*.

Diagnosis

Diagnosis is clinical, ruling out other causes of vulvar pain. X-ray examination, computed tomography (CT), or MRI may be needed.

Treatment

Support is essential. These patients need an understanding and sympathetic physician. Take time to listen to them. Involve other team members (e.g., neurology, gynecology, pain clinic, urology) as appropriate. Biofeedback may be useful here if pelvic floor muscle spasm is a problem. The following medications may be prescribed:

Amitriptyline 10 to 150 mg/day
Carbamazepine 200 to 1200 mg/day
Sertraline 50 to 150 mg/day

DYSESTHETIC (ESSENTIAL) VULVODYNIA

This is a chronic vulvar pain syndrome. It probably originates as a myofascial pain that sets up a sympathetically-mediated and self-perpetuating "pain loop." It is often associated with an overlying psychoneurosis. It is most common in older women.

The etiology is the same as pudendal neuralgia, probably a combination of exaggerated pain response leading to a spasm-pain-spasm-pain loop. Although there may be a coexistent psychoneurosis, depression may be either primary or secondary. In some cases a borderline personality may play a role.

These middle-aged or older women complain of chronic widespread persistent pain. The description of this nonprovoked or spontaneous pain is often dramatic. It is stinging, lancing, and raw like nettles or peppers on the area. Libido is generally low, but sexual intercourse may be possible, inducing burning sensations afterwards for hours or days. There may be associated back pain, bladder, or bowel complaints. Some patients have associated fibromyalgia or interstitial cystitis.

Physical Examination

There are no visible changes. Pain may be evoked by light touch using a cotton-tipped applicator. Some have pain on palpation of the transverse perineal or levator ani muscles, with or without vaginismus. The chronicity and severity of this condition may lead to development of a distinct personality—anxious, angry, obsessive, hostile, and depressed.

Diagnosis

Diagnosis is clinical and requires ruling out other causes of vulvar pain.

Treatment

A dermatologist or gynecologist with interest in this area is needed to coordinate care. Support and understanding are vital. Never say "there is nothing to see" or "it is all in your head." As a physician you must avoid the "neurotic" label. Instruct the patient to avoid painful stimuli such as tight clothing. Physiotherapy is also a necessary aspect of care. This involves a musculoskeletal assessment looking at posture, back, pelvis, and the internal musculature. Initiate exercise, biofeedback, and electrical stimulation to help the patient control the pain.

Medications to be prescribed include the following:

amitriptyline 5 to 150 mg/day
desipramine 25 to 150 mg/day
sertraline 50 to 100 mg/day
fluoxetine 20 to 80 mg/day
pimozide 1 to 3 mg/day or combination of fluoxetine and pimozide

Note: *Start the dosage low and go slow. Remember that is takes at least 3 or up to 6 months for the medication to make a difference. Explain to the patient that "these aren't nerve pills, they are pills for sore nerves."*

ACRODERMATITIS ENTEROPATHICA

Acrodermatitis enteropathica is a rare autosomal recessive or acquired disorder caused by abnormal zinc absorption. Acral dermatitis, diarrhea, and alopecia are the presenting triad. Synonyms for acrodermatitis enteropathica are Danbolt-Closs syndrome, acrodermatitis enteropathica–like zinc deficiency disorders, zinc deficiency syndrome, zinc depletion syndrome, and iatrogenic acrodermatitis enteropathica.

The genetic variant is caused by a deficiency in structure or function of picolinic acid or another zinc-binding ligand resulting in poor zinc absorption. The acquired condition is due to zinc-deficient total parenteral nutrition or malabsorption of zinc (as in Crohn's disease).

Infants present with diarrhea, a persistent "diaper rash," anorexia, alopecia, and irritability. Without supplementation they will die. In adults the condition presents with a chronic erosive perineal dermatitis, diarrhea, irritability, lethargy, and sometimes hair loss.

Physical Examination

In infants the rash is a sharply marginated vesiculobullous, pustular, or erosive eruption covering the perineal and perianal area, spreading up into the gluteal cleft and all around the buttocks (Fig. 20-3, *A*). The same eruption occurs on the face, sometimes around the nose and eyes, in the flexural areas, and in older children it will involve the hands and feet (acrodermatitis) (Fig. 20-3, *B*). These children also suffer from alopecia, growth retardation, and erosions in the mouth. Older lesions may look somewhat psoriasiform and not as eroded. In adults it can be an acneiform perioral eruption of the face.

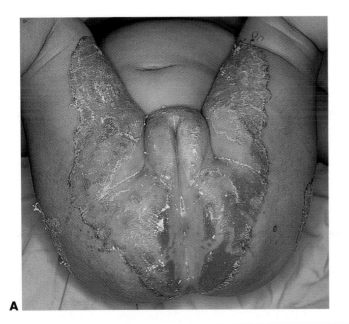

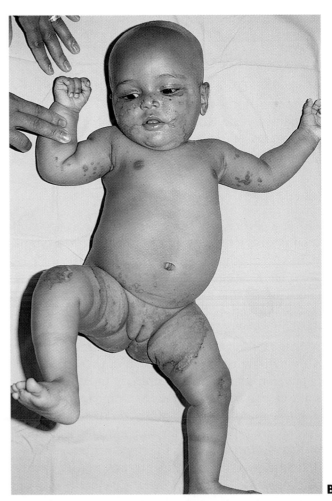

A   B

FIG. 20-3
A, Well demarcated scaling plaques of the whole diaper area with erosion and bleeding perianally in a case of acrodermatitis enteropathica. **B,** Typical perioral dermatitis. There are also some erosions on knees and inner arms in this baby.

Diagnosis

Clinical pattern and low serum zinc levels help determine diagnosis. A clinical trial of oral zinc supplementation can be tried. Differential diagnoses include cystic fibrosis and malabsorption, glucagonoma syndrome, mucocutaneous candidiasis, biotin deficiency, seborrheic dermatitis, and psoriasis.

Treatment

Management includes the medication zinc gluconate 10 to 15 mg tid.

VARICOSE VEINS

Twenty percent of pregnant women develop varicose veins in the vulva during pregnancy. The majority of these resolve spontaneously. Obstruction can also cause vulvar varicosities. Symptoms include pressure and itchiness. Rupture causes bruising and even extensive bleeding (Fig. 20-4).

Treatment

Surgery may be necessary if there is symptomatic thrombosis or bleeding.

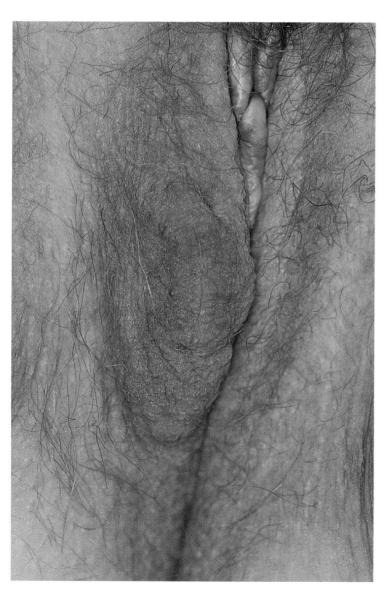

FIG. 20-4
Varicose veins of the right labium major several weeks postpartum.

PERIPHERAL VASCULAR DISEASE

This is a progressive condition in the elderly, primarily as a result of atherosclerosis but exaggerated by microangiopathy in patients with diabetes. Usually the feet and lower legs are involved, less commonly the fingers and hands. Very rarely a patient may suffer from severe generalized atherosclerotic disease. Ischemic cutaneous ulcers can result and can be of sudden onset with considerable pain (Fig. 20-5). Progression is relentless unless revascularization is possible. The area of cutaneous involvement depends entirely on the site of the vascular lesion.

Contributing factors include family history, hypercholesterolemia, diabetes, obesity, inactivity, and vasoconstrictive substances (e.g., nicotine in cigarettes, patches, or gum).

With involvement of the pelvic vascular tree it is possible to develop painful ulcers in the perivulvar area with progressive destructive gangrene and associated incapacitating pain.

Treatment

Requires vascular surgical repair if possible, along with management of pain and chronic wounds.

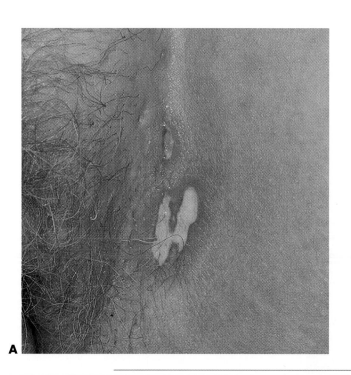

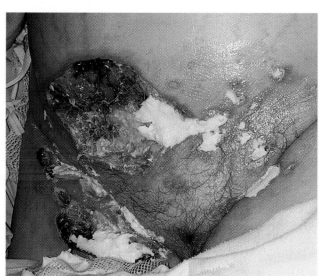

FIG. 20-5

A, Three small exquisitely painful ulcers on the left labiocrural fold that on biopsy showed necrosis only. **B,** Four months after *A,* showing extensive gangrenous necrosis of the abdominal wall and thigh in this severe case of peripheral vascular disease. At this time, this 52-year-old smoker and Nicorette user had dry gangrene of both feet, extending partway up to the knees. Pain was controlled with a morphine pump, and she was nursed on a Clinitron bed until she expired. Investigations showed almost complete vascular occlusion of all the vessels below the renal arteries. No surgical repair was possible.

DARIER'S DISEASE

Darier's disease is an uncommon autosomal dominant disorder of keratinization that presents with keratotic crusted papules. Synonyms for Darier's disease include Darier-White disease and keratosis follicularis. The etiology is a genetic disorder of keratin formation. Onset is usually in late childhood. Complaints are initially of mild irritation. As the condition becomes more pronounced, build-up of keratotic debris favors secondary infection and a resulting odor. Hygiene, especially in the genital area, becomes progressively difficult.

Physical Examination

The condition affects most commonly the neck, central torso, and flexural areas. The genital area is often involved. The lesions are widespread and increase in size and number with age (Fig. 20-6). Typical lesions are greasy, crusted, skin-colored, yellow, or brown papules. With time, they become progressively more verrucous. Secondary infection produces crusting.

Diagnosis

Diagnosis is clinical and histopathologic. Differential diagnoses include acanthosis nigricans, benign familial pemphigus, and impetigo.

Treatment

Hygiene is important to keep the area cool and dry and to avoid secondary infection. Instruct the patient to wear loose cotton clothing and to use thin absorbent cotton strips in the skin folds to stop the surfaces from rubbing together and to decrease moisture. The patient should wash with triclosan solution bid, pat the area dry, and use an absorbent powder like Zeasorb. Appropriate treatment of yeast and bacterial infection, topical and systemic, is also important.

For difficult disease the use of oral retinoids—acitretin (Soriatane) or etretinate (Tegison) or high-dose vitamin A—could be considered in appropriate patients. Local ablation of genital skin using skin grafting and/or a carbon dioxide laser may be necessary.

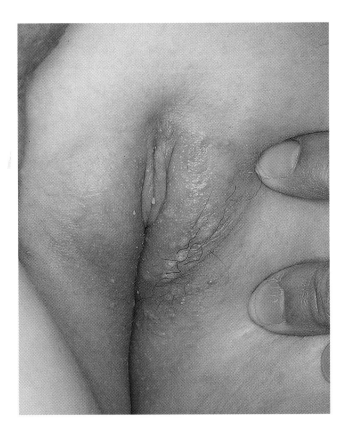

FIG. 20-6
An unusual case of a baby presenting with an increasing number of pink, slightly irritated papules in the groin. This is an extremely early onset. Biopsy showed Darier's disease.

STEROID REBOUND DERMATITIS

A common synonym is steroid rosacea. After moderately potent or stronger topical steroids have been used for more than 6 weeks, their withdrawal may result in rebound dermatitis. Topical steroids are vasoconstrictors. Their vasoconstrictive effect varies directly with their potency. Withdrawal results in a rebound vasodilation and a sensation of burning and irritation. Patients respond by immediately reapplying the same topical to obtain relief, and the cycle continues. With time, atrophy and telangiectasia result. This process, predictably, is more severe with higher potency topical steroids (note that ointments are stronger than creams). Only the mildest formulation (1% hydrocortisone) does not cause this reaction. Fair-skinned individuals are at greater risk for this problem.

Patient history includes use of mid-potency or stronger topical steroids. The patient complains of burning if the product is stopped and notes relief on restarting.

Physical Examination

The labia majora, less commonly the labia minora, and perivulvar skin show a diffuse papular erythema (Fig. 20-7). If there has been long-term use there may be signs of atrophy with telangiectasia.

Differential diagnoses include contact dermatitis, candidiasis, and psoriasis.

Treatment

"Stop the steroid" is the main form of management. This may be easier said than done. For comfort, recommend the use of sitz baths (see Appendix C), cool compresses, and a 1% hydrocortisone in petrolatum ointment or a bland mix of ¼% menthol, ¼% camphor in a petrolatum or Aquaphor base.

Note: *In some cases this problem is iatrogenic, predictable, and unavoidable (e.g., in severe erosive lichen planus).*

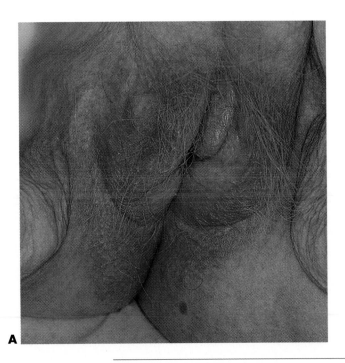
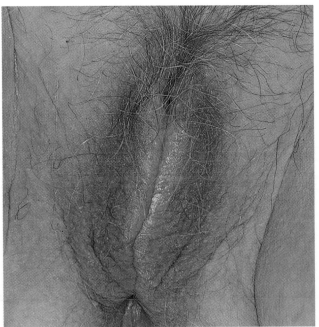

A   B

FIG. 20-7

A, Diffuse papular, fiery-red pattern of extensive rebound steroid dermatitis in an elderly woman with severe erosive vaginal lichen planus. Her vaginal erosive disease settled with 3 months of unavoidable intravaginal superpotent steroid (clobetasol), then her predictable rebound eruption was managed (see text for more information). **B,** Diffuse bright red papular erythema in rebound steroid dermatitis caused by an amcinonide ointment for psoriasis.

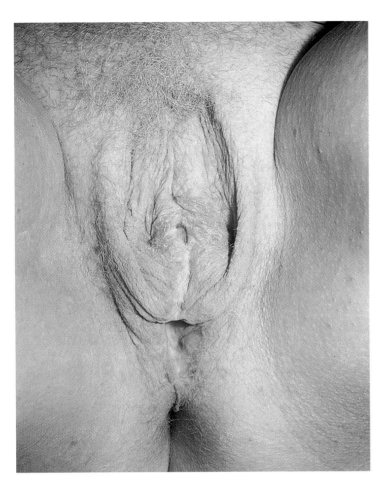

FIG. 20-8
Surgically constructed vulva/vagina in a transsexual.

TRANSSEXUAL SURGERY

Transsexual transformation surgery is done in carefully selected patients. The resulting vulva and vagina are constructed from the empty scrotum and penis (Fig. 20-8).

SUGGESTED READINGS

Vulvar Edema

Kaufman RH, Faro S: *Benign disease of the vulva and vagina,* ed 4, St Louis, 1994, Mosby.

Lynch PJ, Edwards L: *Genital dermatology,* Baltimore, 1995, Churchill Livingstone.

Tovell HMM, Young AW: *Diseases of the vulva in clinical practice,* New York, 1991, Elsevier.

Dysesthetic (Essential) Vulvodynia

Baggish MS, Milkos JR: Vulvar pain syndrome: a review, *Obstet Gynecol Surv* 50(8):618-627, 1995.

Koblenzer CS, Bostrom P: Chronic cutaneous dysesthesia syndrome: a psychotic phenomenon or a depressive symptom? *J Am Acad Dermatol* 30(2): 370-374, 1994.

Meana M, Binik YM: Painful coitus: a review of female dyspareunia, *J Nerv Ment Dis* 182(5): 264-272, 1994.

Paavonen J: Diagnosis and treatment of vulvodynia, *Ann Medicine* 27(2):175-181, 1995.

Paavonen J: Vulvodynia: a complex syndrome of vulvar pain, *Acta Obstet Gynecol Scand* 74(4): 243-247, 1995.

Although a penile biopsy may be thought to be a difficult procedure, it is actually technically easy and frequently helps in diagnosis. Excisional, incisional, punch, or shave biopsies can all be easily performed. ▲ **I prefer an incisional or an excisional biopsy.** ▼ The abundant vascularization of the penis causes extra bleeding in biopsy sites, but being prepared for this fact and using sutures easily deals with the problem.

BIOPSY TECHNIQUE
Instruments

The instruments used in taking a biopsy include the following:

1 mL or 3 mL disposable syringe with a #27 or #30 short needle
#15 scalpel blade and handle
Small curved iris scissors
Small needle holder
Fine-toothed tweezers
#6 Nylon or silk sutures

Procedure

The skin of the penis is very fine and thin, comparable only to the skin of the eyelids. Therefore it should be handled with gentleness and care. Plan the procedure. For small lesions that are going to be excised entirely, try to make an elliptic excision that follows the natural skin folds. This produces the best functional and cosmetic results.

Use 1% or 2% lidocaine with epinephrine. The epinephrine causes localized short-lasting vasoconstriction, which reduces bleeding and thus facilitates the surgical procedure. Some physicians are reluctant to use epinephrine-containing local anesthetics in the penis because of possible vasoconstriction with ensuing local damage. I have never seen this happen. The risk is negligible for procedures on the shaft of the penis and probably minimal if small amounts of anesthetic (0.3 to 0.5 mL) are used on the glans penis. To stay on the safe side, in elderly patients use lidocaine without epinephrine for procedures on the glans penis.

Cleanse the area to be biopsied with 70% alcohol or any suitable local antiseptic. Stabilize the lesion by stretching the skin and holding it down between your thumb and forefinger or between your forefinger and medius finger. Insert your needle very *superficially,* not farther than 1 to 2 mm from the border of the lesion, and start to infiltrate the anesthetic slowly. This raises a bleb whose size is determined by the amount you infiltrate. The ideal amount should give you a bleb just a bit larger than the area you intend to excise. The area then becomes anesthetized within a few seconds. Proceed to cut out the lesion using a superficial elliptic excision of the bleb's roof that includes the lesion. This suffices for the vast majority of lesions that involve the skin only and do not go deeper. It is obvious that when the lesion is deeper or more invasive your incision has to go deeper. ▲ **On those rare occasions when the lesion is quite deep or clearly invasive, I prefer to refer the patient to a plastic surgeon or urologist.** ▼ Closing the wound is no problem, just keep in mind that when the effect of the epinephrine wears off, the lesion may bleed if you do not suture the wound carefully. Use 6-0 nylon or 5-0 silk sutures to close the wound. These can be removed in about 5 days. ▲ **Absorbable 5-0 sutures can be used, but I prefer the nonabsorbable sutures. This gives me the opportunity to see the patient again when he returns for suture removal, and I can inspect the wound.** ▼ Frequently by the time of removal I already have the histology report and can plan further treatment as necessary with the patient.

Clinical Evaluation of Vulvar Patients

HISTORY AND PHYSICAL EXAMINATION

Patients with vulvar disease take time. Most patients have had chronic symptoms and multiple, often ineffective, treatments. It is important that the course of each patient's disease be accurately documented. This must be carried out in a nonjudgmental and a very supportive environment. **Take the time to listen.**

In each patient start from the beginning. Do not allow yourself to be seduced into telephone diagnosis. New or changing symptoms require a new physical examination. Scabies in a patient with vulvar psoriasis is not just a worsening of the psoriasis.

History

A general medical, social, and family history should be obtained from the patient and should include the following:
   Menstrual
   Gynecologic
   Obstetric
   Sexual—sexual practices, sexually transmitted
      diseases (STDs), treatments
   Previous treatments with responses (positive and
      negative)
   Prescription medications
   Over-the-counter products, past and present

Specific Symptoms

The most common complaints in vulvar disease are itch and pain. These may stand alone or in combination and vary in their description and localization. Complaints of burning are also often heard.

Characteristics to be defined in each patient include the following:

   Episodic
   Time of day or month
   Menstrual association
   Factors that help or worsen
   Degree of incapacity

Physical Examination

Examine all surfaces of the external genitalia and do a vaginal examination as needed. Problems with dermatoses, blistering diseases, or infections may involve other body areas. Examine other body surfaces and the oral mucosa. The diagnosis may be more obvious elsewhere.

Visualization

Proper lighting for the physical examination is imperative. The light should be bright but without glare. Full-spectrum incandescent lighting provides the red needed to discern subtle color variations. Magnification needs to be available with either special eyeglasses, loupes, or a magnifier/light source combination. Culposcopy can be very useful.
   Signs of vulvar disease include the following:
   Erythema
   Ulceration
   Whiteness
   Exudation
   Lichenification
   Crusting
   Erosion
   Purpura
   Loss of architecture
   Discharge

Note: *Look for related cutaneous physical signs (e.g., pitted nails and papulosquamous rash on the scalp or body in psoriasis).*

Equipment for Vulvar Diagnosis

10% KOH for microscopic diagnosis of dermatophyte, yeast

Litmus paper for pH determination (pH 4 to 5 in candidiasis, 5 to 7 in trichomoniasis, >4.5 in bacterial vaginosis)

Microscopic slides and cover slips

Microscope

Magnifying glass or specialized eyeglasses/loupes

Culture media for bacteria, fungus and yeast, and herpes simplex (have access to special media for STDs such as chlamydia and gonorrhea)

Vaginal specula—various sizes

Vinegar for acetowhitening

Normal saline and test tubes for wet mounts

Equipment for Local Anesthesia

Lidocaine 2% with and without epinephrine

30-gauge needles

3-cc syringe

Lidocaine/prilocaine cream (EMLA)

Plastic wrap

Equipment for Biopsy

Disposable skin biopsy punches—3 and 4 mm

Cervical biopsy forceps

Small iris scissors

Needle driver

Mosquito hemostat

#15 scalpel plus handle

Monsel's solution

Suture material

Formalin and specialized transport media for immunofluorescence

Note: *For interpretation of histopathology, a dermatohistopathologist is invaluable.*

Equipment for Therapy

Liquid nitrogen and cotton-tipped applicators, probes, and spray units for cryotherapy

Triamcinolone acetonide (Kenalog-10) for intralesional treatment and (Kenalog-40) for intramuscular treatment

Normal saline for injection

Hyfrecator for electrodesiccation

Trichloroacetic acid

Miscellaneous Equipment Needed

Gauze

70% isopropyl alcohol

Cotton-tipped applicators and cotton balls

Gloves

Optional Extras

Culposcope

Camera

Patient information sheets

Lidocaine/Prilocaine (EMLA) Cream

To use EMLA for topical local anesthesia apply a thick layer of cream to the area (expect initial stinging on application) and cover with plastic wrap. The cream should be left in place for 15 to 20 minutes for mucosal surfaces and for 1½ hours for skin surfaces. EMLA can be used for biopsy, destruction of warts, removal of small tumors, drainage of small cysts, and before local injections.

Vulvar Biopsies

Preanesthetize with EMLA, then supplement with lidocaine, used with epinephrine to limit bleeding. Warm the anesthetic solution to body temperature and inject slowly with a 30-gauge needle to minimize pain.

For superficial biopsies, gently "tent" the area to be sampled using the 30-gauge anesthetic needle and use fine iris scissors to undercut the specimen. Avoid crushing tissue with forceps. In some locations, cervical biopsy forceps are useful. For thick or granulomatous lesions, a biopsy punch or excisional biopsy is preferred.

Bleeding from superficial biopsies can be stopped with Monsel's solution and pressure. A suture is necessary for deeper biopsies.

SUGGESTED READINGS

Black MM, McKay M, Braude P: *Color atlas and text of obstetric and gynecologic dermatology,* London, 1995, Mosby.

Tovell HMM, Young AW: *Diseases of the vulva in clinical practice,* New York, 1991, Elsevier.

General Therapy

GENERAL THERAPEUTIC APPROACHES FOR VULVAR CONDITIONS

Instruct the patient to avoid the following:

Irritating soaps

Sanitary napkins

Lotions

Disposable wipes

Feminine deodorant products

Tight synthetic clothing

Some detergents, fabric softeners

Pantyhose and girdles, all but loose cotton panties

To cleanse the vulvar area the patient should do the following:

Avoid soap and use Cetaphil cleanser, Basis body soap, or a Dove (unscented) cleansing bar. In the United Kingdom aqueous cream is available (Box C-1).

Use bare hands only—no face cloths

For infection use triclosan solution 0.5% (Tersaseptic) or chlorhexidine 2% (Hibitane) solution

Pat the area dry; do not rub

Lubricants and Emollients

When the skin is dry and cracked, it must be hydrated by soaking in water in a tub or shower. Excess water is quickly patted off the skin surface and an emollient is applied immediately (within one minute) to "hold in" the moisture and protect the skin. White petrolatum is preferred. In the United Kingdom, emulsifying ointment is used (see Box C-1). It is simple, cheap, and nonsensitizing. Many creams and lotions are drying.

For sexual intercourse, lubricants that can be used include light mineral oil or a dab of olive oil (used sparingly) or Astro-Glide. For a vaginal lubricant, consider Replens.

Sitz Baths for Weeping Irritated Skin or Acute Swelling

Irritated skin or swelling can be treated with Burow's solution 1:40 (mix 1 packet or tablet of Domeboro or Buro-Sol or Bluboro in 500 mL water) in a sitz bath for 5 to 10 minutes 2 to 3 times a day or use a cool compress for 15 minutes 3 to 4 times a day. Use as antiseptic and astringent.

Severe Pruritus

One or several of the following treatments can be used to decrease swelling and pruritus.

Cool sitz baths with or without Burow's solution (use solution if the area is weeping or raw)

Cool gel packs (plastic picnic/freezer packs)—keep in a plastic bag in the refrigerator and apply to the area as required

Plain, cold yogurt on a sanitary napkin as required

Chopped ice in a plastic bag (wrapped in a washcloth to prevent frostbite)

SUGGESTED READINGS

Black MM, McKay M, Braude P: *Color atlas and text of obstetric and gynecologic dermatology,* London, 1995, Mosby.

Tovell HMM, Young AW: *Diseases of the vulva in clinical practice,* New York, 1991, Elsevier.

BOX C-1			
BRITISH EMOLLIENTS, LUBRICANTS, AND PROTECTANTS			
Aqueous cream		**Emulsifying ointment**	
Emulsifying ointment	30g	Emulsifying wax	3 parts
Phenoxyethanol	1g	White soft paraffin	5 parts
Distilled water	69g	Liquid paraffin	2 parts

LOCAL VULVAR CARE FOR EROSIVE AND BLISTERING DISEASES OF THE VULVA

For cooling and drying the sore area—Burow's solution (mix one packet or tablet of Domeboro or Bluboro in 500 mL of water in a sitz bath) or use a cool compress 2 to 3 times a day for 5 to 10 minutes.

For topical pain control—EMLA cream applied in a thick layer under plastic wrap occlusion for 20 minutes to numb the area for 1 to 2 hours.

For antiinflammatory effect

Topical—potent fluorinated corticosteroid: clobetasol or halobetasol 0.05% ointment

Intravaginally with a vaginal applicator

- Clobetasol or halobetasol 0.05% ointment 2 to 4g qhs
- Clobetasol or halobetasol 0.05% ointment mixed 50:50 with a bioadhesive compound
- Replens vaginal moisturizer 2 to 4g, every 2 to 3 nights
- Hydrocortisone acetate in a foam (Cortifoam) using 40 to 80 mg qhs or in suppository form (Cortiment) 20 to 40 mg qhs

Intralesional—triamcinolone acetonide (Kenalog-10) diluted to yield 3.3 to 5 mg/mL is administered with a 30-gauge needle into tissues beneath the ulcers and erosions. This can be repeated every 2 to 4 weeks.

Severe vaginal involvement—a Silastic vaginal mold is used to prevent stenosis, with or without a vaginal dilator to prevent vaginal synechiae.

For dysuria or urinary retention—consider catheterization.

To suppress menses—medroxyprogesterone acetate 150 mg IM every 3 months.

Protective (Barrier) Pastes

Over open painful erosions or vulvar ulcers, barrier pastes can be used to protect the raw surface and decrease pain. After a sitz bath or compress, apply Ihle's paste (25% zinc oxide, 25% starch, 25% anhydrous lanolin, 25% petrolatum) or zinc oxide ointment (25% zinc oxide in petrolatum), or emulsifying ointment (see Box C-1).

Apply the paste in a thick layer over the open areas once or twice a day. To remove the paste, gently dab it away using a liberal amount of light mineral oil on a cotton ball or tissue.

SUGGESTED READINGS

Black MM, McKay M, Braude P: *Color atlas and text of obstetric and gynecologic dermatology,* London, 1995, Mosby.

Tovell HMM, Young AW: *Diseases of the vulva in clinical practice,* New York, 1991, Elsevier.

TOPICAL STEROIDS FOR INFLAMMATORY DERMATITIC VULVAR CONDITIONS

These products are the mainstay of topical treatment for itchy, inflamed dermatoses. There are many types from which to choose. Choose and use three or four ointments of different strengths, making appropriate selections, noting the following:

Ointments are stronger than creams

Ointments stay on longer than creams (creams are diluted or washed away with body fluids)

Ointments are less irritating and have fewer allergens than creams

Patients may find one base irritating so choose another—be flexible

Steroids do not relieve the burning of vulvodynia

Cortisones

Cortisones come in different strengths. The following is a very short list of examples.

Class I	Superpotent	Clobetasol 0.05% ointment and cream Halobetasol 0.05% ointment and cream
Class II	High potency	Halcinonide 0.1% ointment and cream Amcinonide 0.1% ointment
Class III		Betamethasone-17-valerate 0.1% ointment
Class IV	Potent	Triamcinolone acetonide 0.1% ointment
Class V		Prednicarbate 0.1% cream
Class VI	Low potency	Desonide 0.05% ointment and cream
Class VII	Mild	Hydrocortisone 1% or 2.5% ointment and cream

Choose the strength and base that meets the need.

For thick itchy dermatoses (e.g., lichen simplex chronicus, thick psoriasis), use a superpotent steroid, clobetasol 0.05% ointment, twice a day for 2 weeks; then once a day for 2 weeks; and then Monday, Wednesday, Friday for 2 weeks. After that switch to a mild ointment, 1% hydrocortisone in petrolatum or a mixture of 1% hydrocortisone and 1% pramoxine cream (Pramosone or ProctoFoam), as required for maintenance.

For severe ulcerative topical therapy (e.g., ulcerated lichen planus, pemphigus) use a superpotent steroid (e.g., clobetasol 0.05% ointment) as described in the previous paragraph.

Note: *If there is a risk of secondary candidiasis, a nystatin ointment or ketoconazole cream is used under the superpotent steroid to prevent yeast. Apply the products separately—do not mix.*

Topical Cortisone Side Effects

Side effects associated with the use of topical cortisones include the following:

Thin skin with telangiectasia, striae, bruising

Rebound burning and irritation, "steroid rosacea"

Secondary infection with yeast, herpes simplex, bacteria

Systemic absorption (>60g superpotent steroid per week results in adrenal suppression)

Rarely a patient has an allergic contact dermatitis to the topical or systemic steroid

Note: *This treatment can cause subdermal atrophy beneath the infected area.*

Intralesional Treatment

Intralesional treatment is used for thick itchy resistant dermatoses (e.g., lichen simplex chronicus, psoriasis, lichen sclerosus, lichen planus) and for localized or resistant ulcerative diseases (e.g., Crohn's disease, Behçet's syndrome).

Treatment consists of triamcinolone acetonide (Kenalog-10) diluted with saline to be used for injection (1 part triamcinolone acetonide into 2 parts normal saline). Inject the solution with a 30-gauge needle using a 1 cm grid. Repeat the injection every 3 to 4 weeks.

SUGGESTED READINGS

Black MM, McKay M, Braude P: *Color atlas and text of obstetric and gynecologic dermatology,* London, 1995, Mosby.

Tovell HMM, Young AW: *Diseases of the vulva in clinical practice,* New York, 1991, Elsevier.

Differential Diagnosis

ULCERS AND EROSIONS OF VULVA ALONE

1) Infection

Venereal

Chancroid

Granuloma inguinale

Herpes simplex

Lymphogranuloma venereum

Syphilis

Nonvenereal

Candida

Herpes zoster

Impetigo

Varicella

Schistosomiasis

Amebiasis

2) Dermatoses

Bullous

Acute contact dermatitis

Benign familial pemphigus

Bullous pemphigoid

Erythema multiforme

Pemphigus vulgaris

Toxic epidermal necrolysis

Nonbullous

Aphthosis/Behçet's syndrome

Crohn's disease

Lupus erythematosus

Lichen planus

Lichen sclerosus

Pyoderma grenosum

Fixed drug eruption

3) Tumors
Basal cell carcinoma
Extramammary Paget's disease
Squamous cell carcinoma
Vulvar intraepithelial neoplasia

4) Trauma
Blunt/sharp injury
Factitial
Mechanical or chemical trauma

5) Miscellaneous
Acrodermatitis enteropathica
Fixed drug reaction
Necrolytic migratory erythema

Note: *The most common cause of acute vulvar ulceration is herpes simplex.*

EROSIVE/ULCERATIVE DISEASE OF THE VULVA AND VAGINA

Conditions affecting the vulva and vagina resulting in erosions or ulcers that can ultimately lead to scarring and loss of tissue include the following:
Cicatricial pemphigoid
Erythema multiforme (major)
Lichen planus
Lupus erythematosus
Pemphigus vulgaris
Toxic epidermal necrolysis

CAUSES OF VULVAR PRURITUS

Many conditions may cause pruritus. Always consider more than one cause because there may be several factors involved, for example, *Candida* vulvitis with secondary contact dermatitis (allergic or irritant). A list of causes follows:
Infections
Candidiasis
Scabies
Molluscum contagiosum
Tinea cruris
Pediculosis
Varicella
Dermatoses
Atopic dermatitis
Lichen simplex chronicus
Atrophic vulvovaginitis
Lichen sclerosus
Contact dermatitis
Psoriasis
Lichen planus
Urticaria
Neoplasia
Vulvar intraepithelial neoplasia
Paget's disease
Miscellaneous
Factitial
Fox-Fordyce disease
Metabolic—as part of a generalized pruritic condition (diabetes, liver, or kidney disease)
Psychogenic

PATIENT INFORMATION FOR LICHEN SCLEROSUS

Lichen means white and mosslike.
Sclerosus means scarred.

What is lichen sclerosus?

This is a common disease of the genital skin in women. The areas involved are the vulva and perianal area. The vulva is the skin located at the entrance to the vagina. The skin in this area is highly specialized in that it performs many unique functions and to do so contains many glands and nerve endings. The covering skin is specialized also—in some areas thick and resilient, and in others thin and more fragile.

Lichen sclerosus usually occurs on the vulva but can occur anywhere on the body. It can start at any age (even in childhood) but most commonly affects women 40 to 50 years of age.

In this condition the vulvar skin usually becomes thin, white, and fragile. If there has been a lot of scratching, the skin is thick and may be scarred. The cause is unknown. Very rarely there can be a familial occurrence. It is not infectious and not sexually transmitted.

What are the symptoms?

Usually it starts with itching or burning. Other symptoms include painful intercourse, splitting of the skin, and bleeding. With time the vulvar skin changes and becomes progressively more thin and white, and the small lips (the labia minora) begin to shrink and eventually disappear. The clitoris may become buried in the shrinking skin folds, and these folds can close over it. Rarely the vaginal opening gradually shrinks.

If the area is very itchy the skin may be white and very thickened. This itching may be severe enough to wake you up at night. Scratching often can cause bruising. In young children this bruising can result in a mistaken diagnosis of sexual abuse. Scratching or any irritation worsens this condition.

Can lichen sclerosus be treated?

The diagnosis usually must be first confirmed with a biopsy, and then therapy can be started. Treatment usually involves a topical cream or ointment in addition to general measures. A super-strong topical cortisone—clobetasol—is used to stop the inflammation that is attacking the skin cells in this area, causing the whitish discoloration, thinning, splitting, and scarring. The cortisone is often combined with an antiyeast product—nystatin (Mycostatin) or ketoconazole (Nizoral). The ointment(s) are used for 12 to 16 weeks on a regular basis and then further treatments are individualized.

Continued long-term daily treatment with this medication is not possible because it can cause thinning of the skin itself. After 12 to 16 weeks, when the area has improved, treatment is used intermittently 1 to 3 times a week as needed or intermittently only when needed.

What else can I do?

Avoid harsh and irritating soaps, detergents, and tight synthetic clothing that may rub or irritate the area.

To cleanse use a mild cleaning lotion like Cetaphil cleanser or a very mild bar cleanser such as Dove (unscented) or Basis.

Try not to scratch.

Avoid using panty liners.

How long will therapy be needed?

Lichen sclerosus can be controlled. There is no definitive "cure." With the previously described form of therapy, improvement is quite rapid in most cases and some people have been so improved that no further treatment has been needed. It is too early to call those patients cured; only time will tell. Most patients require maintenance treatment using the ointment once a week or on an intermittent basis. Regular follow-up is necessary.

Can I become pregnant and deliver a baby?

Lichen sclerosus does not prevent you from becoming pregnant. It does not affect any of the tissues inside you. You can continue your treatment throughout your pregnancy with the supervision of your doctor. Problems are usually few with vaginal delivery, unless you have a lot of extensive scarring.

Does this condition lead to cancer?

Up to 5% of patients have developed skin cancer in the vulvar area associated wtih lichen sclerosus. Usually they have had the condition untreated for years. We hope that early recognition and aggressive treatment will reduce or eliminate the risk of cancer. That is the reason close follow-up is essential.

GENERAL INSTRUCTIONS FOR ITCHY VULVAR CONDITIONS

Avoid irritating soaps, feminine deodorant products, disposable wipes, regular use of panty liners, girdles (i.e., body shapers), and panty hose.

Wear cotton underwear.

Consider the use of the following:

"Stay-up" hose

Garter belt and stockings

Pantyhose with cut-out crotch

To cleanse:

For severe itch or irritation—Burow's solution 1:40 (mix one packet or tablet of Domeboro or Bluboro in 500 mL of water) in a sitz bath for 5 to 10 minutes 2 or 3 times per day.

For general cleansing—Wash gently with a mild liquid cleanser like Cetaphil cleanser or an unscented cleansing bar like Dove or Basis. Do not use a face cloth. Do not scrub the area. Rinse thoroughly. Gently pat the area dry.

For thick, itchy dermatoses (e.g., thick psoriasis, lichen simplex chronicus):

Use a super-potent steroid, clobetasol or halobetasol .05% ointment twice a day for 2 weeks; then once a day for 2 weeks; and then Monday, Wednesday, and Friday for 2 weeks. After that switch to mild, 1% hydrocortisone in petrolatum or 1% hydrocortisone powder in 1% pramoxine cream.

For secondary yeast, when using a super-potent steroid, add nystatin ointment or ketoconazole cream, applied under the strong ointment.

For marked itching:

Cold gel pack (plastic picnic/freezer pack)—keep in a self-sealing plastic bag in the refrigerator and apply to the area as needed.*

Ice—chopped ice can be used in a plastic bag or plastic glove.*

Dish-washing soap bottle—partially fill it with water and leave it in the freezer until frozen. The bottle is left by the bed when retiring and can be used during the night for relief.*

General Suggestions:

If the area is very swollen use a cool sitz bath with or without the Burow's solution.

Cold gel pack (plastic picnic/freezer pack)—keep in a plastic bag in the refrigerator and apply as needed.*

Plain, cold yogurt from the refrigerator can be spread on a sanitary napkin and applied directly to the painful, raw area as needed.

---

*Note that ice packs or frozen items should not be placed directly on the skin. Use with a cloth as a barrier to prevent frost bite.

May be duplicated for use in clinical practice. From Fisher BK, Margesson LJ: *Genital Skin Disorders: Diagnosis and Treatment,* St Louis, 1998, Mosby.

GENERAL INSTRUCTIONS FOR WEEPING, BLISTERING, OR ULCERATED AREAS OF THE VULVA

Avoid irritating soaps, feminine deodorant products, disposable wipes, the regular use of panty liners, girdles (i.e. body shapers), and panty hose.

Wear cotton underwear.

Consider:

"Stay-up" hose

Garter belt and stockings

Pantyhose with a cut-out crotch

To cleanse and to use as an antiseptic/astringent:

For severe itch or irritation—Burow's solution 1:40 (mix one packet or tablet of Domeboro or Bluboro in 500 mL of water) in a sitz bath for 5 to 10 minutes two or three times per day or use a cool compress for 15 minutes three to four times a day.

To make a compress, use a full-sized handkerchief or a thin cotton cloth moistened in the Burow's solution (damp but not dripping wet). Lay the cloth/tissue over the vulvar area for 1 to 1½ minutes then remove and let the solution evaporate for 1 to 2 minutes and repeat 5 to 10 times each treatment session.

For gentle cleaning when blisters and open areas are healed—Use a mild liquid cleanser like Cetaphil. Do not use a face cloth. Do not scrub. Rinse thoroughly.

After any cleaning routine gently pat the area dry.

Topical Pain Control

EMLA cream—Apply a thick layer of the cream under plastic wrap for 20 minutes to numb the area for 1 to 2 hours. This will initially sting when it is applied.

If the open areas are very painful and raw after the sitz baths or compress, use a protective barrier paste (Ihle's paste (Appendix D) or zinc oxide ointment).

Apply these in a thick layer over the open areas as needed daily.

To remove the sticky paste, gently dab it away using a liberal amount of light mineral oil on a cotton ball or tissue. Pat, not rub, the area dry.

Antiinflammatory Ointments

Strong topical cortisone—clobetasol or halobetasol 0.05% ointment with or without nystatin ointment or ketoconazole cream once or twice a day to all involved areas.

May be duplicated for use in clinical practice. From Fisher BK, Margesson LJ: *Genital Skin Disorders: Diagnosis and Treatment*, St Louis, 1998, Mosby.

Index